Congenital and Paediatric Acquired Heart Disease in Practice

Yiu-fai Cheung

Congenital and Paediatric Acquired Heart Disease in Practice

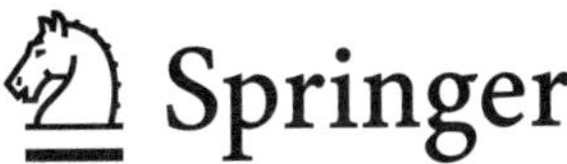

Springer

Yiu-fai Cheung
Bryan Lin Professor in Paediatric Cardiology
Department of Paediatrics and Adolescent Medicine
Hong Kong Children's Hospital
School of Clinical Medicine
LKS Faculty of Medicine
The University of Hong Kong
Hong Kong, China

ISBN 978-981-99-2864-4 ISBN 978-981-99-2862-0 (eBook)
https://doi.org/10.1007/978-981-99-2862-0

This Springer imprint is published by the registered company Springer Nature Singapore Pte Ltd.
The registered company address is: 152 Beach Road, #21-01/04 Gateway East, Singapore 189721, Singapore

Foreword

I write this foreword during my last few months of an incredibly rewarding career in this wonderful field of ours. It is a time for reflection, both personally and professionally, and for looking towards the future.

First some reflections. As Dr. Cheung writes in his preface to this book, our specialty has undergone the most tremendous advances over a few short decades. Inoperable disease has become operable, surgical outcomes have improved beyond the wildest dreams of our early pioneers, entirely new subspecialties have developed, and our understanding of the consequences of our interventions is improving every day. It has been a privilege to have witnessed, and perhaps contributed in a small way, to this extraordinary evolution of our field. Consequently, we are now able to help more children and their families to lead better lives than ever before. This is, of course, the ultimate reward for the clinical, scientific, and educational efforts of all the practitioners, researchers, and teachers that have contributed to our field over the years.

As I look back, there are other rewards. Of them, perhaps the most long-lasting and enriching have been the personal relationships that form across a career. Our mentors are never forgotten; we work day-in day-out with our multi-disciplinary colleagues that become our 'family' but, for me, watching mentees grow into leaders has been particularly gratifying. I have been lucky to have worked with some of the most talented young cardiologists as they develop their careers, the author of this book being one of them. I first met a young Dr. Yiu-fai Cheung almost 25 years ago. Even then it was clear to me that he was going to make a huge contribution to our field. His accomplishments are too numerous to mention, but in many ways the book you hold in your hands is a culmination of them all. As sub-specialization becomes more and more the norm, the breadth of Dr. Cheung's training and practice is on show here. It is a product of the learnings of a clinical and research polymath who has 'walked the walk' throughout his career.

Let there be no mistake, the production of a monograph such as we have in *Congenital and Paediatric Acquired Heart Disease in Practice* is a monumental task. It is a practical, comprehensive, contemporary, and beautifully illustrated text that will become a 'must have' for practitioners learning our field. As someone who has edited multi-author texts, I can only imagine the many hundreds of hours that

Dr. Cheung has dedicated to producing the book, each and every word and illustration of which he has singularly written and produced for you. Although Dr. Cheung has many more contributions to make, enjoy this synthesis of all that he has learned so far.

Looking to the future……you are the future of our field. As you learn and assimilate the contents of this book, you embark on a career that I hope will be as fulfilling and rewarding as my own. What is almost mind-boggling is that you will witness a similar transformation to the practice and outcomes of treatment for congenital and paediatric heart disease that Dr. Cheung and I have seen over the past three decades. I envy you that privilege a little, but how exciting it is to imagine the heights that will be achieved for our patients in the future!

Andrew N. Redington

Heart Institute
Cincinnati Children's Hospital Medical Center
Cincinnati, OH, USA

Department of Pediatrics
University of Cincinnati
Cincinnati, OH, USA

Preface

Advances in paediatric cardiology and cardiac surgery can only be described as phenomenal over the past half-century. The evolution of and refinements in the practice of paediatric cardiology in the past three decades, based on important works of predecessors in this field, have made a tremendous impact on the survival and quality outcomes of congenital heart patients and children and adolescents with acquired heart disease.

It is my fortune to not only have witnessed the staggering advances but also be engaged in different aspects of paediatric cardiology over the past one-and-a half score and in the years to come. I have been blessed with the opportunities to come across and work with great teachers, mentors, friends, and colleagues from all parts of the world, and from whom I have learnt so much about cardiac morphology, genetics, pathophysiology, clinical evaluation, imaging and other investigation modalities, medical therapies, catheter interventions, surgery, intensive care, and research. As we cross our paths, my life career in paediatric cardiology has been very much enlightened. At this phase, I feel obliged to share my knowledge and skills, albeit far from perfect, with young people who help shape the future of paediatric cardiac care.

This book aims to equip medical undergraduates and trainees in paediatric cardiology, cardiac surgery, cardiac intensive care, and cardiac nursing staff with up-to-date knowledge and practical skills to manage and to care for children with congenital and acquired heart disease. Each of the chapters is written in a concise and practical manner for use in the ward and clinic with up-to-date information on congenital and paediatric acquired heart disease. Key features of this book include comprehensive coverage of the spectrum of congenital and paediatric acquired heart disease, extensive use of coloured figures, tables, and boxes to illustrate structural cardiovascular conditions, clinical manifestations, investigations, and management approach, and incorporation of contemporary updates on aetiology, pathophysiology, and management of paediatric cardiac conditions including emerging ones related to the COVID-19 pandemic.

Quoting from Rabindranath Tagore, 'I leave no trace of wings in the air, but I am glad I have had my flight. The fireflies, twinkling among leaves, make the stars wonder'. I am grateful that I have had my flight and elated to be able to continue to fly for as long as I can. I hope though to share with you a trace of my reflection on the practice of paediatric cardiology.

Yiu-fai Cheung

Acknowledgements

I gratefully thank Professor Chap-yung Yeung for recruiting me as a young faculty member into the Department of Paediatrics immediately upon my graduation from the university and supporting me unreservedly through all these years, Professor Maurice Leung who picked (not sure being cherry-picked though) me to join the marvellous arena of paediatric cardiology and groomed me to become a member of this community, and Professor Andrew Redington for his mentoring during my days of training in England and being such a great role model as a sharp clinician, a distinguished researcher, and a world leader in this field.

I thank my colleagues at the Hong Kong Children's Hospital, Dr. Kwok-lap Chan, Dr. Pak-cheong Chow, Dr. Kevin Fung, Dr. Sit-yee Kwok, Dr. Carol Ng, Dr. Julia Shi, Dr. Sabrina Tsao, Dr. Clement Yu, and Ms. Yvonne Yip, who helped retrieve archived images and shared with me their image and ECG collections. I would also like to thank Mr. Ray Cheung, Mr. Spencer Ng, and Dr. Wilfred Wong for the wonderfully drawn illustrations.

Finally, I express my deepest gratitude to all my patients and their families who have taught me so much on how to practice clinical medicine with all our heart and to remain humane and humble.

Contents

Part II Acyanotic Congenital Heart Disease

Part VII Systemic and Pulmonary Venous Anomalies

Part VIII Coronary Arterial Anomalies

Part I

The Basics

1 Clinical Presentation

Children with heart disease may be asymptomatic and present with incidental finding of a cardiac murmur during medical consultation for other reasons, abnormal cardiac contours on the chest radiograph, or abnormal electrocardiograms. Infants, children, and adolescents with heart disease may present with symptoms of heart failure or cyanosis. Older children and adolescents with heart disease may occasionally present with chest pain, syncope, or palpitations. While uncommon, shock is a life-threatening presentation in infants with critical congenital heart disease and in older children with acquired heart disease and cardiomyopathies. Rarely, sudden cardiac arrest is the initial presentation and the underlying cardiac cause is diagnosed in survivors after successful resuscitation.

1.1 Incidental Finding of a Cardiac Murmur

1.1.1 Innocent Murmurs

Innocent murmurs are not associated with heart disease and are found at sometime during childhood in up to 50% of children. Innocent murmurs can be systolic or continuous, but never diastolic, in nature (Table 1.1).

1.1.2 Pathological Murmurs

Pathological heart murmurs are due to underlying heart conditions, which can be diagnosed based on further history taking and physical examination (Table 1.2).

Y.-f. Cheung, *Congenital and Paediatric Acquired Heart Disease in Practice*, https://doi.org/10.1007/978-981-99-2862-0_1

Table 1.1 Types of innocent murmurs

Type	Nature	Location	Origin
Still's murmur	Ejection systolic murmur	Left lower sternal border	Turbulence in the left ventricular outflow or vibration of fibrous bands in the left ventricle
Pulmonary flow murmur	Ejection systolic murmur	Left upper sternal border	Ejection vibration in main pulmonary artery
Peripheral pulmonary stenosis of newborn	Ejection systolic murmur	Left and right upper sternal border with radiation to the axilla and back	Relatively small size of branch pulmonary arteries
Supra-clavicular bruit	Ejection systolic murmur	Base of the neck on either side, suprasternal notch	Turbulent flow in the major brachiocephalic arteries
Venous hum	Continuous	Just above or below either clavicle	Turbulent flow in major veins at the thoracic inlet

Table 1.2 Features differentiating innocent from pathological murmurs

Innocent murmurs	Pathological murmurs
Asymptomatic	Symptomatic
Quiet praecordium	Abnormal signs
Normal heart sounds	Abnormal heart sounds
No added sounds	Added sounds
Soft, short, systolic murmur	Presence of a thrill
Localized murmur	Radiation of murmur
Variation with posture	Diastolic murmur

1.2 Heart Failure

1.2.1 Concept of Heart Failure

The term 'heart failure' is a misnomer. 'Heart failure' may simply be interpreted to mean failure of the heart to fulfil its function as a pump (contractile function) or as a suction chamber to receive the venous return (diastolic function). However, in the majority of infants and children with clinical manifestations of heart failure, the myocardium is not failing. In essence, failure of the myocardium is only one of the two components that leads to the 'clinical syndrome of heart failure'.

Optimal cardiovascular performance requires normal functioning of the heart to meet the demand of the body and the workload posed on the heart. Hence, 'the syndrome of heart failure' represents an imbalanced state, in which the heart fails to provide an adequate output at a rate to meet the demand of the body. This may be due to (a) impaired contraction or relaxation of the myocardium, and/or (b) extra demand posed by an abnormal haemodynamic load and by other body systems.

Impaired contraction of the ventricles (systolic dysfunction) reduces cardiac output. This occurs in children with disease of the myocardium (myocarditis, dilated cardiomyopathy) and myocardial ischaemia (coronary artery stenosis or occlusion after Kawasaki disease). Rarely, impaired diastolic ventricular filling (diastolic dysfunction) leads to reduction of cardiac output, an example is restrictive cardiomyopathy. Secondary causes of myocardial dysfunction may occur in neonates with asphyxia, sepsis, hypoglycaemia or hypocalcaemia. Overall, cardiac dysfunction is not the most common cause of heart failure in children.

Most commonly, heart failure in children is related to structural congenital heart disease that poses an abnormal load on the heart, albeit the ventricular contractility remains normal. In 'volume overloading' conditions, the ventricle is dilated as in the presence of large left-to-right shunts (ventricular septal defect, persistent arterial duct) or valvar regurgitation (aortic regurgitation, mitral regurgitation). In 'pressure overloading' conditions, the afterload to the ventricle is increased as in ventricular outflow obstruction (aortic stenosis, coarctation of the aorta).

In hyperthyroidism and anaemia, the heart is required to pump an abnormally large volume of blood to meet the metabolic demand of the body. This is referred to as the 'high-output' failure.

1.2.2 Causes of Heart Failure

In infants and children, the timing of onset of heart failure provides an important clue to the underlying aetiology (Table 1.3). Structural cardiac lesions that cause severe obstruction of the left ventricular outflow (e.g. critical aortic stenosis,

Table 1.3 Causes of heart failure in infants and children

Neonatal period	Infancy	Older children and adolescents
Structural heart defects • severe left ventricular outflow obstruction • persistent arterial duct in premature infants	Structural heart defects • large left-to-right shunts	Unoperated structural heart defects Repaired or palliated congenital heart disease
Myocardial dysfunction • myocarditis • secondary to asphyxia, sepsis, hypoglycaemia or hypocalcaemia	Myocardial dysfunction • cardiomyopathies	Acquired heart disease • cardiomyopathies (primary and secondary e.g. iron overloading, post chemotherapy, neuromuscular disease) • infection-related (myocarditis, endocarditis)
Arrhythmias • congenital heart block • upraventricular tachycardia		

coarctation of the aorta, interrupted aortic arch) are the most important causes of heart failure in early neonatal period. Structural heart lesions that cause significant left-to-right shunting of blood (e.g. ventricular and atrioventricular septal defects) typically present in young infancy at 2–3 months of age. This timing corresponds to the postnatal fall in pulmonary vascular resistance with consequent increase in pulmonary flow. In older children and adolescents, by contrast, heart failure is usually related to diseases of the myocardium (myocarditis, cardiomyopathy) or ventricular dysfunction in association with complex congenital heart disease despite surgery.

1.2.3 Clinical Manifestations of Heart Failure

The history is important in the diagnosis of heart failure. Physical examination shows signs of pulmonary arterial and venous congestion, systemic venous congestion, and, in decompensated state, signs of diminished cardiac output. Symptoms and signs of heart failure in children and adolescents are shown in Table 1.4.

1.2.4 Quantifying Severity of Heart Failure

For older children and adolescents, the class measure developed by the New York Heart Association is useful in quantifying the severity of heart failure (Table 1.5). The Ross Classification has been used for scoring heart failure primarily in infants with heart failure (Table 1.6). Subsequent modifications of the Ross Classification

Table 1.4 Symptoms and signs of heart failure

Symptoms	Signs
Infants	Compensatory mechanisms
Poor feeding	Tachycardia
Failure to thrive	Cardiomegaly
Shortness of breath	Pulmonary vascular congestion
Excessive sweating	Tachypnoea
Recurrent lower respiratory tract infection	Subcostal insucking
Older children and adolescents	Laboured breathing
Malaise	Wheezing in infants
Shortness of breath on exertion	Systemic venous congestion
Decreased exercise tolerance	Hepatomegaly
Weight gain (fluid retention)	Distension of neck veins (difficult to observe in infants)
Rarely orthopnoea (due to left ventricular systolic and/or diastolic dysfunction)	Ankle oedema
	Diminished cardiac output
	Cool extremities
	Decreased pulse volume
	Prolonged capillary refill

Table 1.5 New York Heart Association Functional Class

Functional class	Description
Class I	No limitation of physical activity, no symptoms with normal physical activity
Class II	Slight limitation of physical activity, presence of symptoms with ordinary physical activity
Class III	Marked limitation of physical activity, presence of symptoms with less than ordinary physical activity
Class IV	Inability to carry on any physical activity without discomfort, symptoms even at rest

Table 1.6 Ross classification

Functional class	Description
Class I	No limitation or symptoms
Class II	Mild tachypnoea or sweating with feedings in infants, or dyspnoea on exertion in older children, no growth failure
Class III	Marked tachypnoea or sweating with feedings or exertion and prolonged feeding times with growth failure
Class IV	Symptoms at rest with tachypnoea, retraction, grunting or excessive sweating

take into account of age-dependent changes in heart rate and respiratory rate, peripheral perfusion status, ventricular ejection fraction, atrioventricular valvar regurgitation, and circulating N-terminal pro-brain natriuretic peptide level. The New York University Paediatric Heart Failure Index uses signs and symptoms of heart failure, use of heart failure medications, and single ventricular physiology to generate a score that ranges from 0 (no heart failure) to 30 (severe heart failure). In clinical practice, the paediatric classification systems are not widely used.

1.3 Shock

Shock is a state in which there is significant reduction in tissue perfusion, which results in impairment of delivery of oxygen to peripheral tissues. Activation of homeostatic mechanisms of the body may compensate to a certain extent to maintain systemic blood pressure and tissue perfusion (compensatory shock). However, if left undiagnosed and unmanaged, hypotension, severely compromised tissue perfusion, and progressive organ dysfunction result in cardiovascular collapse and death.

1.3.1 Clinical Recognition of Shock

Early clinical recognition of shock, its underlying cause, and immediate institution of treatment is the key to successful management (Box 1.1)

Box 1.1 Clinical Recognition of Shock

- tachycardia
- hypotension (a late sign due to the initial compensatory response)
- in cardiogenic and hypovolaemic shock, evidence of peripheral shutdown (cool extremities, mottling of skin, and prolonged capillary refill), except in distributive shock
- in distributive shock, flushing of skin, hyperaemic and warm peripheries
- oliguria
- lactic acidosis

1.3.2 Types of Shock

History and physical examination provide clues to the type of shock, which falls under either of the three categories: (a) hypovolaemic, (b) distributive, and (c) cardiogenic.

Hypovolaemic shock is the most common type of shock seen in children. Fluid loss (usually extravascular loss from diarrhoea and vomiting, and less commonly intravascular loss from bleeding) leads to hypovolaemia, which reduces cardiac preload and hence cardiac output.

Distributive shock is related to severe peripheral vasodilation, which decreases systemic vascular resistance and redistributes blood flow with reduced tissue perfusion. The heart usually attempts to compensate by increasing the cardiac output. Causes of distributive shock include sepsis (the commonest cause of distributive shock in children), anaphylaxis, and neurogenic shock (with sudden loss of venous tone).

Cardiogenic shock is discussed in the following section. It is important to note that the types of shock can overlap and may have a causal relationship (e.g. sepsis leading to myocardial dysfunction and cardiogenic shock).

1.3.3 Cardiogenic Shock

Cardiogenic shock is caused by conditions that lead to inadequacy of the cardiac output due to obstruction of ventricular outflow, impairment of cardiac contractility or filling, cardiac arrhythmias, metabolic disturbance, or increase in metabolic demand of the body (Table 1.7).

Red herring and clues when approaching a child with shock are highlighted in Box 1.2. Point-of-care ultrasound assessment is helpful in these situations.

Table 1.7 Causes of cardiogenic shock in children

Primary cardiac causes	Non-cardiac causes
Obstruction of left ventricular outflow	Sepsis
Critical aortic stenosis	Septic shock with myocardial depression
Coarctation or interrupted aortic arch	Metabolic disturbance
Hypoplastic left heart syndrome	Acidosis
Impaired cardiac contractility or filling	Hyperkalaemia
Cardiomyopathies	Hypocalcaemia
Myocarditis	Thyrotoxicosis
Cardiac tamponade	Phaeochromocytoma
Tension pneumothorax	
Myocardial ischaemia	
Anomalous origin of left coronary artery	
Thrombosis of coronary artery aneurysm due to previous Kawasaki disease	
Cardiac arrhythmias	
Supraventricular tachycardia	
Ventricular tachycardia	
Complete heart block	

Box 1.2 Red Herring and Clues When Approaching Shock

- a child with fever and shock may not always have septic shock
- severe left ventricular outflow obstructive lesions must be excluded in neonates and infants with shock
- in a child with shock presenting even with predominant gastrointestinal or respiratory symptoms, cardiac causes must be excluded
- absence of cardiomegaly does not exclude cardiogenic shock
- sinus tachycardia in an afebrile child with shock suggests cardiogenic shock

1.4 Cyanosis in the Newborn

Newborn babies with cyanotic heart disease present usually with bluish discoloration of the lips and the perioral area soon after birth. Central cyanosis is caused by arterial hypoxaemia and manifests as bluish discoloration of the lips, extremities, tongue, and other mucosal membranes. It is apparent when >3 g/dL of desaturated haemoglobin is present. Hence, anaemia may mask clinical cyanosis, while polycythaemia may cause apparent cyanosis. Peripheral cyanosis refers to bluish discoloration only limited to the extremities. It is caused by vasoconstriction secondary to hypothermia or a low cardiac output rather than arterial hypoxaemia.

1.4.1 Causes of Cyanosis

Cyanosis in the newborn is primarily caused by respiratory and cardiovascular pathologies (Table 1.8). Neurological conditions leading to hypoventilation and haematological abnormalities are less common causes of cyanosis.

1.4.2 Clinical Approach

Central cyanosis is confirmed by a reduced oxygen saturation measured using a pulse oximeter. Measurement of both preductal (right hand, unless the right subclavian artery is arising aberrantly from the descending aorta) and post-ductal (foot) provides clue to right-to-left shunting at the level of the persistent arterial duct. A normal preductal with reduced postductal saturation suggests persistent pulmonary hypertension of the newborn or severe coarctation or interruption of the aorta.

History and examination findings provide clues to possible aetiologies, while further investigations help to confirm the diagnosis.

1.4.2.1 History Taking

The following information should be gathered:

- antenatal diagnosis of congenital heart disease
- maternal conditions associated with fetal cardiac malformations (e.g. congenital infection syndromes, poorly controlled diabetes mellitus, drug intake)
- polyhydramnios (associated with airway abnormalities and neurological conditions) or oligohydramnios (associated with pulmonary hypoplasia)
- family history of congenital heart disease or haemoglobinopathy
- clues to increased risk of sepsis (peripartum maternal fever, prolonged rupture of membrane, fetal distress)
- presence of meconium-stained liquor

Table 1.8 Causes of central cyanosis in the newborn

Systems	Conditions
Respiratory	Congenital pneumonia
	Meconium aspiration syndrome
	Transient tachypnoea of the newborn
	Respiratory distress syndrome (preterm babies)
Cardiovascular	Cyanotic heart disease
	Persistent pulmonary hypertension of the newborn
Neurological	Asphyxia
	Drugs (maternal drug addiction, pethidine use before delivery)
	Brain pathologies
Haematological	Congenital methaemoglobinaemia

1.4.2.2 Physical Examination

Respiratory assessment provides important clues to the cause of central cyanosis. Shallow breathing and apnoea suggest a neurological cause. Respiratory distress, as reflected by tachypnoea, subcostal insucking and nasal flaring, suggests respiratory pathologies. When the breathing pattern is normal, cyanotic congenital heart disease is likely.

While a detailed examination of the cardiovascular system is required, it is important to note that the absence of heart murmurs does not exclude congenital heart disease as the diagnosis (e.g. cardiac murmurs in pulmonary atresia conditions and transposition of the great arteries are typically soft and non-specific or absent).

1.4.2.3 Investigations

Initial investigations usually include sepsis screening (complete blood count and blood culture) and a chest radiograph. The need for an arterial blood gas depends on findings of respiratory assessment.

An initial chest radiograph is taletelling. Hazy lung fields are typical of lung parenchymal disease, while dark oligaemic lung fields indicate reduced pulmonary blood flow, which is present in most types of cyanotic congenital heart disease. The exception is total anomalous pulmonary venous connection with obstructed pulmonary venous return (Chap. 37), in which the lung fields have a hazy, indistinct, ground-glass appearance.

Echocardiography is performed in many centres as part of the initial assessment of cyanotic neonates. While persistent cyanosis not responsive to supplemental oxygen and/or ventilatory support is a conventional indication of echocardiography, in the current era, the threshold for echocardiographic assessment is low. The wide availability of bedside and point-of-care echocardiography facilitates early exclusion or confirmation of critical congenital heart disease in these neonates.

Hyperoxic or nitrogen washout test has traditionally been used to differentiate between respiratory and cardiac cause of cyanosis. It involves the assessment of partial pressure of oxygen of arterial blood (PaO_2) obtained from the right radial artery after administration of 100% oxygen for 10 min. While the PaO_2 usually exceeds 15 kPa (>110 mmHg) in lung disease after oxygen administration, it remains relatively the same in cyanotic heart disease. However, given the concern of promoting ductal closure in duct-dependent circulation by a high inhaled oxygen concentration and increasing availability of bedside echocardiography, this test is seldom performed nowadays.

In an apparently cyanotic neonate but with cyanotic heart disease and respiratory conditions being excluded, the rare condition of congenital methaemoglobinaemia should be considered. Methaemoglobin is an oxidized form of haemoglobin, with the heme iron being in the ferric 3+ state instead of the usual ferrous 2+ state. It is incapable of carrying oxygen and can further decrease oxygen delivery to the tissues through increasing the oxygen affinity of the normal ferrous hemes residing within the same tetrameric haemoglobin molecule.

Congenital methaemoglobinaemia is due to cytochrome b5 reductase deficiency or haemoglobin M (an abnormal haemoglobin that is more susceptible to oxidation) disorder. The clues to this diagnosis are (a) a low oxygen saturation (methaemoglobin causes error in estimating the percentages of reduced haemoglobin and oxyhaemoglobin), (b) normal PaO_2 (the calculated oxygen saturation is falsely elevated in the presence of methaemoglobin), and (c) an arterial blood sample that has a chocolate-brown colour and does not turn red when exposed to air. Diagnosis is confirmed by direct measurement of methaemoglobin using co-oximetry in the blood gas analyzer.

1.5 Chest Pain

Chest pain is a common symptom in children and adolescents. This presentation causes anxiety to patients and family and may lead to restriction of exercise. The underlying causes are mostly benign. Nonetheless, in a minority of patients, the underlying causes are potentially more serious or even life-threatening.

1.5.1 Causes of Chest Pain

In up to 99% of children and adolescents, the underlying causes of chest pain are non-cardiac in origin. Cardiac conditions causing chest pain are usually related to left ventricular outflow obstruction, congenital or acquired coronary arterial abnormalities or inflammation of the pericardium (Table 1.9). Rarely aortic dissection in children with inherited connective tissue disease is the cause. Palpitations cause chest discomfort rather than pain.

Table 1.9 Causes of chest pain in children and adolescents

Cardiac conditions	Non-cardiac conditions
Left ventricular outflow obstruction	Idiopathic
Aortic stenosis	Musculoskeletal conditions
Hypertrophic cardiomyopathy	Muscle strain
Coronary arterial abnormalities	Costochondritis
Kawasaki disease	Slipping rib syndrome
Anomalous origin or course of coronary arteries	Psychogenic
Coronary arterial spasm induced by recreational drug use (e.g. cocaine, amphetamines)	Anxiety
Pericardial inflammation	Panic disorder
Pericarditis	Somatic symptom disorder
Myopericarditis	Respiratory
Others	Pneumonia with pleuritis
Aortic dissection	Spontaneous pneumothorax
Pulmonary hypertension	Gastrointestinal
Tachyarrhythmias	Gastritis
	Peptic ulcer
	Breast
	Gynaecomastia in adolescent boys
	Thelarche in adolescent girls

1.5.2 Clinical Approach

1.5.2.1 History Taking

The importance of careful history taking in children and adolescents presenting with chest pain cannot be over emphasized.

During history taking, the following information should be gathered:

- detailed description of chest pain (nature, frequency, location, radiation, precipitating and relieving factors, associated symptoms as dizziness, sweatiness, syncope, palpitation)
- respiratory and gastrointestinal symptoms
- family history of sudden death
- constitutional symptoms
- recent illness (viral prodrome), past medical history (Kawasaki disease, history of cardiac surgery), use of drugs including recreational ones (cocaine, amphetamines, marijuana, and synthetic cannabinoids)
- recent vaccination (mRNA COVID-19 vaccine) (Chap. 61)

Alarming symptoms and history suggestive of significant underlying cardiac condition are highlighted in Box 1.3.

Box 1.3 Alarming Symptoms and History in Children and Adolescents with Chest Pain

- excruciating pain that radiates to the back (aortic dissection)
- anginal pain (coronary anomalies causing myocardial ischaemia)
- pain on exertion (left ventricular outflow obstruction, coronary arterial anomalies)
- associated syncope (left ventricular outflow obstruction, coronary arterial anomalies, pulmonary hypertension)
- past medical history: congenital heart disease (left ventricular outflow obstruction, coronary arterial anomalies, pulmonary hypertension), Kawasaki disease (coronary artery aneurysm and stenosis), autoimmune disease (pericarditis), inherited disorders of connective tissue disease (aortic dissection)
- family history of sudden death (inherited disorders of connective tissue disease, hypertrophic cardiomyopathy)

1.5.2.2 Physical Examination

While most of children and adolescents are not in distress at the time of presentation, the presence of respiratory distress and shock-like features demand urgent assessment and treatment.

During physical examination, the following signs should be assessed:

- general well-being
- fever (may be present in pericarditis or perimyocarditis) and other vital signs

- phenotypic features of syndromic disorders and inherited disorders of connective tissue disease associated with aortic dissection
- cardiovascular examination: signs of cardiogenic shock, tachycardia, pulse volume, signs of pulmonary hypertension, signs of left ventricular outflow obstruction, pericardial rub
- respiratory examination: distress, signs of injury, deformities, localized tenderness, assess for slipping rib syndrome by hooking fingers under the ninth and tenth ribs and pulling the ribs anteriorly
- breast examination if necessary
- abdominal examination

1.5.2.3 Further Investigations

Further assessments are not required in most of the children and adolescents with chest pain, in whom history and physical findings are suggestive of either idiopathic or musculoskeletal pain. The need for respiratory and gastrointestinal studies is guided by history and examination findings. In patients with suspected underlying cardiac conditions, further investigations may include chest radiograph, electrocardiogram, echocardiogram, treadmill exercise testing, and ambulatory electrocardiographic monitoring.

1.6 Syncope

Syncope refers to temporary loss of consciousness and postural tone secondary to transient inadequacy of cerebral blood perfusion. This alarming symptom understandably causes anxiety to patients and family. Whereas majority of syncopal episodes are benign, a minority are caused by potentially serious or even life-threatening conditions. It is important therefore to determine the cause of syncope, to identify and treat potentially life-threatening causes, and to prevent future occurrence.

1.6.1 Causes of Syncope

Syncope is a common in children and adolescents. At least 15% of children have been reported to have experienced syncope before the end of adolescence and about 50% of college students having a history of fainting.

Vasovagal syncope (also called simple faint, vasodepressor syncope, and neurocardiogenic syncope) is the most common cause in children. The proposed mechanism is a vagally mediated reflex initiated by cardiac mechanoreceptors. In this condition, syncope occurs when the child is sitting or standing upright and has a characteristic prodrome (dizziness, light-headedness, nausea, sweating, pallor, and blurred vision). Other common causes of reflex-mediated syncope include orthostatic hypotension and, in toddlers, breath holding spells. Certain factors precipitate occurrence of vasovagal and other reflex mediated syncope (Box 1.4)

Box 1.4 Factors Precipitating Occurrence of Vasovagal Syncope and Other Reflex-Mediated Syncope

- prolonged standing, especially in confined spaces with warm temperature, with increased venous pooling
- fasting
- pain and emotion
- lack of sleep and fatigue
- febrile illnesses and menstruation
- medications affecting vascular volume or vascular tone

The potentially serious and life-threatening conditions can be cardiac and non-cardiac in origin (Table 1.10). Cardiac causes include reflex-mediated syncope, cardiac arrhythmias, structural heart and coronary artery disease, and myocardial disease and dysfunction. Non-cardiac causes include neurologic, psychogenic, and metabolic conditions.

1.6.2 Clinical Approach

1.6.2.1 History Taking

The importance of careful history taking in children and adolescents presenting with syncope again cannot be over emphasized.

Table 1.10 Causes of syncope in children and adolescents

Cardiac	Non-cardiac
Reflex-mediated	Neurologic or psychogenic causes
Vasovagal syncope	Seizure or epilepsy
Breath holding spell	Brain tumours
Orthostatic hypotension	Atypical migraine
Cardiac arrhythmias	Hyperventilation
Long or short QT syndrome	Hysteria
Brugada syndrome	Metabolic causes
Catecholaminergic polymorphic	Hypoglycaemia
Ventricular tachycardia	Hypoxaemia
Preexcitation syndromes	Severe anaemia
Bradyarrhythmias	Hypovolaemia
Structural or functional cardiac abnormalities	
Acute myocarditis	
Cardiomyopathies	
Arrhythmogenic right ventricular dysplasia/cardiomyopathy	
Coronary arterial anomalies	
Valvar aortic stenosis	
Pulmonary arterial hypertension	

During history taking, the following information should be gathered:

- a detailed description of the syncopal episode by the witness
- previous syncopal episodes
- precipitating factors
- prodromal symptoms
- recent illness, past medical history, medications

Alarming symptoms and history suggestive of significant underlying cardiac condition are highlighted in Box 1.5.

Box 1.5 Alarming Symptoms and History

- history atypical of vasovagal syncope
- syncope when supine
- syncope during exercise
- syncope in response to loud noise, fright, or extreme emotional stress
- syncope preceded by chest pain or palpitations
- past medical history: cardiac arrhythmias, congenital and acquired heart disease
- family history of sudden death in young relatives, cardiomyopathy, and cardiac arrhythmias (a family history of vasovagal syncope is common)

1.6.2.2 Physical Examination

A general examination followed by targeted cardiovascular and neurologic examination should be performed. Cardiovascular signs of interest include the pulse rhythm, signs of left and right ventricular outflow obstruction, and evidence of postural hypotension (a decrease in systolic blood pressure of 20 mmHg or a decrease in diastolic blood pressure of 10 mmHg within 3 min of standing when compared with blood pressure from the sitting or supine position). Neurologic examination should identify focal neurological signs and hyperventilation may reproduce the symptoms if history is suggestive of this being the cause.

1.6.2.3 Further Investigations

Further assessments are indicated if warning bells are present in the history, syncope is recurrent, convulsion occurs during syncope, and physical findings are abnormal. The initial investigation is usually an electrocardiogram to assess for arrhythmias, preexcitation, corrected QT interval, evidence of Brugada syndrome, and voltage criteria for ventricular hypertrophy. In an acute setting, haemoglobin, glucose, and electrolytes are usually checked, though rarely abnormal. Other investigations are guided by history and examination findings. Cardiac investigations include an echocardiogram, ambulatory electrocardiographic monitoring, exercise testing (for assessing changes in QT interval and arrhythmias), and tilt table testing (for assessing recurrent unexplained syncope). Neurologic investigations include electroencephalogram and brain imaging.

1.7 Sudden Cardiac Arrest

Sudden cardiac arrest is a rare presentation of cardiac disease in children. A mortality rate of about 90% has been reported in children presenting with sudden cardiac arrest. Survivors of sudden cardiac arrest require extensive workup for the underlying cardiac abnormality.

1.7.1 Causes of Sudden Cardiac Arrest

While the cause may remain unknown despite extensive assessments in some of the survivors, identifiable causes include arrhythmic and non-arrhythmic ones (Table 1.11).

1.7.2 Clinical Approach

1.7.2.1 History Taking

Although cardiac arrest as a presentation may often seem to develop suddenly without antecedent complaints, warning symptoms and a significant family history are not infrequently noted during history taking in survivors after successful resuscitation (Box 1.6).

Table 1.11 Causes of sudden cardiac arrest in children and adolescents

Arrhythmic	Non-arrhythmic
Primary arrhythmias	Structural or functional cardiac abnormalities
Brugada syndrome	Cardiomyopathies
Catecholaminergic polymorphic ventricular tachycardia	Myocarditis
Long or short QT syndrome	Congenital heart disease
Preexcitation syndromes	Pulmonary hypertension
Arrhythmias associated with underlying heart disease	Coronary artery abnormalities
Cardiomyopathies	Anomalous origin of coronary artery
Myocarditis	Thrombosis of coronary artery aneurysm after Kawasaki disease
Congenital heart disease	Premature coronary artery disease
	Others
	Aortic dissection (e.g. Marfan syndrome)
	Commotio cordis
	Drug-induced

Box 1.6 Warning Symptoms and Significant History in Survivors of Sudden Cardiac Arrest

- chest pain on exertion
- excessive fatigue and/or shortness of breath after exertion
- syncope or near fainting, especially after exertion
- dizziness
- palpitations
- symptoms suggestive of recent viral infection
- family history of sudden death in young relatives

1.7.2.2 Physical Examination

Initial examination should target at the assessment of the clinical manifestations of post-cardiac arrest syndrome. These include evidence of brain injury (encephalopathy and seizure), myocardial dysfunction (low cardiac output syndrome), and systemic ischaemia and reperfusion injury (fever, hypotension, and multiorgan dysfunction). After initial stabilization, cardiovascular signs of importance include the pulse rhythm and signs suggestive of myocarditis and cardiomyopathies, left and right ventricular outflow obstruction and other structural heart lesions, and pulmonary hypertension.

1.7.2.3 Further Investigations

Comprehensive cardiovascular assessments are indicated in survivors of sudden cardiac arrest. Initial investigations should include an electrocardiogram to assess for arrhythmias, preexcitation, corrected QT interval, evidence of Brugada syndrome, and voltage criteria for ventricular hypertrophy, and an echocardiogram for structural and functional assessment of the heart. Further investigations are guided by history and examination findings and may include an exercise stress testing (for assessing changes in QT interval and arrhythmias), adrenaline provocation test (for diagnosis of long QT syndrome and catecholaminergic polymorphic ventricular tachycardia), flecainide challenge test (for unmasking of the ECG pattern in Brugada syndrome), ambulatory electrocardiographic monitoring, computed tomography coronary angiography, and cardiac magnetic resonance imaging. Genetic testing using targeted panels (cardiac arrhythmias and cardiomyopathies) is based on the diagnosis of an identifiable disease phenotype by initial investigations and informs the need for cascade evaluation. Emerging data also support the use of genetic testing in survivors with sudden cardiac arrest that remains unexplained despite extensive assessment.

1.8 Palpitations

Palpitations describe an uncomfortable sensation of feeling that the heart is beating strongly, fast, or irregularly. In children and adolescents, palpitations are most commonly due to physiological stimuli (anxiety, fever, exercise, hyperventilation, caffeine, and anaemia). Non-cardiac causes of palpitations in childhood include thyrotoxicosis, phaeochromocytoma, and hypoglycaemia.

Cardiac causes of palpations in children and adolescents are premature atrial and ventricular contraction, more significant cardiac arrhythmias (e.g. supraventricular and ventricular arrhythmias), and mitral valve prolapse. Supraventricular and ventricular arrhythmias can occur in isolation or in association with congenital (both before and after surgery) and acquired heart disease. Nonetheless, palpitations are not the usual complaints on initial presentation of congenital and acquired heart disease in children and adolescents.

1.9 Newborn Screening

Newborn screening using pulse oximetry aims to identify neonates with critical congenital heart defects before development of symptoms or signs and before they are discharged from the hospital.

1.9.1 Targeted Critical Congenital Heart Defects

Critical congenital heart defects are those that present with hypoxaemia at some or most of the time and require intervention in the first year of life. These include all of the cyanotic congenital heart defects described in Part III (Chaps. 16–22), double-outlet right ventricle (Chap. 23), critical aortic stenosis and coarctation and interruption of the aorta (Chap. 13), and critical pulmonary stenosis (Chap. 12). The sensitivity of pulse oximetry for their detection differs, however, among defects (Table 1.12).

Additionally, conditions other than critical congenital heart defects, which may present with hypoxaemia (e.g. pneumonia, pneumothorax, meconium aspiration, persistent pulmonary hypertension of the newborn, sepsis), may also be detected.

Table 1.12 Sensitivity of pulse oximetry for detection of critical congenital heart disease

High (>85%)	Medium (60–80%)	Low (<60%)
Pulmonary atresia	Tricuspid atresia	Coarctation of the aorta
Critical pulmonary stenosis	Double-outlet right ventricle	Interrupted aortic arch
Transposition of the great arteries	Critical aortic stenosis	Tetralogy of Fallot
Truncus arteriosus		Ebstein anomaly
Total anomalous pulmonary venous drainage		
Functional single ventricles		
Hypoplastic left heart syndrome		

Based on Martin et al. Pediatrics 2020:146:e20191650

1.9.2 Strategies for Pulse Oximetry Screening

The screening involves that measurement of the oxygen saturation (SpO2) in the right hand (preductal oxygen saturation) and either foot (postductal oxygen saturation) using a motion-tolerant pulse oximeter at around 24 h of age or earlier if being discharged.

1.9.2.1 Screening Algorithm

The screening algorithm in the United States has been updated in 2018. The differences from the 2011 American Academy of Pediatrics algorithm include (a) the requirement of ≥95% in both (formerly either) the right hand and foot to be considered a pass, (b) having only 1 retest instead of 2, and (c) the acknowledgement that earlier screening within the first 24 h is acceptable (Fig. 1.1).

1.9.2.2 Assessment of Newborns with Failed Screening

Newborns who failed the screening (positive screen) should be evaluated to identify the cause of hypoxaemia. Initial evaluation should include complete history taking and physical examination to determine noncardiac and cardiac causes of

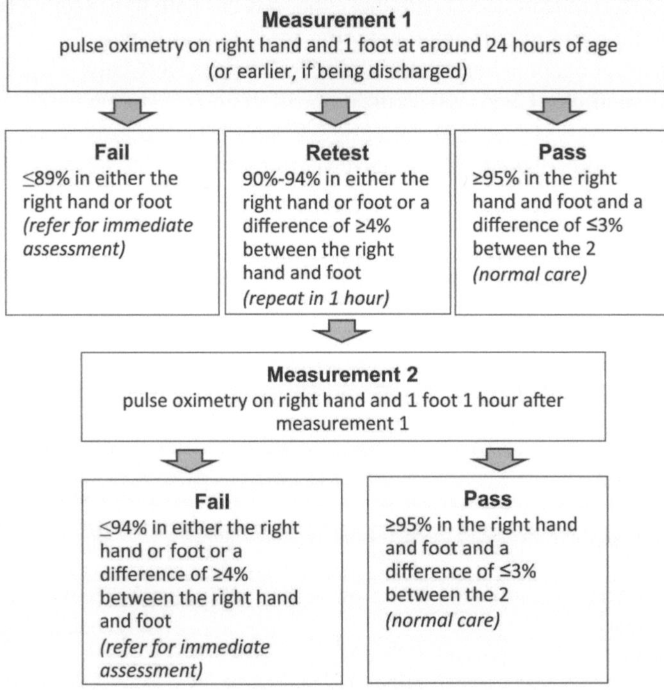

Fig. 1.1 2018 updated algorithm in the United States for screening of critical congenital heart disease with pulse oximetry. (Adapted with modifications from Martin et al. Pediatrics 2020:146:e20191650)

hypoxaemia. Further investigations include usually blood tests to screen for sepsis, a chest radiograph to assess respiratory conditions, and an echocardiography to diagnose critical congenital heart disease and persistent pulmonary hypertension of the newborn. The false positive rate of pulse oximetry screening for critical congenital heart disease has been reported to be 0.06%.

1.9.2.3 Newborns with Negative Screening

While majority of newborns with negative screening do not harbour critical congenital heart disease, it is important to note that a negative screen does not rule out congenital heart disease. Newborns and infants with a negative screen can still have acyanotic congenital heart disease and even critical congenital heart disease as hypoxaemia may not always be present. The suspicion of congenital heart disease based on history and physical examination should supersede a negative pulse oximetry screening in guiding the need for further evaluation.

History Taking

2

History taking is an active and goal-oriented process by which relevant information is gathered for hypothesis generation and irrelevant information is filtered. History taking is an art and requires good verbal and non-verbal communications skills and listening skills (Table 2.1).

Table 2.1 Communication skills

Verbal	Non-verbal	Listening
• greet and introduce yourself	• put the informant at ease	• listen and observe actively for verbal and non-verbal cues
• gather appropriate information in a sensitive manner	• maintain eye contact	• avoid unnecessary interruptions
• pace questions in a coherent manner	• be sensitive and respond to verbal and non-verbal cues	• observe interaction between parents and child
• use appropriate tone	• use appropriate body language	
• avoid the use of jargons, explain where necessary	• show an appropriate level of confidence	
• use language deemed appropriate for the informant		

Y.-f. Cheung, *Congenital and Paediatric Acquired Heart Disease in Practice*, https://doi.org/10.1007/978-981-99-2862-0_2

2.1 Framework of Paediatric History Taking

Paediatric history taking differs from adult history taking (Box 2.1). This step represents the first encounter with the patient and parents and formal establishment of a doctor-patient relationship. Through history taking, rapport between doctors and the family is beginning to establish.

Box 2.1 Points to Note on Paediatric History Taking

- involvement of child and family in history taking
- parents are the primary informants
- unique information to be gathered: antenatal, perinatal and birth history, development, immunization, emphasis on family and social history
- age and development to be considered when generating hypothesis

2.1.1 Introduction

- self-introduction
- note the name, age, sex, and ethnicity of the child
- note the relation to the carer(s) who bring him/her for the consultation
- establish rapport by playing with infants and young children and talking to older children and adolescents
- observe the interaction between the parents (carers) and the child

2.1.2 Presenting Complaints

- reason(s) for the present consultation
- duration of the presenting complaint(s)

2.1.3 History of Presenting Problems

This is the most important part of history taking. One should always begin with open questions to allow the parents and the older children to describe the history of the presenting complaint(s) in their own way. Avoid frequent interruptions to facilitate a good flow of information from patients and parents. Fill in the details afterwards with closed (specific) questions.

Note the chronology and severity of presenting and associated symptoms, previous consultations, explore concerns of parents and carers, and identify important medical and psychosocial problems. Ask goal-directed closed questions to facilitate hypothesis generation (formulation and exclusion of differential diagnoses). There is nothing as a routine set of questions. There must be a reason for each of the questions, open or closed, being asked.

For children with presentations that may suggest an underlying heart disease (Chap. 1), one may wish to enquire about further:

- the occasion in which cardiac murmur was detected
- presence of associated cardiac symptoms (heart failure, cyanosis)
- exercise tolerance and capacity
- previous consultation and presumptive diagnosis
- previous investigations performed and the findings
- medical and surgical treatments received and current medications

2.1.4 Systemic Enquiry

A blind systemic review of symptoms is counterproductive. A general enquiry of symptomatology of all body systems is unnecessary. One should only focus on the relevant ones:

- general activity and playfulness
- diet, appetite and growth
- behaviour
- respiratory system (cough, wheezing, shortness of breath, recurrent chest infections)
- gastrointestinal system (gastroesophageal reflux, vomiting, diarrhoea, constipation)
- genitourinary system (dysuria, frequency)
- neurological system (seizures, stroke, abnormal movements)

2.1.5 Antenatal and Perinatal History

- parity, gestation, birth weight
- fetal ultrasound examination
- maternal medical problems (e.g. gestational diabetes, systemic lupus erythematosus, phenylketonuria)
- antenatal infection (e.g. rubella)
- maternal use of teratogenic medications, alcohol and smoking habit during pregnancy
- birth and perinatal problems

2.1.6 Past Medical History

- other medical problems
- use of medications
- drug and food allergies
- previous hospital admissions

2.1.7 Developmental History

Developmental delay may occur in infants and children with congenital heart disease due to prolonged hospitalization, emotional deprivation, associated brain abnormalities and syndromic disorders, morbidities related to poor haemodynamics (e.g. severe heart failure, intense cyanosis), and history of cardiopulmonary bypass. A detailed developmental history is important for infants and young children, although it is probably less relevant for the older children and adolescents.

- developmental milestones (gross motor, fine motor, language, social development, vision, hearing)
- predisposing risk factors in those with evidence of developmental delay

2.1.8 Immunization History

In general, heart disease in children is not a contraindication to immunization. The immunization record should be checked. Influenza and pneumococcal vaccinations are recommended, in particular for children with heart failure, those with cyanotic congenital heart defects, and those with congenital asplenia that occurs in association with heterotaxy syndrome (Chap. 20). Influenza vaccination is also recommended for children on long-term aspirin therapy (e.g. in Kawasaki disease patients with coronary artery aneurysms). In children presenting with chest pain, enquiry about recent mRNA COVID-19 vaccination is required.

2.1.9 Contact and Clustering History

Febrile illnesses may precipitate heart failure in infants with large left-to-right shunts and in children with cardiomyopathies. Febrile illness with skin rash may be infectious in origin or can be due to Kawasaki disease.

2.1.10 Family History

The risk of congenital heart disease in siblings and offspring of patients is greater than that in the general population (Chap. 62). There is an association between congenital cardiac malformations and consanguineous marriage. Cardiomyopathies has usually an autosomal dominant inheritance pattern, although autosomal recessive, X-linked, and mitochondrial patterns of inheritance are also possible (Chap. 44).

- family history of congenital and acquired heart disease
- construction of a pedigree
- consanguineous marriage

2.1.11 Social History

The importance of the social history cannot be overemphasized. Paediatric heart disease is a chronic childhood condition that may require long-term medications, multiple catheter interventions and operations, and long-term follow-up.

- parental occupation
- housing
- social and financial status
- the main caretaker
- schooling

2.2 Outcomes After History Taking

At the end of the history taking, one should summarize the history, identify the problem(s) of the patient, reason the implications of the information gathered, and proceed with targeted physical examination and investigations (Box 2.2).

Box 2.2 Outcomes of History Taking

- identify and summarize the important medical and psychosocial problems
- understand the concerns of parents and carers
- formulate and prioritize differential diagnoses
- exclude the less likely differential diagnoses
- ascertain severity of the problems and their impact on child and family
- use the information gathered to guide physical examination, investigations, and management

3 Paediatric Cardiovascular Examination

Like history taking, physical examination is an art. It should be goal-oriented and aim to provide additional information to help to confirm or reject hypothesis. It may be tempting for diagnose a cardiac condition based on cardiac murmurs alone. Nonetheless, auscultatory findings are neither sensitive nor specific in the diagnosis of paediatric cardiac conditions as described later in this Chapter.

3.1 Framework of Paediatric Cardiovascular Examination

Examination of the cardiovascular system in children differs from that in adults (Box 3.1). A complete cardiovascular examination includes (a) general inspection, (b) pulse examination, (c) praecordial inspection, (d) praecordial palpation, (e) auscultation, and (f) examination of other systems (chest and abdomen).

Box 3.1 Points to Note on Paediatric Examination

- depending on whether the child is cooperative or not, the sequence of examination may need to be altered
- assessment of jugular venous pressure is difficult, if not impossible, in infants and young children (but not usually useful for the initial diagnosis of heart disease in children)
- age of patient needs to be considered when interpreting pulse rate, respiratory rate, and blood pressure

Y.-f. Cheung, *Congenital and Paediatric Acquired Heart Disease in Practice*, https://doi.org/10.1007/978-981-99-2862-0_3

3.1.1 General Inspection

3.1.1.1 Growth

The general well-being, nutritional status, and physical growth of the child should be noted. The weight, height, and head circumference should be measured and plotted onto standard growth charts.

Failure to thrive is common in heart failure due to poor nutritional intake and increased energy expenditure. The weight percentile drops first, followed by the height percentile. The increase in head circumference is usually spared. Short stature is seen for example in Turner syndrome, which is associated with coarctation of the aorta and bicuspid aortic valve. On the other hand, tall stature is seen in Marfan syndrome, which is associated with mitral valve prolapse, aortic root dilation, and aortic regurgitation.

3.1.1.2 Dysmorphism

Congenital malformation syndromes and genetic disorders are associated with dysmorphic facial features and congenital heart disease (Chap. 62). The presence of characteristic phenotypic abnormalities of these syndromic and genetic disorders should prompt one to examine for associated cardiac abnormalities.

3.1.1.3 Cyanosis

Central cyanosis is assessed usually by examination of the colour of the tongue (Fig. 3.1a). The conjunctiva may be congested due to secondary polycythaemia. When the bluish discoloration is limited to the extremities, this is referred to as peripheral cyanosis. Peripheral cyanosis is due to vasoconstriction secondary to hypothermia or a low cardiac output.

3.1.1.4 Hand and Feet

Chronic hypoxaemia, even of a subclinical degree, results in clubbing of fingers and toes (Fig. 3.1b). Clubbing manifests initially as an increase in convexity of the nails,

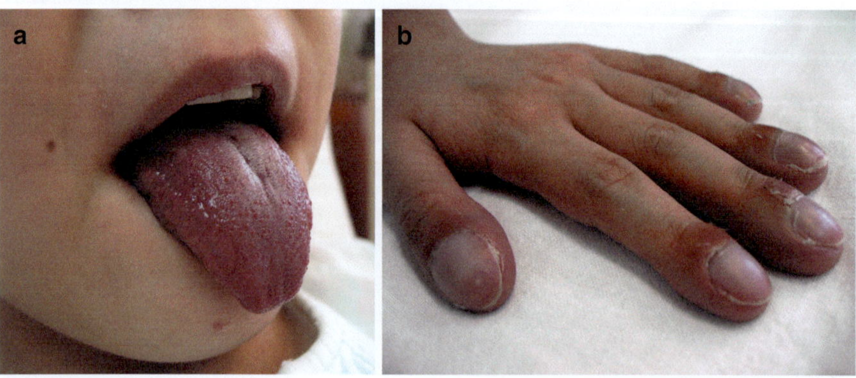

Fig. 3.1 Central cyanosis and clubbing. (**a**) Central cyanosis. (**b**) Finger clubbing

with further extension of the convexity to include the base of the nail, and eventually elimination of the angle between the base of the nail and contiguous soft tissue. On applying light pressure to the nail base, a spongy texture may be detected.

Infective endocarditis may complicate congenital heart disease and congenital and acquired valvar abnormalities. Clinical manifestations on the hands and feet include (a) splinter haemorrhages in the nail beds, which can be subtle, (b) Osler nodes: tender, erythematous, raised areas in the pulps of the fingers and toes and on the thenar and hypothenar eminence of the palms and the soles, (c) Janeway lesions: painless haemorrhagic cutaneous lesions on the palms and soles, and (d) finger clubbing.

The fingers are long, slender (arachnodactyly) and hyperextensible in Marfan syndrome (Fig. 3.2a–c). Increased space between the fourth and fifth fingers, incurving of the short fifth finger (clinodactyly), a single transverse palmer crease, and sandal gap between the first and second toes are present in Down syndrome (Fig. 3.2d, e). Polydactyly of the hands is seen in Ellis-van Creveld syndrome, which is associated with a common atrium with absence of the atrial septum. On the other hand, the thumb is absent or hypoplastic in Holt-Oram syndrome, which is associated commonly with secundum atrial septal defect.

3.1.1.5 Dependent Oedema

Fluid retention is a feature of heart failure. In heart failure related to impaired contraction or relaxation of the ventricles, imbalance of Starling forces with an increase in intravascular hydrostatic pressure results in leakage of fluid from the vascular to the interstitial compartment. The clinical manifestation is pitting and dependent oedema over the ankle and feet (in the upright position) or sacrum (in the supine

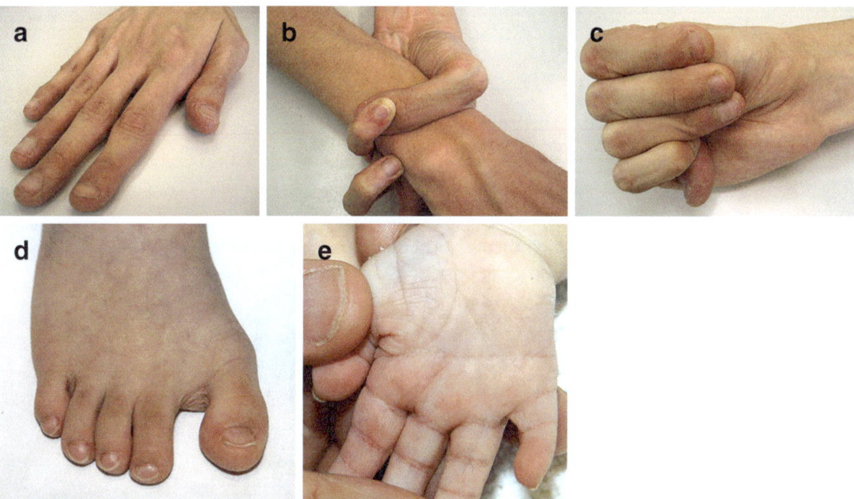

Fig. 3.2 Hand and feet examination. (**a**) Arachnodactyly. (**b**) Wrist sign. (**c**) Thumb sign. (**d**) Sandal gap between the first and second toe. (**e**) Single palmar crease and clinodactyly

position). In infants with heart failure, most commonly due to large left-to-right shunts, dependent oedema is unusual as ventricular contraction and intravascular hydrostatic pressure remain normal.

3.1.2 Pulse Examination

After general inspection, one should proceed to examine the pulses of the upper and lower limbs. The following features of the pulses should be noted: rate, rhythm, character, volume, and presence or absence of radio-femoral pulse volume discrepancy or delay.

In older children and adolescents, the radial arterial pulse is assessed for pulse characteristics. In small infants, the brachial arterial pulse is preferred, as the brachial artery is larger and closer to the central arteries, hence allowing for more accurate assessment of the pulse characteristics.

After examining the upper limb pulses, the femoral arterial pulse should be examined. Diminished femoral pulse volume is a sign of coarctation or interruption of the aorta. However, the radio-femoral pulse 'delay' found in older children and adults with aortic coarctation may be difficult to detect due to the short aortic length in infants and small children.

Abnormalities of the pulse character and volume provide clue to underlying cardiac abnormalities (Table 3.1). A bounding pulse, which is exaggerated by elevation of the forearm and felt with the distal palmar surface of the hand, is due to a large persistent arterial duct or severe aortic regurgitation. The pulse appears collapsing in nature as the increase in left ventricular volume causes a rapid upstroke, while diastolic runoff to respectively the pulmonary artery and the left ventricle leads to a rapid descent of the pulse. Weak or absent femoral pulses in the presence of strong upper limb pulses suggest aortic coarctation or interruption. In severe aortic

Table 3.1 Pulse character and cardiac abnormalities

Pulse character	Cardiac abnormalities
Large volume, strong pulses	Persistent arterial duct
	Systemic arteriovenous fistula
	Significant aortic regurgitation (aortic valve pathologies, aortic root dilation)
	Hyperdynamic circulation (anaemia, thyrotoxicosis)
Small volume, weak pulses	Aortic stenosis
	Low cardiac output syndrome (cardiogenic, hypovolaemic or cold septic shock)
Absent or weak lower limb pulses only	Coarctation of the aorta
	Interrupted aortic arch
Pulsus bisferiens	Aortic regurgitation with or without stenosis
	Hypertrophic cardiomyopathy
Pulsus paradoxus	Constrictive pericarditis
	Cardiac tamponade

stenosis, all of the arterial pulses are weak and slow rising. Pulsus bisferiens refers to a double-peaked arterial pulse with a mid-systolic dip and is most commonly detected in severe aortic regurgitation. Pulsus paradoxus describes the marked fall in pulse volume and systemic arterial pressure during inspiration and is found in cardiac tamponade.

3.1.3 Praecordial Inspection

The child should be undressed to expose the praecordium and the chest for inspection of the following features: signs of respiratory distress, Harrison's sulcus, chest deformities, surgical scars, and cardiac pulsation. Inspection of the jugular venous pulse is challenging, if not impossible, in infants and young children.

3.1.3.1 Respiratory Distress

Signs of respiratory distress include tachypnoea, subcostal and suprasternal insucking, and use of accessory respiratory muscles. In children with heart disease, these signs are due to pulmonary arterial congestion (increased pulmonary arterial flow in large left-to-right shunts) and/or pulmonary venous congestion (reduced left ventricular compliance in volume overloaded left ventricle, increased left ventricular end-diastolic pressure in dilated cardiomyopathy, mitral stenosis, pulmonary venous obstruction).

3.1.3.2 Harrison's Sulcus

Repetitive traction on the diaphragmatic insertions of the rib cage during growth results in Harrison's sulcus, which is recognized by a depression in the lower rib cage. This is found in infants and young children with chronic respiratory distress due to pulmonary vascular congestion or obstructive airway disease.

3.1.3.3 Chest Deformities

Bulging of the praecordium is seen in infants and children with cardiomegaly. It is most prominent when the right ventricle is dilated. Pectus excavatum and carinatum are features of Marfan syndrome.

3.1.3.4 Surgical Scars

A mid-sternotomy scar (Fig 3.3a) suggests previous open heart surgery (e.g. patch closure of ventricular septal defect, repair of tetralogy of Fallot, arterial switch operation for transposition of the great arteries). A thoracotomy scar (Fig. 3.3b) may indicate previous systemic-to-pulmonary arterial shunt insertion (e.g. palliation of pulmonary atresia with ventricular septal defect) or surgical repair of coarctation of the aorta.

3.1.3.5 Cardiac Pulsation

The cardiac pulsation may be visible in children with a thin chest wall. However, an obvious pulsation may signify volume or pressure overload of either the left or the

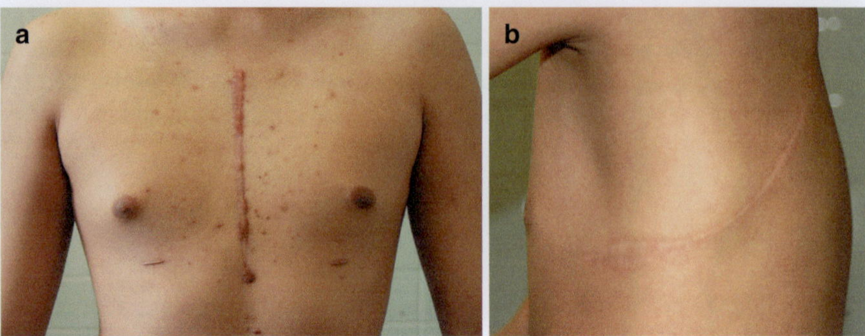

Fig. 3.3 Surgical scars. (**a**) Mid-sternotomy scar. (**b**) Lateral thoracotomy scar

right ventricle, depending on the site of pulsation. In the normal heart, the left ventricle occupies the apex, while the right ventricle is anteriorly located and lies beneath the left lower sternal border at the fourth and fifth intercostal spaces.

3.1.3.6 Jugular Venous Pulse

Evaluation of jugular venous pulsation with positioning of the patient at 45° by elevating the head of the bed is challenging, if not impossible, in infants and young children. Assessment of jugular venous pressure is not usually useful for initial diagnosis of heart disease in children. It is more indicated in older children and adolescents with conditions associated with right ventricular systolic and diastolic dysfunction (e.g. cardiomyopathy, repaired tetralogy of Fallot) and significant tricuspid regurgitation.

3.1.4 Praecordial Palpation

After inspection of the praecordium, palpation should be performed to locate the cardiac apex, assess abnormally strong cardiac impulses, detect praecordial thrills, and feel for suprasternal pulsation.

3.1.4.1 Localization of Cardiac Apex

In the normal heart, the left ventricle is at the apex. The position of the apex beat is defined by the lowest and outermost point of distinct cardiac pulsation. Its location is described in terms of the intercostal space and distance from the mid-clavicular line. In children, it is best identified using the tips of the index and middle fingers. It is normally located in the fourth intercostal space in infants and the fifth intercostal space in older children at or medial to the mid-clavicular line.

3.1.4.2 Assessment of Cardiac Impulse

Abnormal cardiac impulses are related to either pressure or volume overloading of the ventricles (Table 3.2).

As the left ventricle is at the cardiac apex, a strong apical cardiac impulse suggests left ventricular pressure or volume overloading. In pressure overloading conditions, the cardiac apex is usually not displaced. By contrast, volume

Table 3.2 Praecordial impulse and cardiac abnormalities

Impulse	Cardiac abnormalities
Left ventricular (apical) impulse	Volume overloading of left ventricle: large left-to-right shunts (ventricular septal defect, atrioventricular septal defect, persistent arterial duct, aortopulmonary window), left-sided valvar regurgitation (mitral regurgitation, aortic regurgitation)
	Pressure overloading of left ventricle: aortic stenosis (valvar, subvalvar and supravalvar), coarctation of the aorta, systemic hypertension, hypertrophic obstructive cardiomyopathy
	Left ventricular dilation due to impaired myocardial function: dilated cardiomyopathy
Right ventricular (left parasternal) impulse	Volume loading of right ventricle: large left-to-right atrial shunt (atrial septal defect), right-sided valvar regurgitation (tricuspid regurgitation, pulmonary regurgitation)
	Pressure overloading of right ventricle: pulmonary stenosis (valvar, subvalvar and supravalvar), branch pulmonary arterial stenosis, pulmonary hypertension

overloading of the left ventricle results in lateral displacement of the cardiac apex.

The body of the right ventricle underlies the left lower sternal border at the fourth and fifth intercostal spaces. A left parasternal impulse suggests therefore right ventricular hypertrophy or dilation. It may be felt by placing the heel of the hand (distal metacarpals) firmly over the praecordium just to the left of the sternum. In infants and small children, palpation along the left sternal border with the fingertips may be useful for the detection of mildly increased right ventricular impulse.

3.1.4.3 Detection of Praecordial Thrill

A thrill is a palpable murmur with an intensity of at least grade 4/6. The location and timing in relation to the cardiac cycle of a thrill help in the diagnosis of the underlying heart disease. Thrills should be sought over the praecordium, at the suprasternal region, and over the carotid arteries. The presence of carotid thrills suggests aortic stenosis.

3.1.4.4 Feel for Suprasternal Pulsation

The great arteries lie in proximity to the suprasternal area. The main pulmonary artery is beneath the left second intercostal space, and the aortic root is convex to the right of the sternum in the second intercostal space. Prominent suprasternal pulsation with or without thrills occurs in aortic stenosis, pulmonary stenosis and, less commonly, coarctation of the aorta and persistent arterial duct.

3.1.5 Auscultation

3.1.5.1 Use of Stethoscope

The stethoscope has a diaphragm and a bell. Diaphragm picks up high-pitched sounds and murmurs better. Splitting of the second heart sound and the blowing diastolic murmur in aortic regurgitation are best heard with the diaphragm. The bell is used to pick up low-pitched sounds and heart murmurs. Diastolic heart sounds (third and fourth heart sounds) and diastolic murmurs through the atrioventricular

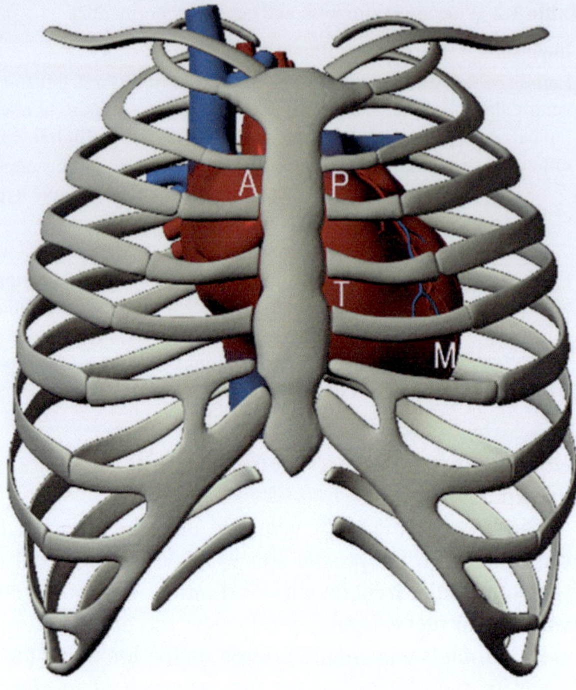

Fig. 3.4 Auscultatory areas. A, aortic area (right upper sternal border in the second intercostal space), P, pulmonary area (left upper sternal border in the second intercostal space), T, tricuspid area (left lower sternal border), M, mitral area (apex)

valve (e.g. the rumbling diastolic murmur in mitral stenosis) are best heard with the bell. In children with heart disease, the diaphragm is more commonly used for auscultation than the bell.

3.1.5.2 Auscultatory Areas

In general, one starts by listening to the four cardinal auscultatory areas with the diaphragm. These cardinal areas have been customarily called by the name of the valve from which murmurs and sounds arise (Fig. 3.4). These terms may not be applicable to children with complex congenital heart disease. Furthermore, sounds and murmurs heard in a particular area may not necessarily arise from that particular valve. Hence, the areas for auscultation are best described by the location on the praecordium.

Apart from listening to the praecordium, one should also place the stethoscope over the carotid arteries as systolic murmurs of aortic in origin may radiate to the carotid arteries. Furthermore, murmurs should also be sought from the posterior chest wall. Murmurs arising from stenotic branch pulmonary arteries radiate to the back. Soft, continuous murmurs of collaterals (in association with aortic coarctation or pulmonary atresia and ventricular septal defect) are also heard on the back.

3.1.5.3 Repositioning of Patient

With the patient leaning forward in a sitting positioning and breathing out, the high-pitched diastolic murmur of aortic regurgitation at the left sternal edge, best heard

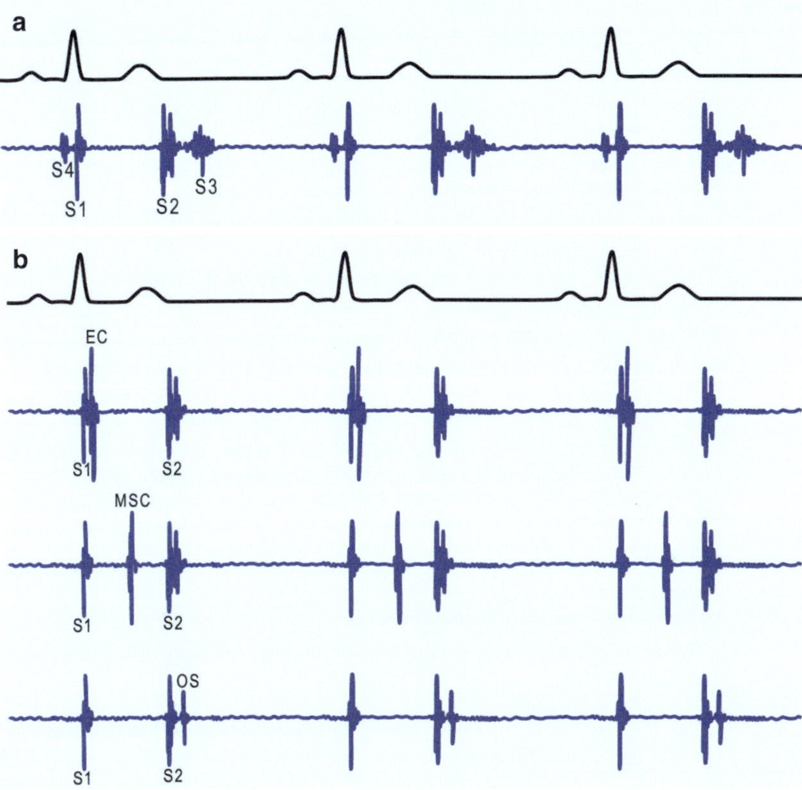

Fig. 3.5 Heart sounds and added sounds. (**a**) Timing of the four heart sounds. (**b**) Added sounds: *EC* ejection click, *MSC* mid-systolic click, *OS* opening snap

using the diaphragm, is accentuated. Turning of the patient to the left lateral decubitus position brings the left ventricle closer to the bell of the stethoscope and facilitates auscultation of diastolic flow murmur across the mitral valve.

3.1.5.4 Heart Sounds and Added Sounds

The timing of the four heart sounds and added sounds are illustrated in Fig. 3.5 and their origins and interpretation are described in Table 3.3.

3.1.5.5 Heart Murmurs

Turbulent blood flow within the heart or blood vessels produces vibrations and audible as murmurs. Turbulence occurs when (a) flow volume increases (e.g. in hyperdynamic circulation, increased pulmonary flow in atrial septal defect), (b) flow velocity increases across stenosis (e.g. valvar stenosis) or cardiac chambers with different pressures (e.g. ventricular septal defect), and (c) blood flows into a vessel with an abrupt increase in calibre (e.g. in post-stenotic aortic dilation, idiopathic dilation of the main pulmonary artery).

Table 3.3 Heart sounds and added sounds

Sound	Origin and interpretation
Heart sounds	
S1	Closure of mitral and tricuspid valves, usually single and best audible at the cardiac apex and left lower sternal border
S2	Closure of aortic and pulmonary and aortic valves, aortic component slightly earlier than pulmonary component (higher aortic pressure)
	Physiological splitting: widening of splitting of S2 during inspiration
	Wide and fixed splitting of S2: atrial septal defect
	Single S2: absent or soft P2 due to pulmonary stenosis or atresia
	Loud P2: pulmonary hypertension
S3	Audible at diastole due to sudden cessation of ventricular distension, contributes to the so-called gallop rhythm, occurs in conditions with dilated and poorly compliant ventricle (e.g. dilated and hypertrophic cardiomyopathies, large ventricular septal defect), may be audible in healthy children
S4	Pathological and generated during atrial filling of poorly compliant ventricles (e.g. left ventricular hypertrophy, hypertrophic cardiomyopathy, endocardial fibroelastosis)
Added sounds	
Ejection click	High frequency sound occurring at early systole, due to valvar pulmonary stenosis (at left mid-sternal border), valvar aortic stenosis (at apex), or dilation of the great arteries (aorta or main pulmonary artery)
Mid-systolic click	High frequency sound occurring at mid systole and audible at apex, due to mitral valve prolapse
Opening snap	High frequency sound occurring at diastole and audible at left lower sternal border, due to mitral stenosis

Table 3.4 Grading of cardiac murmurs

Grade	Description
1	Barely audible
2	Soft
3	Easily audible
4	Loud with a thrill
5	Very loud with a thrill, audible even with stethoscope partly off the chest
6	Very loud with a thrill, audible with the stethoscope off the chest

Heart murmurs should be analyzed and described in terms of the nature, location, intensity (Table 3.4), timing in the cardiac cycle, radiation, and variation with posture.

While the intensity of cardiac murmurs is conventionally graded as shown in Table 3.4, the intensity of diastolic murmurs has also been described in four grades: grade 1, barely audible, grade 2, audible but soft, grade 3, easily audible, and grade 4, loud.

The different types of cardiac murmurs (Fig. 3.6) and their possible causes are described in Table 3.5.

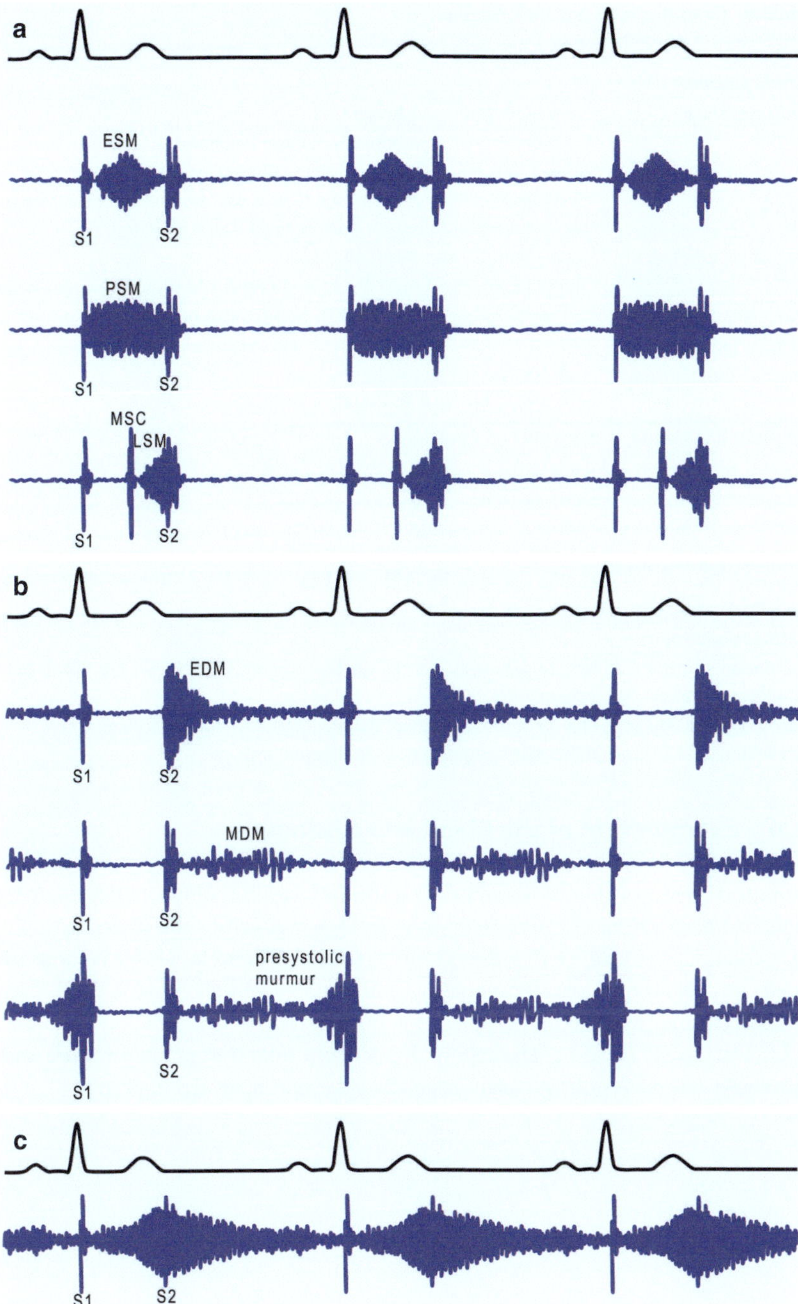

Fig. 3.6 Types of cardiac murmurs. (**a**) Systolic murmurs: *ESM* ejection systolic murmur, *LSM* late diastolic murmur, *PSM* pansystolic murmur. (**b**) Diastolic murmurs: *EDM* early diastolic murmur, *MDM* mid-diastolic murmur. (**c**) Continuous murmur

Table 3.5 Heart murmurs and their origins

Murmur	Nature and origin
Systolic murmurs	
Ejection systolic murmur	Crescendo-decrescendo murmur
	An interval is present between S1 and its onset
	Related to turbulent flow across the obstructed left or right ventricular outflow or increased flow across normal semilunar valve (e.g. increased pulmonary flow in atrial septal defect)
Pansystolic murmur	Begins with S1 and end with S2
	Due to ventricular septal defect and mitral and tricuspid regurgitation
Late-systolic murmur	Due to mitral regurgitation with mitral valve prolapse
Diastolic murmurs	
Early diastolic murmur	High-pitched decrescendo murmur
	Occurs in aortic or pulmonary regurgitation
Mid-diastolic murmur	Low-pitched frequency
	An interval is present between S2 and its onset
	Due to turbulent flow across stenotic mitral or tricuspid valve or increased flow across normal atrioventricular valve (e.g. increased mitral flow in large ventricular septal defect)
Presystolic (late diastolic) murmur	Due to mitral or tricuspid stenosis
Continuous murmurs	
Continuous murmur at infraclavicular area	Due to persistent arterial duct, modified Blalock-Taussig shunt, or venous hum
Continuous murmur in other areas	Due to coronary arterial fistulas, aortopulmonary collaterals, pulmonary arteriovenous malformations

3.1.6 Examination of the Chest and Abdomen

Respiratory distress due to increased pulmonary arterial flow in large-left-right shunts has been discussed. Increased lung fluid as a result of the increased pulmonary venous congestion (e.g. reduced left ventricular compliance in volume overloaded left ventricle, cardiomyopathy, pulmonary venous obstruction) causes so-called cardiac wheeze and crepitations on respiratory examination. Abdominal examination may reveal hepatomegaly due to fluid retention in heart failure and/or an increase central venous pressure secondary to right heart dysfunction.

4 Chest Radiograph

The chest radiograph provides information on haemodynamics (magnitude of left-to-right shunt, severity of valvar regurgitation, adequacy of pulmonary blood flow in cyanotic heart lesions, and evidence of left ventricular inflow obstruction and diastolic filling abnormalities), serial changes in heart size on follow-up of heart failure, and results of surgical or catheter interventions.

From the chest radiograph, the following should be assessed: (a) heart size, (b) cardiac contours, (c) pulmonary vascularity, (d) bony abnormalities, and (e) position of the heart and abdominal organs.

4.1 Heart Size

Heart size is quantified by determining the cardiothoracic ratio (transverse diameter of the heart/width of the thoracic cavity) from the standard frontal film. The heart is enlarged if the cardiothoracic ratio is larger than 0.5 for adults and older children or 0.6 for infants. However, the thymus in infants and young children may simulate cardiomegaly. During expiration and on lying supine, the heart also appears larger.

4.2 Cardiac Contours

The borders of the cardiac silhouette are formed by cardiac chambers and blood vessels (Fig. 4.1). The size and shape of the cardiac silhouette provide clues for underlying cardiac conditions. Enlargement or hypertrophy of different cardiac chambers produces specific changes in the contours of the cardiac silhouette (Table 4.1 and Fig. 4.2).

Y.-f. Cheung, *Congenital and Paediatric Acquired Heart Disease in Practice*, https://doi.org/10.1007/978-981-99-2862-0_4

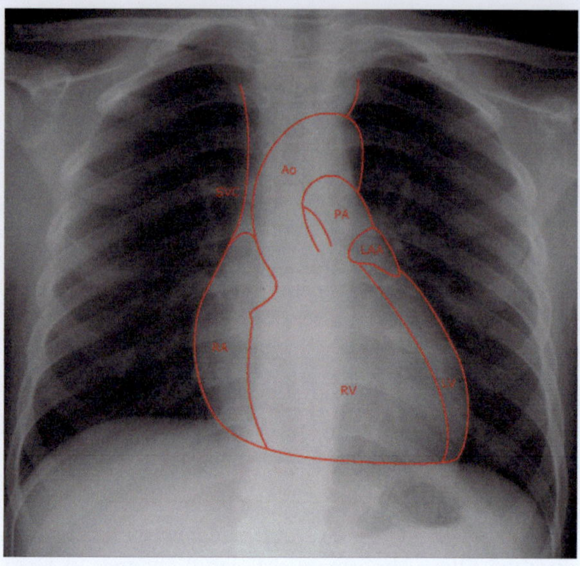

Fig. 4.1 Cardiac silhouette. *Ao* aorta, *LAA* left atrial appendage, *LV* left ventricle, *PA* pulmonary arterial trunk, *RA* right atrium, *RV* right ventricle, *SVC* superior caval vein

Table 4.1 Changes in the contours of the cardiac silhouette

Cardiac chamber dilation or hypertrophy	Contour
Right atrial dilation	Right cardiac border becomes more convex and bulges into the right lung
Right ventricular dilation	Increased cardiothoracic ratio with upward tilting and lateral displacement of cardiac apex
Right ventricular hypertrophy	Upward tilting cardiac apex but with no displacement
Left atrial dilation	A small bulge is present on the left cardiac border, inferior to the shadow of the main pulmonary trunk
Left ventricular dilation	Lateral extension and downward pointing of cardiac apex
Left ventricular hypertrophy	The cardiac size and contour are usually normal

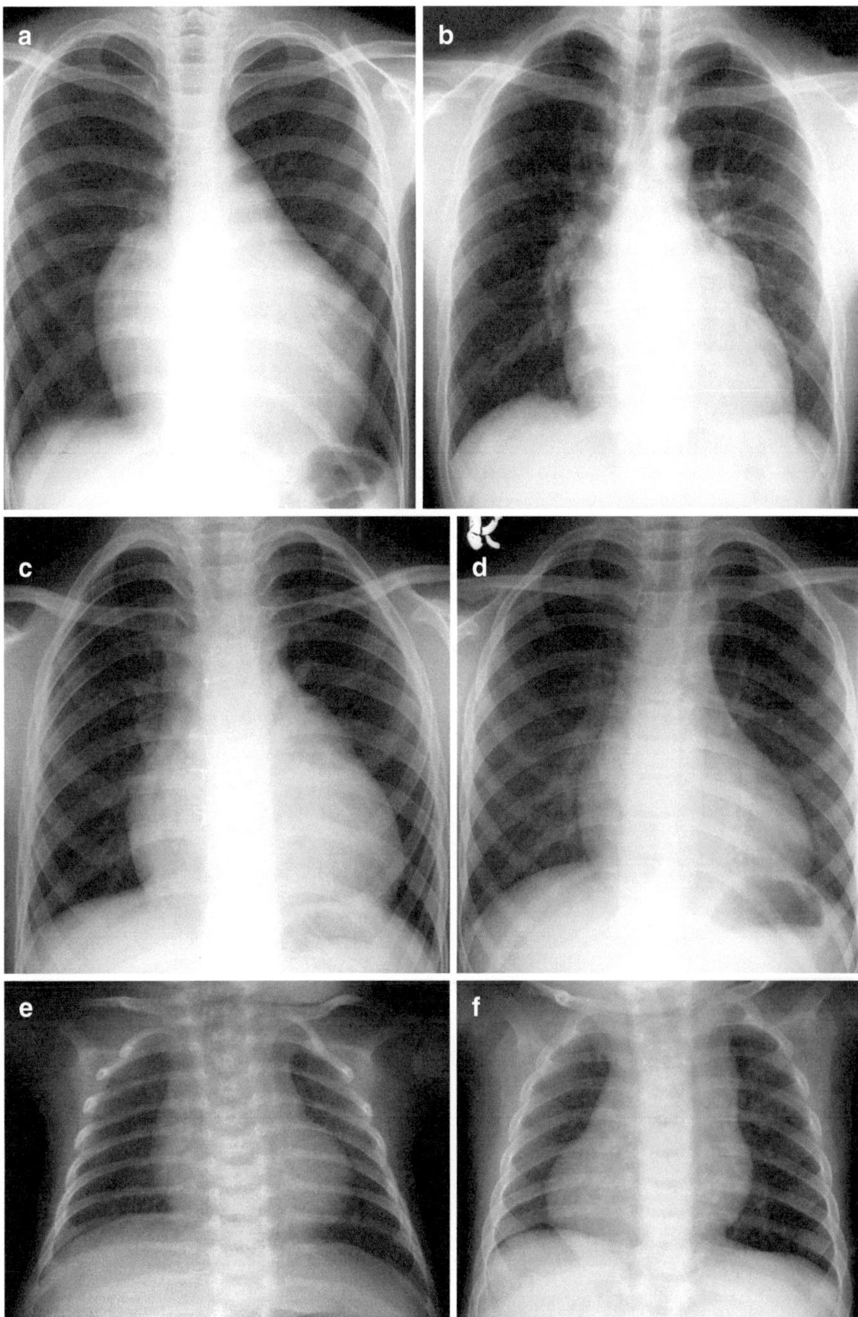

Fig. 4.2 Cardiac contours. (**a**) Right atrial dilation. (**b**) Left atrial dilation. (**c**) Right ventricular dilation. (**d**) Left ventricular dilation. (**e**) Right ventricular hypertrophy. (**f**) Dextrocardia

4.3 Pulmonary Vasculature

The pulmonary vascularity provides information on the amount of pulmonary arterial blood flow and evidence of pulmonary venous obstruction (Fig. 4.3).

In large left-to-right shunts, increased pulmonary vascular markings (pulmonary plethora) with increased cardiothoracic ratio due to volume overloading of the left (e.g. in ventricular septal defect and persistent arterial duct) or the right (e.g. in atrial septal defect) ventricle are characteristic.

Increased pulmonary vascular markings in the presence of a normal-sized heart suggest pulmonary venous congestion due to pulmonary venous obstruction, mitral stenosis, restrictive cardiomyopathy, and conditions causing of left ventricular systolic and diastolic dysfunction. Pulmonary venous markings appear hazy and indistinct, as contrast to the distinct pulmonary arterial markings.

Reduced pulmonary vascular markings (pulmonary oligaemia) causes dark lung fields and is found in cyanotic heart disease with pulmonary outflow obstruction. The degree of pulmonary oligaemia reflects the severity of pulmonary outflow obstruction.

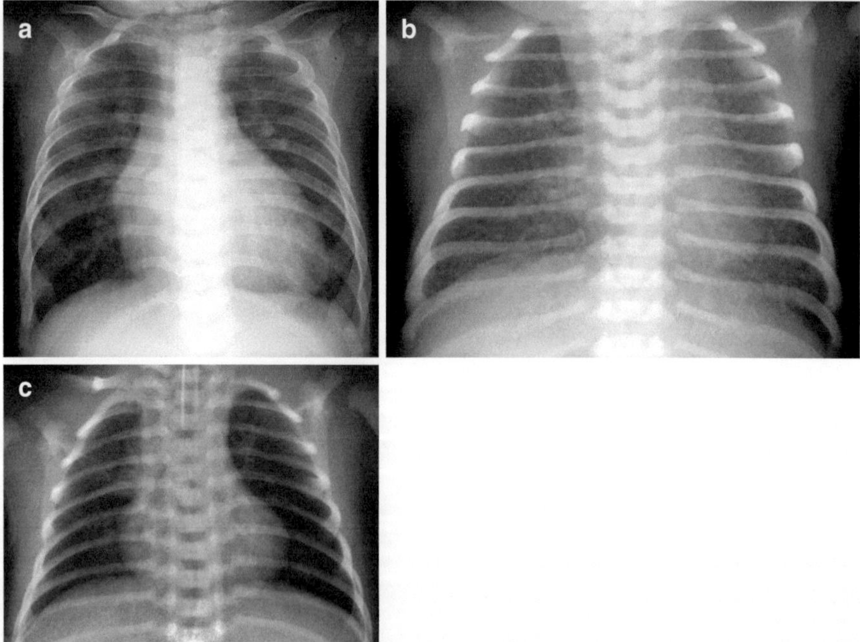

Fig. 4.3 Pulmonary vasculature. (**a**) Plethora lung fields due to increased pulmonary arterial flow and congestion. (**b**) Hazy lung fields due to pulmonary venous congestion. (**c**) Oligaemic lung fields due to reduced pulmonary blood flow

4.4 Bony Abnormalities

Scoliosis and vertebral anomalies due to underlying genetic and other syndromic disorders may be present in patients with congenital heart disease. Scoliosis and other skeletal abnormalities are associated with Marfan syndrome and other inherited disorders of connective tissue disease (Chap. 33). Hemivertebrae and butterfly vertebrae may be present in Alagille syndrome (Chap. 62), which is associated with peripheral branch pulmonary arterial stenosis.

4.5 Position of Heart and Abdominal Organs

Dextrocardia occurs when the greater part of the heart is in the right hemithorax. The abdominal visceral arrangement is assessed by identifying the gastric air bubble and the position of the liver. Dextrocardia in association with abdominal situs inversus suggests mirror-imaged dextrocardia, while dextrocardia in association with a normal left-sided gastric bubble or a central liver and gastric air bubble suggests probable complex congenital cardiac malformation. A central liver suggests heterotaxy syndrome (Chap. 20). Dextrocardia also occurs when the right lung is hypoplastic, which can be associated with partial anomalous pulmonary venous connection in scimitar syndrome (Chap. 37).

5 Electrocardiogram

Electrocardiography provides evidence of hypertrophy or enlargement of cardiac chambers due to an abnormal load in congenital and acquired heart disease in children. Hypertrophy and dilation of a cardiac chamber cause similar electrocardiographic abnormalities. Electrocardiographic (ECG) findings of altered ST segment and T wave changes provide diagnostic clues to pericardial and/or myocardial inflammation and myocardial ischaemia. In conjunction with other investigation modalities, electrocardiography helps in the diagnosis of the underlying congenital and acquired cardiac lesions.

5.1 Age-Related Changes

In interpreting the electrocardiogram of a child, age-related changes in electrocardiographic features must be considered. Continuous changes in ECG variables during childhood (Box 5.1) require the use of different cutoff values (available conveniently nowadays on smartphone apps). Recently, a z-score-based approach to interpret ECG variables has been proposed.

Box 5.1 Change in ECG Variables with Age

- change of right ventricular dominance in infants to left ventricular dominance in older children and adults
- increase in RR interval (decrease in heart rate)
- increase in PR interval, QRS duration, and QT and corrected QT intervals
- increase in praecordial R and S wave amplitudes
- T waves are upright in right praecordial leads in the first week of life, become inverted until 8 years old, and appear upright thereafter (in some adolescents, the juvenile T wave pattern may still be present)

Y.-f. Cheung, *Congenital and Paediatric Acquired Heart Disease in Practice*, https://doi.org/10.1007/978-981-99-2862-0_5

5.2 ECG Features of Ventricular Dominance

In fetuses, the right ventricle is thicker and has a larger stroke volume than the left ventricle as it supplies blood to the descending aorta through the arterial duct. Postnatally, the left ventricular mass progressively increases to cope with the systemic circulation, while the right ventricular mass decreases as the pulmonary vascular resistance drops.

In newborns and infants, the electrocardiographic features of right ventricular dominance include (a) a right QRS axis (mean of 125° in the newborn), (b) tall R waves in right praecordial leads (V1 and V2), and (c) tall S waves in left praecordial leads (V5 and V6). With increasing age, the QRS axis shifts leftward (mean of 90° at 1 month and 60° at 1 year) and an adult R/S progression is seen (dominant S waves in right praecordial leads and dominant R waves in left praecordial leads).

5.3 Hypertrophy or Dilation of Cardiac Chambers

5.3.1 Atrial Hypertrophy or Dilation

The P wave amplitude, duration, and shape provide clues to atrial hypertrophy or dilation (Fig. 5.1a).

Right atrial dilation or hypertrophy produces tall and peaked P waves. A typical example is the 'giant' P waves found in Ebstein anomaly due to gross dilation of the right atrium.

Left atrial dilation or hypertrophy prolongs the P wave duration and the P wave may be notched or biphasic. This is commonly seen in children with volume overloading of the left atrium due to large left-to-right shunts (ventricular septal defect, persistent arterial duct) or mitral regurgitation. A less common cause is left ventricular inflow obstruction, as in congenital or acquired mitral stenosis.

5.3.2 Ventricular Hypertrophy or Dilation

Ventricular dilation or hypertrophy causes abnormalities in ventricular depolarization (QRS axis), amplitude of the QRS complex (QRS voltages and R/S ratio), and ventricular repolarization ('strain' pattern) (Fig. 5.1b, c).

Left ventricular dilation or hypertrophy results in left axis deviation, increased R wave voltage in leads V6, increased S wave voltage in V1, and sometimes a strain pattern (inverted T waves in V6 or I). In children, these abnormalities are commonly seen in large left-to-right shunts (left ventricular volume overload), significant aortic stenosis (left ventricular pressure overload), and cardiomyopathies.

Right ventricular hypertrophy results in right axis deviation, increased R wave voltage in V1 and increased S voltage in V6, and Q wave (qR pattern) in V1. An upright T wave in V1 of children between 3 days and 6 years of age suggests right ventricular hypertrophy. These features occur in children with pulmonary stenosis

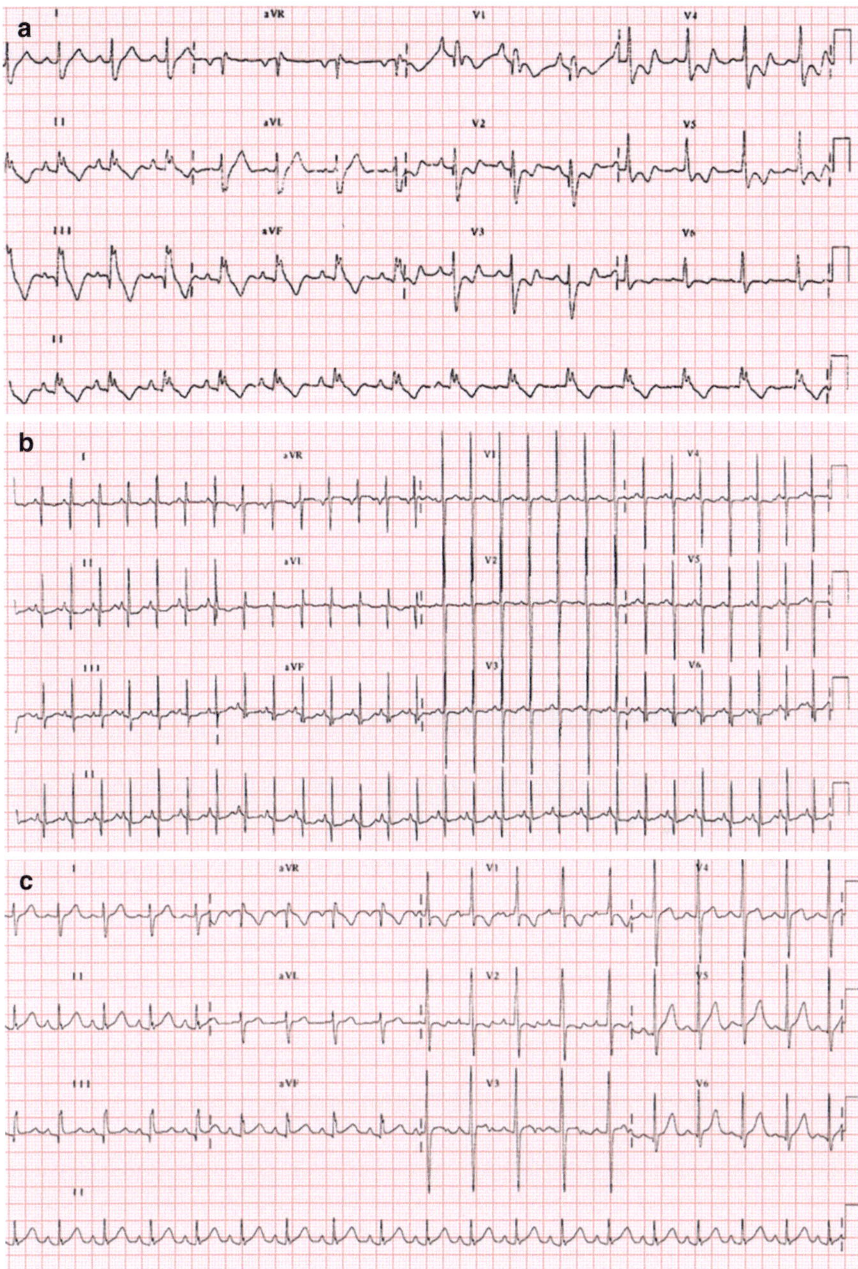

Fig. 5.1 Electrocardiographic findings of chamber hypertrophy or dilation. (**a**) Tall P waves in Ebstein anomaly. (**b**) Electrocardiographic evidence of biventricular ‘hypertrophy’ in large ventricular septal defect. (**c**) Electrocardiographic evidence of right ventricular enlargement in large atrial septal defect

and pulmonary hypertension (right ventricular pressure overload). In right ventricular volume overload, an rsR′ pattern in V1 is commonly observed, as in children with a large atrial septal defect.

Congenital heart disease may cause volume and/or pressure overloading of both ventricles in various combinations. Pulmonary hypertension in association with a large ventricular septal defect, for example, result in right ventricular pressure overload and left ventricular volume overload. Biventricular loading is suggested by the presence of criteria for both left and right ventricular 'hypertrophy' or large equiphasic QRS complexes in the mid-praecordial leads (V2 through V5) (Katz-Wachtel phenomenon).

5.4 Pericardial and Myocardial Disease and Coronary Insufficiency

In healthy subjects, the ST segment is isoelectric. Changes in ST segment and T waves provide clue to pericardial and myocardial disease and myocardial ischaemia. ST segments should not usually be elevated >1 mm or depressed >0.5 mm in any of the leads. Elevation or depression of ST segment, determined in relation to the isoelectric line (TP segment), can be non-pathological or pathological (Fig. 5.2).

5.4.1 Non-pathological Changes in ST Segment

Two common types of ST segment changes are regarded as non-pathological: (a) J point (junction between QRS complex and ST segment) depression without sustained ST depression (so-called upsloping ST depression), and (b) early repolarization pattern as diagnosed in the presence of J point elevation ≥1 mm in ≥2 contiguous inferior and/or lateral leads of a 12-lead ECG (this should be distinguished from 'early repolarization syndrome', which is diagnosed in patients resuscitated from unexplained ventricular fibrillation or polymorphic ventricular tachycardia in the presence of these findings).

5.4.2 Pathological Changes in ST Segment and T Wave

Pathologic horizontal or downsloping depression of the ST segment together with flattening or inversion of T wave can be found in myocarditis, cardiomyopathies, myocardial ischaemia due to congenital coronary anomalies or Kawasaki disease, severe ventricular hypertrophy (strain pattern), and digoxin toxicity.

ST elevation occurs in pericarditis and in acute myocardial infarction (e.g. coronary thrombosis of giant coronary artery aneurysms complicating Kawasaki disease). ST segment elevation in myocardial infarction occurs usually in association with reciprocal ST depression in the ECG leads in which the axis is opposite in direction to those with ST elevation.

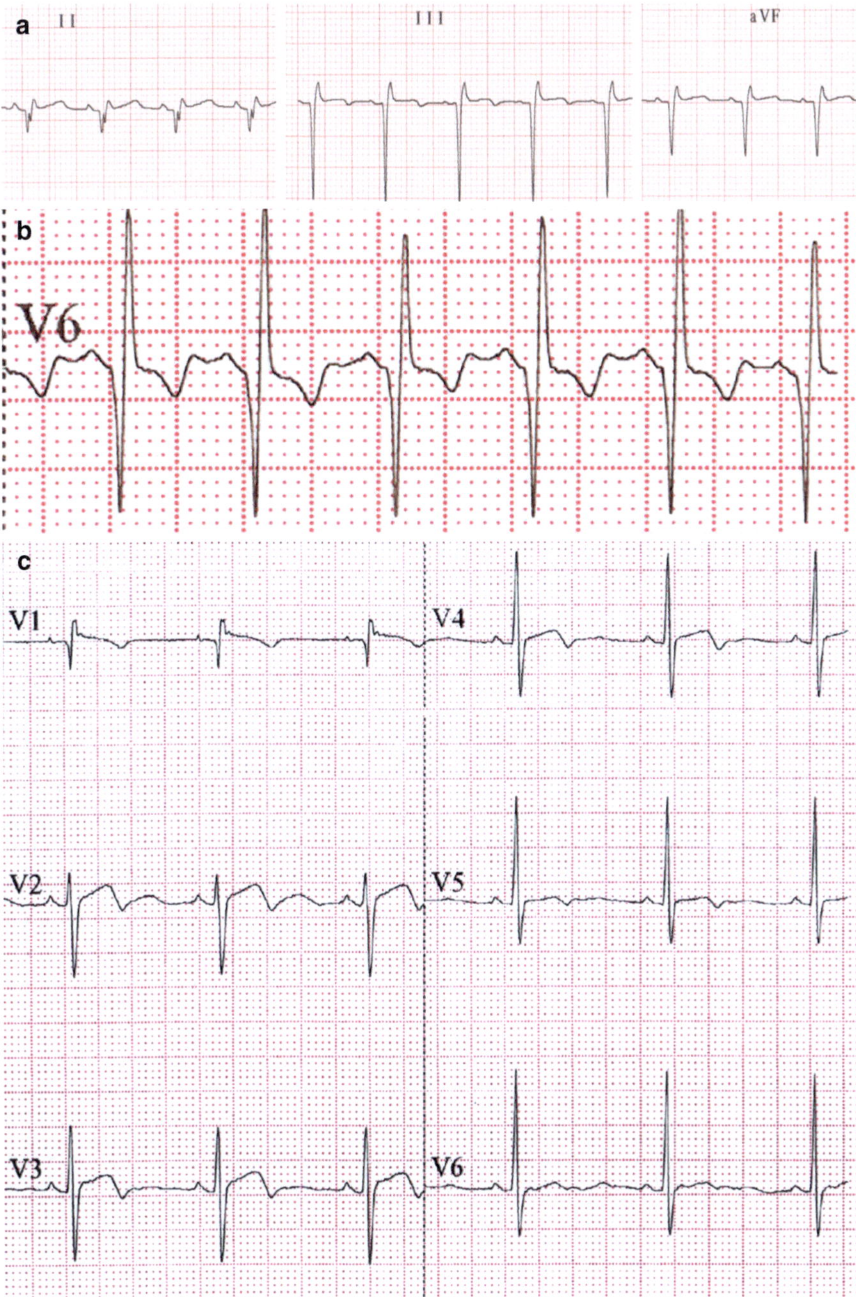

Fig. 5.2 Q wave and changes in ST segment and T wave. (**a**) Q waves in II, III, and aVF due to acute thrombotic occlusion of the right and left coronary artery aneurysms in an infant with Kawasaki disease. (**b**) Q waves in an infant with anomalous origin of the coronary artery from the pulmonary artery. (**c**) ST elevation and T wave inversion in an adolescent with myopericarditis

5.4.3 Q Wave

Q waves are normally seen in I, II, III, aVF, V5, and V6 with duration <0.03 s and depth <5 mm (may be up to 8 mm in children younger than 3 years old). The presence of Q wave in V1 (qR pattern) suggests severe right ventricular hypertrophy, while deep Q wave in V5 or V6 suggests severe left ventricular hypertrophy. Wide and deep Q waves are seen in myocardial infarction.

Echocardiography

6

Echocardiography utilizes ultrasound to image cardiac structures, assess cardiac motion, and interrogate intracardiac and vascular blood flow. This imaging modality is regarded as the gold standard for noninvasive assessment of children with congenital and acquired heart disease. In these patients, echocardiography plays an important role in diagnosis, understanding of the pathophysiology, planning and monitoring of surgical and transcatheter interventions, and evaluation of long-term outcomes and complications.

The types of echocardiography performed in children include: (a) transthoracic echocardiography, which is usually sufficient in infants and children with good acoustic windows, (b) transesophageal echocardiography, which may be considered when transthoracic echocardiographic imaging is unsatisfactory (other options are cardiovascular magnetic resonance or computed tomography), but more commonly, it is used for the intraprocedural monitoring of surgical, transcatheter, or hybrid interventions, and (c) intracardiac echocardiography, which has been used in some centres to monitor transcatheter interventions (primarily occlusion of atrial septal defect) in adolescents and adults.

6.1 Structural Imaging

Echocardiographic transducers emit and receive ultrasound to generate images. The frequencies of sound wave used in clinical echocardiography range from 2 to 12 MHz. The ultrasound transducer houses piezoelectric crystals that serve two functions: (a) in the transmission mode, application of a varying voltage vibrates the crystals to generate ultrasound, and (b) in the receiving mode, the reflected ultrasound from the body tissue distorts the crystals to generate electrical signals to produce images. Based on the time required for the ultrasound reflected from the

Y.-f. Cheung, *Congenital and Paediatric Acquired Heart Disease in Practice*, https://doi.org/10.1007/978-981-99-2862-0_6

tissue to return to the transducer, the tissue depth is displayed on the monitor, and based on the intensity of the reflected ultrasound, the shade of greyness of the image is determined.

6.1.1 M-Mode Echocardiography

M-mode (motion-based) echocardiography is based on real-time tracking of a one-dimensional image along the time axis by placing an M line on a two-dimensional image. It has a high temporal resolution and remains to be used in the current era for assessment of left ventricular dimensions (systolic and diastolic diameters, wall thickness) and systolic function (shortening fraction) and right ventricular systolic function (tricuspid annular plane systolic excursion) (Fig. 6.1a, b).

6.1.2 2D Echocardiography

Two-dimensional images are generated based on information obtained through processing of the multiple scan lines, which are generated by sweeping the ultrasound scan line across an arc. Positioning of the ultrasound transducer at various locations on the praecordium enables the acquisition of different echocardiographic planes (Table 6.1) for evaluation of different cardiac and vascular structures (Fig. 6.1c–j).

6.1.3 3D Echocardiography

Development of matrix-array transducers, which house thousands of piezoelectric crystals, together with advances in computer technology have enabled the application of 3D echocardiography in the clinical arena (Fig. 6.2c). Three-dimensional echocardiography is useful in the following areas: (a) quantification of left ventricular, left atrial, and right ventricular volumes, (b) assessment of valves based on the en face view, (c) evaluation of congenital cardiac anatomy using unique views (Box 6.1), and (d) evaluation of cardiac dyssynchrony.

Box 6.1 Congenital Heart Conditions That May Benefit from Additional 3D Echocardiographic Assessment

- complex atrial and ventricular septal defects
- complete atrioventricular septal defect
- Ebstein anomaly
- mitral valve abnormalities and mechanism of mitral regurgitation
- aortic valve abnormalities and mechanism of aortic regurgitation
- left ventricular outflow tract obstruction

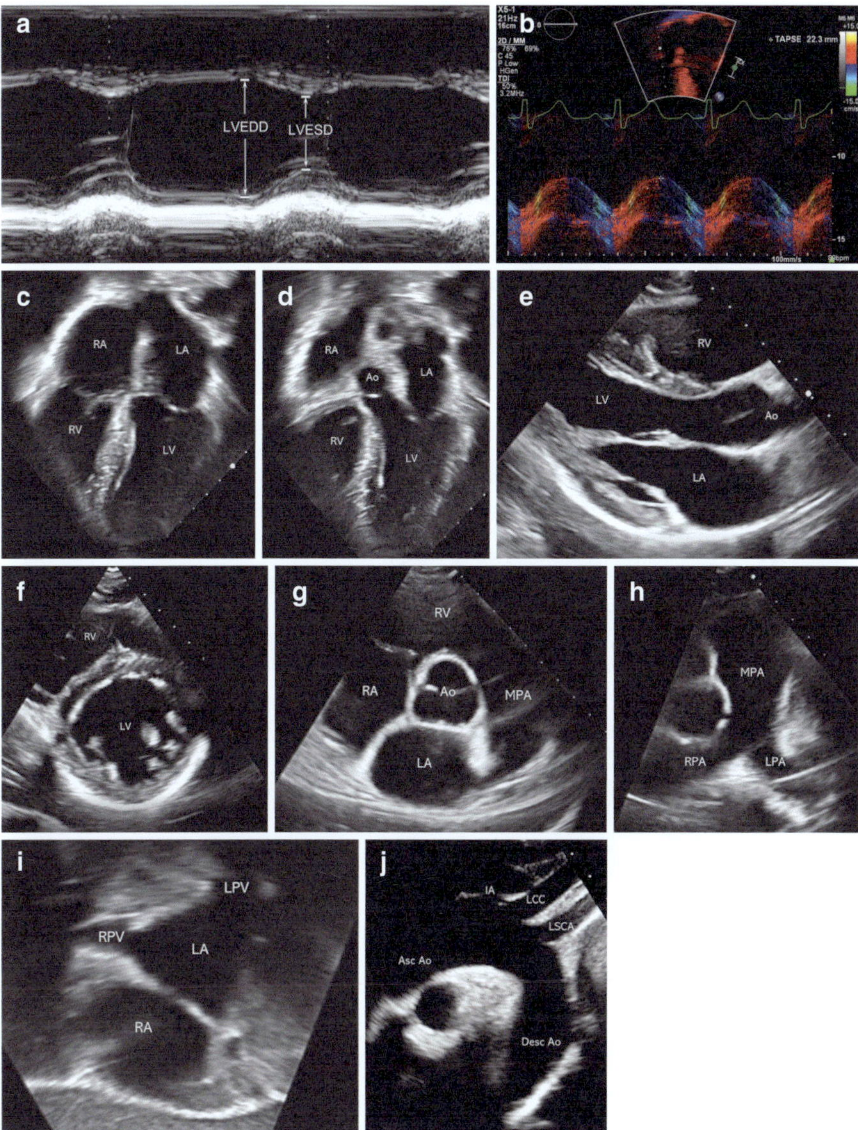

Fig. 6.1 M mode and 2D echocardiographic assessments. (**a**) M-mode assessment of left ventricular systolic function. (**b**) M-mode assessment of tricuspid annular plane systolic excursion. (**c**) Apical four-chamber view. (**d**) Apical five-chamber view. (**e**) Parasternal long-axis view. (**f**) Parasternal short-axis view at papillary muscle level. (**g**) Short axis view at cardiac base. (**h**) Short-axis view showing pulmonary artery bifurcation. (**i**) Subcostal view. (**j**) Suprasternal view

Table 6.1 Transthoracic echocardiographic views

View	Cardiac and vascular structures imaged
Apical four-chamber view	Four cardiac chambers, mitral and tricuspid valves, pulmonary venous return to the left atrium, ventricular septum
Apical five-chamber view	Four cardiac chambers, left ventricular outflow, aortic valve, and proximal aorta (Ao)
Apical long-axis (apical three-chamber) view	Left atrium (LA), mitral valve, left ventricular outflow, aortic valve, and ascending aorta (similar to the parasternal long-axis view, but allow for better alignment of Doppler interrogation of left ventricular outflow)
Parasternal long-axis view	Left atrium, mitral valve, left ventricular outflow, aortic valve, ascending aorta, ventricular septum
Parasternal right ventricular inflow tract view	Right atrium (RA), tricuspid valve, right ventricle (RV)
Parasternal short-axis view	(a) Base of heart: tricuspid valve, right ventricular outflow, pulmonary valve, main pulmonary artery (MPA), left (LPA) and right (RPA) pulmonary arteries, arterial duct, aortic valve and sinus, coronary arteries; (b) mid: mitral valve, papillary muscle, dimensions and wall thickness of left ventricle (LV), ventricular septum; (c) apical: left ventricular trabeculation, ventricular septum
Suprasternal view	Ascending aorta, aortic arch, descending aorta, cranial arteries (IA, innominate artery, LCC, left common carotid artery, LSCA, left subclavian artery), right pulmonary artery, aorto-pulmonary collaterals, arterial duct, innominate vein, superior caval vein, pulmonary veins (crab view)
Subcostal view	Inferior and superior caval veins, abdominal aorta, hepatic veins, left (LPV) and right (RPV) pulmonary veins, atrial septum, four cardiac chambers, right and left ventricular outflow

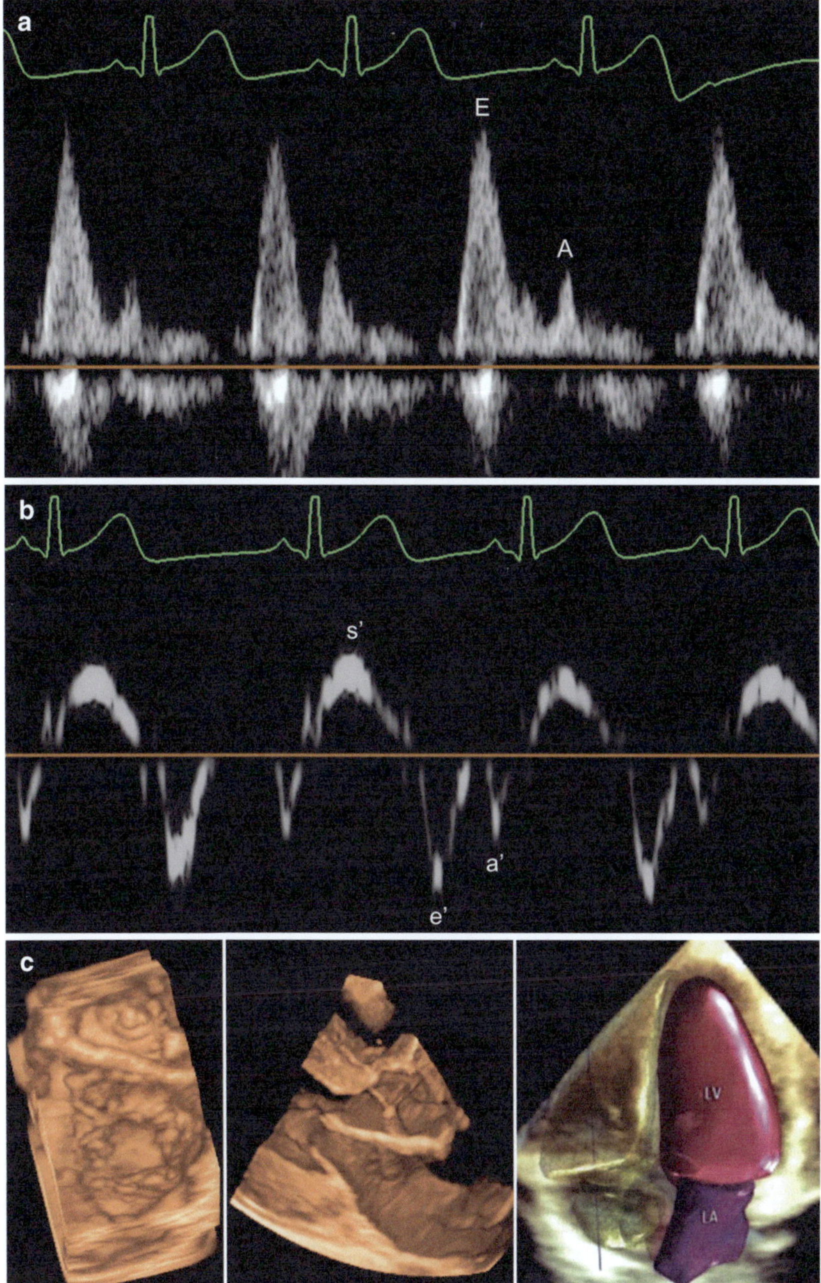

Fig. 6.2 Doppler and 3D echocardiography. (**a**) Transmitral pulsed Doppler assessment: A, late diastolic inflow velocity, E, early diastolic inflow velocity. (**b**) Pulsed tissue Doppler assessment of tricuspid annular velocities: a′, late diastolic annular tissue velocity, e′, early diastolic tissue annular velocity, s′ systolic annular tissue velocity. (**c**) 3D echocardiographic assessment of tricuspid valve (left), left ventricular outflow (central) and left ventricular and left atrial volumes (right)

6.2 Evaluation of Blood Flow

Doppler echocardiography provides an assessment of haemodynamics based on its ability to determine velocity of blood flow and to estimate pressure gradient between cardiac chambers and across sites of stenosis. This technique is based on the Doppler effect (Box 6.2).

Box 6.2 Doppler Echocardiography

Doppler effect

The frequency of sound wave shifts in the presence of relative movement between the sound source and the receiver (e.g. the pitch of the ambulance siren is higher as the ambulance is approaching and is lower as it is leaving)

Doppler formula for assessment of velocity (V) of blood flow

$\mathbf{F_d = 2F_oV\cos\theta/c}$

Hence, $\mathbf{V = cF_d/2F_o\cos\theta}$

F_d is frequency shift (difference between the transmitted and reflected frequency), F_o is transmitted frequency, V is velocity of blood, θ is angle of intercept between the ultrasound beam and flow direction, c is sound velocity (θ should be minimized, to zero degree if possible, by aligning the ultrasound beam with the direction of blood flow to avoid underestimation of velocity)

6.2.1 Continuous Wave Doppler Echocardiography

In continuous wave Doppler echocardiography, two piezoelectric crystals are used, one generating and the other receiving continuously the reflected ultrasound. It measures the maximum blood flow velocity along the entire ultrasound beam. The phenomenon of aliasing (as discussed below) does not occur. Hence, continuous wave Doppler is used to assessing a high-velocity flow (e.g. flow across stenotic valves).

Pressure gradients between cardiac chambers and across sites of stenosis can be determined using the modified Bernoulli equation (Box 6.3).

Box 6.3 Applications of the Modified Bernoulli Equation

Modified Bernoulli equation: $\mathbf{\Delta P = 4\,(v_2^2 - v_1^2)}$

- ΔP is pressure gradient
- v_1 is velocity proximal to the valvar orifice or vascular stenosis
- v_2 is velocity distal to the valvar orifice or vascular stenosis

As v_1 is usually $\ll v_2$, the equation can be simplified to $\Delta P = 4v_2^2$ (however, in the presence of proximal acceleration of velocity, the full equation needs to be used)

Assessment of valvar or vascular stenosis

$$\Delta P = 4v^2$$

v is derived from continuous wave Doppler along the direction of blood flow across the stenotic valve or vessel (this is the peak instantaneous gradient and overestimates the catheter-derived peak-to-peak gradient)

Assessment of right ventricular (RV) and pulmonary arterial (PA) pressure

(a) based on tricuspid regurgitant jet

RV systolic pressure = $4v^2$ + right atrial pressure (5–10 mmHg)

(v is derived from continuous wave Doppler assessment of the tricuspid regurgitant jet)

PA systolic pressure = *RV systolic pressure* (in the absence of pulmonary stenosis)

(b) based on left-to-right shunts

RV (or PA) systolic pressure = systolic blood pressure − $4v^2$

(v is derived from continuous wave Doppler assessment of transventricular or transductal jet)

6.2.2 Pulsed Wave Doppler Echocardiography

In pulsed wave Doppler echocardiography, short bursts of ultrasound are sent and received by the same piezoelectric crystal. These bursts are emitted at a specific pulse repetition frequency (PRF) to a defined small area at a specified depth (based on the position of the sampling volume) from the transducer. This allows the determination of blood flow velocity at a specific location of interest within a small sample volume.

The maximum velocity that can be measured by pulsed Doppler is, however, limited by the Nyquist limit (= PRF/2), which is the maximum Doppler shift frequency without the occurrence of aliasing. Aliasing occurs with undersampling due to the limited PRF and manifests as change in direction of blood flow in high-velocity flow areas (frequency-shift reversal with apparent reversal of blood flow). Hence, pulsed wave Doppler can only be used to measure low velocities of blood flow in defined region of interest (e.g. transmitral early and late diastolic inflow velocities and pulmonary venous inflow velocities) (Fig. 6.2a).

6.2.3 Doppler Colour Flow Mapping

With Doppler colour flow mapping, the direction and velocity of blood flow is displayed in colour and superimposed on two-dimensional images. Red colour represents flow towards the ultrasound transducer, while blue colour denotes flow away from the transducer. The shade of colour indicates the velocity of blood flow, and a mosaic colour pattern is suggestive of turbulent flow (e.g. in the presence of valvar or vascular stenosis).

6.3 Evaluation of Myocardial Tissue Motion and Deformation

6.3.1 Tissue Doppler Imaging

Tissue Doppler imaging utilizes Doppler effect to assess velocities of myocardial tissue motion, which are lower than those of blood flow. This can be performed in pulsed wave and colour modes and is most useful for interrogation of myocardial tissue motion in the longitudinal axis, which is parallel to the direction of the ultrasound beam from the four-chamber view.

In pulsed wave tissue Doppler imaging, the sampling volume is positioned usually at the left and right ventricular free wall-annular junction for measurement of systolic and diastolic annular velocities as measures of ventricular systolic and diastolic function, respectively (Fig. 6.2b). With colour tissue Doppler imaging, the colour-coded myocardial velocities (red represents myocardial tissue moving towards the ultrasound transducer, while blue denotes myocardial tissue moving away from the transducer) are superimposed on two-dimensional images for evaluation of velocity and direction of motion of different myocardial segments simultaneously.

6.3.2 Myocardial Deformation Imaging

Conventional indices of cardiac function based on assessment of changes in the size of cardiac chambers and blood flow are regarded as indirect measurements consequential to myocardial shortening and lengthening throughout the cardiac cycle. Technological advances have enabled direct assessment of myocardial deformation, which allows the evaluation of global and regional myocardial function. There are data to suggest that myocardial deformation imaging may be more sensitive than the conventional echocardiographic indices (e.g. ejection fraction) in the early detection of subclinical myocardial dysfunction.

Two-dimensional speckle tracking has emerged as the most commonly used modality clinically for the assessment of myocardial deformation (Fig. 6.3). This technique tracks the movement of speckles in the myocardium, which are natural acoustic markers present in two-dimensional greyscale images, and evaluates their spatial displacement for direct quantification of myocardial strain (the shortening or lengthening of the myocardium) and strain rate in the longitudinal, circumferential, and radial dimensions. Recently, three-dimensional speckle tracking, which applies speckle tracking technology to three-dimensional echocardiographic dataset, has also been developed.

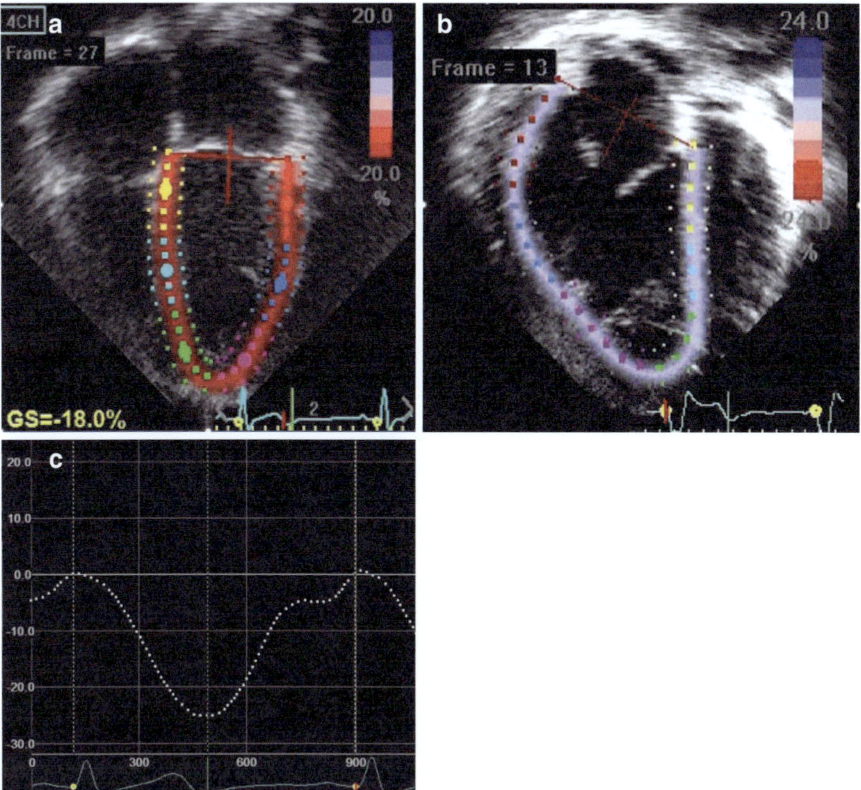

Fig. 6.3 Two-dimensional speckle tracking echocardiography. (**a**) Speckle tracking of left ventricular contour. (**b**) Speckle tracking of right ventricular contour. (**c**) Strain curve depicting longitudinal shortening of the ventricular myocardium (negative strain by convention) during systole

6.4 Functional Assessment

6.4.1 Assessment of Cardiac Function

Systolic (Table 6.2) and diastolic (Table 6.3) function of the right and left ventricles and ventricular dyssynchrony (Table 6.4) can be assessed by two- and three-dimensional, M mode, conventional Doppler and tissue Doppler imaging, and speckle tracking echocardiography.

6.4.2 Stress Echocardiography

Stress echocardiography can be performed in children to assess (a) abnormal regional wall motion abnormalities due to myocardial ischaemia in at-risk paediatric cardiac patients (including patients with history of Kawasaki disease and

Table 6.2 Echocardiographic assessment of systolic function

Echo imaging	LV parameters	RV parameters
2D		Fractional area change
M mode	LV end-diastolic dimension	Tricuspid annular plane systolic excursion
	LV end-systolic dimension	
	Shortening fraction	
	Paradoxical septal motion	
Doppler/TDI	s′	s′
	Doppler-derived MPI	Doppler-derived MPI
	TDI-derived MPI	TDI-derived MPI
2D speckle tracking	Global longitudinal strain	Global longitudinal strain (RV free wall and septum)
	4-chamber longitudinal strain	RV free wall longitudinal strain
3D echo	LV end-diastolic volume	RV end-diastolic volume
	LV end-systolic volume	RV end-systolic volume
	Ejection fraction	Ejection fraction

Table 6.3 Echocardiographic assessment of diastolic function

Echo imaging	LV parameters	RV parameters
Doppler	E	E
	A	A
	E/A	E/A
	MPI	MPI
		Antegrade diastolic pulmonary flow
TDI	Lateral and septal e′	e′
	Lateral and septal a′	a′
	e′/a′	e′/a′
	E/e′	E/e′
	MPI	MPI
LA size	LA lateral and AP diameters	
	LA area/volume	
Doppler assessment of TR	Assessment of pulmonary arterial pressure	

coronary artery aneurysms, patients after surgeries that require coronary artery reimplantation, and those after heart transplantation), (b) dynamic pressure gradient across site of stenosis (e.g. left ventricular outflow in hypertrophic cardiomyopathy, residual coarctation of the aorta), (c) subclinical myocardial dysfunction is childhood survivors, and (d) right ventricular contractile reserve in patients with pulmonary hypertension.

Table 6.4 Assessment of dyssynchrony

Echo imaging	Parameter
Atrioventricular dyssynchrony	
Transmitral pulsed wave Doppler	Diastolic filling time/RR interval
	E and A wave assessment
Interventricular dyssynchrony	
Aorta and main pulmonary artery pulsed wave Doppler	Δ time of onset of LV and RV ejection
Intraventricular dyssynchrony	
Colour TDI wall motion assessment	Septal flash and/or apical rocking
M mode	Septal-to-posterior wall motion delay
TDI	Δ time to s′ between septal and lateral wall (apical four-chamber view)
2D radial strain	Δ time to peak radial strain between anteroseptal and posterior segments
Longitudinal strain assessment of all LV segments	Mechanical dispersion index (SD of LV segmental time-to-peak longitudinal strain)

Abbreviations for Tables 6.2, 6.3, and 6.4: *AP* anteroposterior, *LA* left atrial, *LV* left ventricular, *MPI* myocardial performance index, *RV* right ventricular, *TDI* tissue Doppler imaging, *TR* tricuspid regurgitation

The stressor is either exercise (usually supine bicycle testing in older children) or a pharmacologic agent (usually an escalating dose of intravenous dobutamine infusion in children of different age groups). Incorporation of tissue Doppler and myocardial deformation imaging in addition to qualitative assessment of regional wall motion abnormalities has enabled quantitative analysis of regional and global myocardial function.

To date, however, there are no specific guidelines on the application of stress echocardiography in children. The clinical interpretation of changes in haemodynamic and functional data during stress also remains uncertain.

6.5 Monitoring of Surgical and Transcatheter Interventions

6.5.1 Transesophageal Echocardiography

Transesophageal echocardiography is widely used for the monitoring of children undergoing cardiac surgery. Common indications in the operation room include: (a) delineation of cardiac anatomy, valve abnormalities, and cardiac function prior to surgery, (b) determination of adequacy of deairing prior to coming off cardiopulmonary bypass, (c) assessment of surgical results and residual lesions, and (d) evaluation of ventricular function.

In the paediatric cardiac catheterization laboratory, transesophageal echocardiography provides guidance for placement of occlusion device, transseptal puncture, creation of atrial communication and Fontan fenestration, and monitoring of valve interventions.

6.5.2 Contrast Echocardiography

Transesophageal or transthoracic contrast echocardiography using agitated saline or saline-blood mixture is a sensitive and convenient means to ascertain intracardiac right-to-left shunting, intrapulmonary shunting, or systemic venous anomalies as a cause of unexplained hypoxaemia.

Saline with or without mixture of blood taken from the patient is vigorously agitated by transferring back and forth between two syringes connected to a three-way stopcock. The agitated saline and blood mixture is injected into a peripheral vein in either the upper or the lower limb (depending on the suspected site of right-to-left shunting). Appearance of microbubbles in the left atrium and left ventricle within two cardiac cycles indicates an intra-cardiac right-to-left shunt, while the appearance of microbubbles within three to four cardiac cycles suggests intrapulmonary shunting.

Computed Tomography

7

Technological advances in cardiovascular computed tomography (CT) have significantly improved the spatial and temporal resolution of images, reduced the dose of radiation required, and lessened the need for sedation given the ability to acquire data based only a portion of the cardiac cycle.

Cardiovascular CT is increasingly used as an adjunct imaging modality to echocardiography in paediatric cardiac patients, especially when cardiac magnetic resonance imaging is contraindicated or unlikely to provide satisfactory images for clinical decision making. In these patients, cardiovascular CT plays an important role in diagnosis, planning of surgical and transcatheter interventions, and evaluation of outcomes and long-term complications of congenital and acquired disease. Advantages and limitations of cardiovascular CT are shown in Table 7.1.

Table 7.1 Advantages and limitations of cardiovascular CT

Advantages	Limitations
High spatial resolution for assessment of cardiovascular anatomy	Requires the use of radiation
Concurrent evaluation of extracardiac anatomy and relationship with neighbouring non-cardiac structures	Requires the use of iodinated contrast
Evaluation of stents and conduits	Assessment of cardiac function requires higher dose of radiation and usually not routinely performed
Better assessment of calcification	Fails to quantify shunt or valvar regurgitation
Sedation is often not required	Poor myocardial tissue characterization

Y.-f. Cheung, *Congenital and Paediatric Acquired Heart Disease in Practice*, https://doi.org/10.1007/978-981-99-2862-0_7

7.1 Structural Imaging

The ability of cardiovascular CT to (a) image cardiac structures, coronary arteries, neighbouring non-cardiac structures (airway, lung parenchyma, and skeletal anatomy), and implanted stents and conduits, (b) generate three-dimensional data for visualization and 3D printing, and (c) image patients with implanted pacemakers and defibrillators are of immense importance in evaluating paediatric cardiac patients.

In the current era, cardiovascular CT is widely used for evaluation of children with congenital cardiac malformations of varying complexities, congenital and acquired coronary arterial anomalies, and extracardiac vascular abnormalities (e.g. in patients with inherited disorders of connective tissue disease) (Fig. 7.1).

Common paediatric cardiac applications of cardiovascular CT are shown in Box 7.1.

Box 7.1 Applications of Cardiovascular CT in Paediatric Cardiac Patients

Evaluation of anatomy

- coronary artery imaging
- complex cardiovascular anomalies (with 3D printing)
- evaluation of extra-cardiac anomalies that may be associated with congenital heart defects (e.g. airway, lung parenchyma, skeletal abnormalities)
- pre-operative assessment in patients with prior sternotomy requiring cardiac reoperation (risk of injury to underlying conduits, coronary artery, etc.)

Assessment of calcification

- evaluation of calcification in vessels and conduits prior to transcatheter intervention

When cardiac magnetic resonance is not possible or contraindicated

- critical patients tolerating only short duration of scan
- patients with increased risk of sedation or general anaesthesia
- presence of device or implants incompatible with cardiac magnetic resonance
- anticipated artifact
- severe claustrophobia of patients

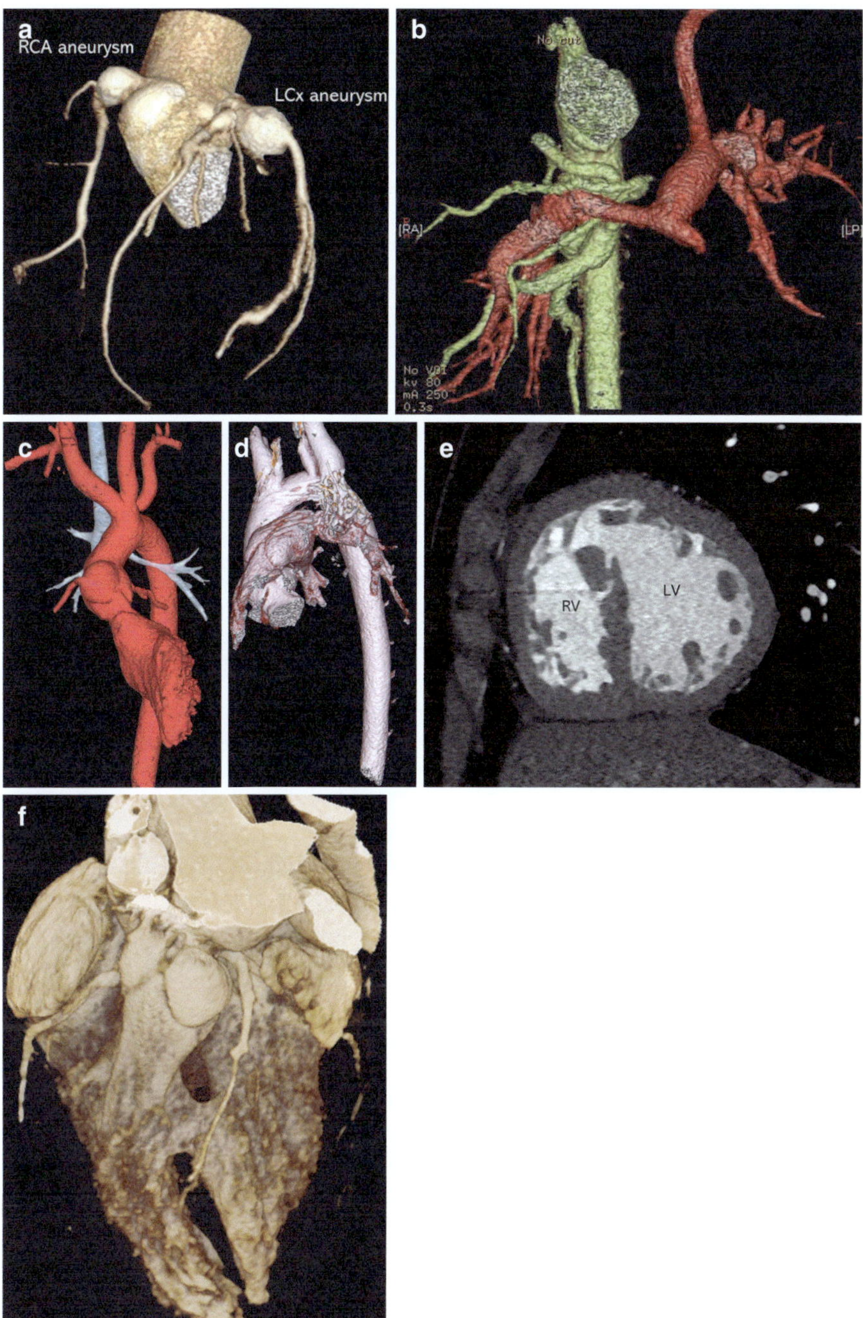

Fig. 7.1 Cardiovascular CT in children with different cardiac conditions. (**a**) Coronary artery aneurysms in Kawasaki disease. (**b**) Multiple aortopulmonary collaterals in pulmonary atresia with ventricular septal defect. (**c**) Repaired interrupted aortic arch. (**d**) Stented coarctation of the aorta. (**e**, **f**) Multiple ventricular septal defects (*LCx* left circumflex artery, *LV* left ventricle, *RCA* right coronary artery, *RV* right ventricle)

7.2 Functional Assessment

Echocardiography and cardiac magnetic resonance imaging remains to the most important non-invasive modalities for assessment of cardiac function in paediatric patients. Although cardiovascular CT may provide an option for assessment of function when there are contraindications to or limitations on the use of other modalities, several caveats of CT should be noted: (a) low temporal resolution, (b) failure to visualize or assess regurgitant or stenotic jets of blood flow, and (c) the need for retrospective ECG-gated protocols with higher radiation dose required.

7.3 Risks of Cardiovascular CT

While cardiovascular CT is regarded as non-invasive, this imaging modality does incur certain risks (Box 7.2).

Box 7.2 Risks of Cardiovascular CT

- ionizing radiation
- iodinated contrast (contrast reaction, contrast-induced nephropathy, possibility of hypothyroidism)
- local complications related to power injection of contrast
- risk of sedation or anaesthesia in some patients
- risk of beta blockade (used to reduce heart rate) in some patients

The importance of using the lowest possible radiation dose cannot be overemphasized. This relies on a comprehensive understanding of the cardiac anatomy, unique congenital cardiac physiology, technical aspects of the scanner and protocols, and personalized pre-scan planning.

8 Cardiovascular Magnetic Resonance

Significant progress in cardiovascular magnetic resonance (CMR) has enabled this imaging modality to provide important information on cardiac anatomy, function, flow, and myocardial tissue properties in children with congenital and acquired heart disease. In these patients, CMR plays an important role in diagnosis, understanding of pathophysiology, planning of surgical and transcatheter interventions, and evaluation of outcomes and long-term complications of congenital and acquired disease. Advantages and limitations of CMR are shown in Table 8.1.

Table 8.1 Advantages and limitations of CMR

Advantages	Limitations
Assessment of ventricular function possible	Sedation more likely required
Quantification of flow and valvar regurgitation	Longer time required for imaging
Characterization of myocardial tissue for oedema, scarring, and diffuse fibrosis	Contraindicated in the presence of some pacemakers and other incompatible devices
No exposure to ionizing radiation	Susceptible to metallic artifacts
Use of contrast agent not required for some assessments	

Y.-f. Cheung, *Congenital and Paediatric Acquired Heart Disease in Practice*, https://doi.org/10.1007/978-981-99-2862-0_8

8.1 CMR Imaging Sequence

Different CMR sequences are used to assess (a) cardiac and vascular anatomy, (b) cardiac function, (c) blood flow, and (d) myocardial perfusion and tissue properties (Table 8.2).

Table 8.2 Imaging techniques commonly used in CMR

Imaging sequence	Utility
Black blood	Displaying static anatomic images
Cine steady-state free precision (SSFP)	Displaying images in cineloop for functional assessment
Velocity-encoded phase contrast imaging	Quantification of blood flow
Magnetic resonance angiogram (contrast agent required)	Delineation of vascular anatomy
Late gadolinium enhancement (contrast agent required)	Imaging of myocardial scars or fibrosis
T1-mapping (contrast agent required for assessment of extracellular volume)	Assessment of myocardial oedema and diffuse fibrosis
T2-weighted imaging	Quantification of myocardial iron load

8.2 Structural Imaging

Structural imaging of the heart can be achieved with the use of black blood sequence (spin-echo imaging, with blood appearing dark) and 2D steady-state free precession (SSFP) acquisition (with blood appearing bright) (Fig. 8.1a, b). By displaying images in cineloop fashion, 2D SSFP provides qualitative assessment of cardiac function and valve motion. The use of 3D SSFP (with or without contrast agents)

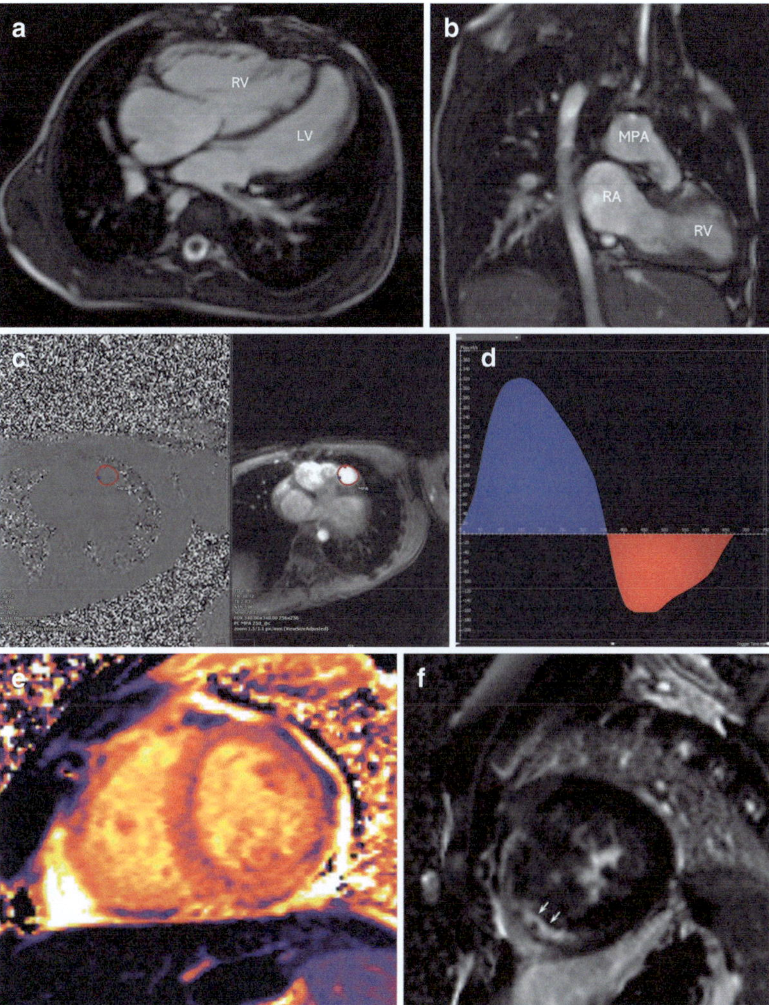

Fig. 8.1 Cardiac magnetic resonance in paediatric cardiology. (**a**, **b**) CMR assessment of ventricular volume and function after repaired of tetralogy Fallot. (**c**) Velocity-encoded phase contrast imaging. (**d**) Quantification of pulmonary regurgitant flow (blue, antegrade flow, red, regurgitant flow). (**e**) Late gadolinium enhancement (arrows). (**f**) T1 mapping in a boy with systemic sclerosis (*LV* left ventricle, *MPA* main pulmonary artery, *RV* right ventricle)

produces a complete 3D cardiovascular dataset for visualization of anatomy and 3D printing. To define vascular anatomy, magnetic resonance angiography with intravenous administration of gadolinium-based contrast agents enables the acquisition of high-resolution images. The full-volume dataset can be volume-rendered into a 3D image.

8.3 Functional Assessment

Acquisition of a stack of 2D SSFP cine slices of the entire heart enables quantification of ventricular systolic and diastolic volumes and calculation of ejection fraction. Recently, feature tracking has been applied to SSFP images for assessment of global and regional myocardial deformation (strain and strain rate) in the longitudinal, circumferential, and radial dimensions (Chap. 6).

8.4 Quantification of Blood Flow

Velocity-encoded phase-contrast imaging enables the measurement of blood flow across the blood vessel of interest. The slice is placed to intersect perpendicularly the blood vessel of interest for quantification of volume of blood flow (the product of velocity and cross-sectional area of the blood vessel) (Fig. 8.1c, d). This is used to evaluate regurgitant, shunt, and collateral flow volumes in congenital heart disease.

Recently, 4D flow CMR, which involves the use of phase-contrast CMR to encode flow in three dimensions with addition of the time dimension throughout the cardiac cycle, has been introduced as a research tool. Four-dimensional flow CMR allows visualization of flow disturbance in valvar disease, vascular stenosis, and complex congenital heart disease and has the potential to increase the understanding of the pathophysiologic impact of altered fluid mechanics on the heart and blood vessels. Its clinical usefulness requires further evaluation.

8.5 Evaluation of Myocardial Perfusion and Tissue Properties

8.5.1 CMR Myocardial Perfusion Imaging

CMR myocardial perfusion imaging is performed based on the first pass perfusion of the myocardium using gadolinium-based contrast agents. Well perfused tissues show enhanced signal on T1-weighted images, while poorly perfused regions will remain dark. This is performed as part of the stress testing (Chap. 10) for identification of myocardial ischaemia and infarction.

8.5.2 Late Gadolinium Enhancement

Late gadolinium enhancement imaging demonstrates the accumulation of gadolinium-based contrast agent late after injection of the contrast agent (Fig. 8.1e). This is the standard CMR technique for imaging of myocardial scar and focal fibrosis. Scars and areas of focal fibrosis appear bright, while non-scarred areas appear dark. Specific patterns of late gadolinium enhancement are described in congenital heart conditions after surgery and cardiomyopathies and carry prognostic implications. Late gadolinium enhancement may, however, fail to detect diffuse fibrosis due to limited spatial resolution and the absence of normal reference myocardium for the purpose of comparison.

8.5.3 T1 Mapping

T1 mapping enables direct quantification of T1 (time after which the longitudinal magnetization of tissue has returned to 63% of its original value after an inversion or saturation pulse) and detection of diffuse myocardial structural alterations (Fig. 8.1f). It is feasible even in patients with severe renal dysfunction.

Two T1 mapping-derived parameters are used to characterize the alteration of myocardial tissue properties: (a) native myocardial T1 time: this represents a composite signal from cardiomyocytes and extracellular volume and is prolonged by oedema (e.g. in myocarditis), increased fibrosis, and protein deposition (e.g. in amyloidosis), and (b) extracellular volume (ECV): this parameter is derived from the myocardial and blood T1 values before and after administration of contrast agents and the haematocrit of the patient. Increased ECV is related to excessive collagen deposition or amyloidosis.

8.6 Paediatric Cardiac Applications of CMR

Common examples of paediatric cardiac applications of CMR are shown in Box 8.1.

Box 8.1 Common Paediatric Cardiac Applications of CMR

Imaging of anatomy

- pulmonary arteries and veins
- aorta and aortic arch anomalies
- proximal coronary arteries (usually with evaluation of myocardial perfusion)
- complex cardiovascular anomalies (with 3D printing)
- evaluation of extra-cardiac anomalies that may be associated with congenital heart defects (e.g. in heterotaxy syndrome)

Assessment of function and haemodynamics

- quantification of ventricular volumes and ejection fraction of the right, left, and functional single ventricles
- assessment of regurgitation fraction (e.g. pulmonary regurgitant fraction in repaired tetralogy of Fallot)
- quantification of intracardiac and extracardiac (e.g. aortopulmonary collaterals) shunt flow

Evaluation of myocardial perfusion and tissue properties

- stress myocardial perfusion imaging in children at risk of myocardial ischaemia (e.g. congenital coronary arterial anomalies, coronary artery aneurysm formation complicating Kawasaki disease)
- late gadolinium enhancement imaging and T1 mapping for assessment of myocardial fibrosis (e.g. myocarditis, cardiomyopathies, repaired tetralogy of Fallot, myocardial infarction complicating Kawasaki disease)

8.7 Risk of CMR

In general, CMR is safe in children. Adequate shielding from the noise generated during imaging to prevent damage to hearing is important. The use of gadolinium-derived contrast agents can be associated with side effects including extravasation of the contrast agent, mild allergic reaction with skin rash, and rarely, anaphylactic shock with cardiovascular collapse. Nephrogenic systemic fibrosis is a rare complication in patients with impaired renal function after exposure to gadolinium-derived contrast agents. It is characterized by thickening of the skin and subcutaneous tissue and fibrosis of the skeletal muscle, liver, heart, and lungs. The use of gadolinium-derived contrast agents is hence contraindicated in children with end-stage renal failure.

Cardiac Catheterization

9

Cardiac catheterization provides information on the anatomy and haemodynamics of congenital and acquired cardiac conditions in children. With significant advances in echocardiography, cardiovascular computed tomography, and cardiac magnetic resonance, the role cardiac catheterization has evolved from a diagnostic to primarily an interventional one.

9.1 Diagnostic Catheterization

Placement of a catheter in the cardiac chambers and blood vessels under fluoroscopic guidance enables direct measurement of pressure and sampling of blood for oximetry measurements. Angiographic evaluation with injection of iodinated contrast delineates the intracardiac and vascular anatomies prior to surgical or transcatheter intervention. Pure diagnostic catheterization is much less frequently performed in the current era (Box 9.1).

Box 9.1 Indications of Diagnostic Catheterization

Evaluation of anatomy

- define coronary arterial anatomy (e.g. Kawasaki disease, coronary arterial fistula)
- delineate complex anatomy that may be difficult to be imaged in totality by other noninvasive modalities (e.g. aortopulmonary collaterals, pulmonary arteriovenous malformations)

Y.-f. Cheung, *Congenital and Paediatric Acquired Heart Disease in Practice*, https://doi.org/10.1007/978-981-99-2862-0_9

Assessment of anatomy and haemodynamics

- as the initial assessment prior to transcatheter interventional procedure
- assessment of postoperative patients with significant residual lesions for planning of further management

Assessment of haemodynamics

- prior to bidirectional Glenn shunt and Fontan operation
- evaluation of pulmonary vasoreactivity in patients with pulmonary arterial hypertension
- differentiation between restrictive cardiomyopathy and constrictive pericarditis
- pre and post (with endomyocardial biopsy) heart transplant assessment

9.1.1 Haemodynamic Assessment

The pressure and oximetry measurements enable the assessment of ventricular filling pressure and pressure waveforms, severity of stenotic lesions (with derivation of peak-to-peak pressure), quantification of shunts (Boxes 9.2 and 9.3), and assessment of systemic and pulmonary vascular resistance (Box 9.4).

Box 9.2 Calculation of Shunt in Biventricular Circulation

$$\mathbf{Qs = VO2 / (SA\ O2\ content - MV\ O2\ content)}$$

$$\mathbf{Qp = VO2 / (PV\ O2\ content - PA\ O2\ content)}$$

VO2 is oxygen consumption (usually estimated from reference chart)
MV, mixed venous, SA, systemic arterial, PA, pulmonary arterial
PV, pulmonary venous
oxygen content = 1.34 × Hb (g/dL) × oxygen saturation (×10 to convert mL/dL to mL/L) + dissolved oxygen
dissolved oxygen = 0.003 × PaO2 (×10 to convert mL/dL to mL/L)
mixed venous oxygen saturation = (3 × SVC O2 + 1 × IVC O2)/4

$$\begin{aligned}\mathbf{Qp : Qs} &= \mathbf{(SA\ O2\,content - MV\ O2\,content) / (PV\ O2\,content - PA\ O2\,content)} \\ &= \mathbf{(SA\ O2sat - MV\ O2sat) / (PV\ O2sat - PA\ O2sat)} \\ &\quad \mathbf{(when\ dissolved\ oxygen\ is\ negligible)}\end{aligned}$$

$$Q_{effective} = VO2/(PV\,O2\ content - MV\,O2\ content)$$

(effective flow = fraction of mixed venous returning to the lung or oxygenated blood to systemic circulation excluding the contribution of shunt flow)

$$left-to-right\ shunt = Qp - Q_{effective}$$
$$right-to-left\ shunt = Qs - Q_{effective}$$

Box 9.3 Estimation of Qp:Qs in Single Ventricular Circulation

Post modified Blalock-Taussig shunt/Norwood surgery with Sano shunt

$$Qp:Qs = (SA\,O2sat - SVC\,O2sat)/(PV\,O2sat - SA\,O2sat)$$

Post cavopulmonary shunt

$$\begin{aligned} Qp:Qs &= (SA\,O2sat - IVC\,O2sat)/(PV\,O2sat - IVC\,O2sat) \\ &= (SA\,O2sat - SVC\,O2sat)/(PV\,O2sat - SVC\,O2sat) \end{aligned}$$

Post Fontan operation

$$Qp:Qs = (SA\,O2sat - SVC\,O2sat)/(PV\,O2sat - PA\,O2sat)$$

Box 9.4 Calculation of Pulmonary and Systemic Vascular Resistance

Pulmonary vascular resistance = (mean PAP – mean LAP or PAWP)/Qp

LAP, left atrial pressure, PAP, pulmonary arterial pressure, PAWP, pulmonary arterial wedge pressure

Systemic vascular resistance = (mean aortic pressure – mean RAP)/Qs

RAP, right atrial pressure

9.1.2 Myocardial Biopsy

In selected paediatric patients with acute onset unexplained heart failure, myocarditis, or dilated cardiomyopathy, catheterization with haemodynamic assessment and endomyocardial biopsy may be considered.

9.2 Interventional Catheterization

The field of paediatric interventional cardiac catheterization has expanded significantly over the past few decades. Advances in device designs, techniques, and imaging modalities have allowed catheter interventions to be performed even in premature and low-birthweight babies.

Transcatheter intervention has made significant impact on the management strategy of congenital heart disease and has become the procedure of choice or a treatment option for many congenital heart conditions (Table 9.1). Interventions involve (a) dilation of stenotic valves or vessels, (b) stenting of vascular stenosis, (c) device closure of shunts, (d) creation of communications, (e) implantation of valves, and (f) removal of intravascular and intracardiac foreign bodies.

Table 9.1 Transcatheter interventional procedures for paediatric cardiac conditions

Procedure	Conditions
Balloon atrioseptostomy	Complete transposition of the great arteries
Balloon valvoplasty	Valvar pulmonary, aortic, mitral, and tricuspid stenosis
Balloon angioplasty	Pulmonary arterial and venous stenosis, right ventricle-to-pulmonary arterial conduit stenosis, aortic (re)coarctation, systemic venous stenosis, intraatrial baffle stenosis after atrial switch, shunt stenosis
Stenting	Pulmonary arterial and venous stenosis, right ventricle-to-pulmonary arterial conduit stenosis, aortic (re)coarctation, systemic venous stenosis, intraatrial baffle stenosis after atrial switch, shunt stenosis, arterial duct-dependent conditions
Device closure of left-to-right and left-to-left shunts	Atrial septal defect, ventricular septal defect, persistent arterial duct, aortopulmonary window, aortopulmonary collaterals, coronary arterial fistula, pulmonary arteriovenous malformations
Perforation of valve and other structures	Pulmonary atresia with intact ventricular septum, transseptal puncture, creation of Fontan fenestration
Valve intervention	Pulmonary valve implantation, device closure of paravalvar leak
Removal of foreign bodies	Device embolization, broken central catheters

9.3 Hybrid Procedures

Collaboration between cardiac surgeons and paediatric interventional cardiologists has led to the birth of hybrid procedures (Table 9.2), which are performed in venues designed to accommodate both open heart surgery and transcatheter interventions.

Table 9.2 Hybrid procedures for paediatric cardiac conditions

Conditions	Procedure
Muscular ventricular septal defect	Perventricular closure with surgical access through the surface of the right ventricle followed by transcatheter deployment of the occluding device
Hypoplastic left heart syndrome	Bilateral pulmonary arterial banding with stenting of the arterial duct as an initial palliative procedure
Right ventricular outflow or conduit stenosis and/or regurgitation	Surgical access through the right ventricle for pulmonary valve implantation
Branch pulmonary arterial stenosis	Intraoperative stenting of branch pulmonary arteries
Critical aortic stenosis	Carotid cutdown to facilitate balloon aortic valvoplasty
Duct-dependent circulation	Carotid cutdown to facilitate ductal stenting

9.4 Risks of Cardiac Catheterization

Despite the technical improvements in paediatric cardiac catheterization, complications may occur after diagnostic and/or interventional catheterization in children (Box 9.5).

Box 9.5 Complications of Paediatric Cardiac Catheterization

- arterial thrombosis, perforation, and avulsion
- venous thrombosis and perforation
- bleeding and haematoma formation at puncture site
- bleeding at other sites (e.g. lungs)
- cardiac arrhythmias
- direct catheter-related complications: staining of myocardium, cardiac perforation and tamponade, thromboembolism, air embolism
- related to interventional procedures: device embolization, balloon rupture, cardiac perforation, vascular tear and dissection
- cardiac arrest and death

Stress Testing 10

Stress testing is commonly performed in children with congenital and acquired heart disease with the general aims of evaluating exercise capacity, determining the impact of stress (exercise or pharmacologic agents) on cardiac haemodynamics and rhythm, and providing functional data for management planning.

10.1 Exercise Laboratory

The paediatric exercise laboratory should provide a controlled environment for the purpose and be spacious to accommodate the equipment required (Box 10.1).

Box 10.1 Paediatric Exercise Laboratory
Environment

- spacious
- temperature between 20 and 24 °C
- relative humidity between 50% and 60%

Equipment

- mouthpiece and facemask
- blood pressure cuff
- ECG monitoring
- pulse oximeter

Y.-f. Cheung, *Congenital and Paediatric Acquired Heart Disease in Practice*, https://doi.org/10.1007/978-981-99-2862-0_10

- treadmill
- cycle ergometer
- metabolic cart (breath-by-breath assessment of end-tidal PCO2 and PO2, and basic spirometry)
- resuscitation trolley
- echocardiography (for stress echocardiography)

10.2 Indications and Contraindications

Common indications of stress testing in paediatric cardiac patients are (a) objective assessment of exercise capacity, (b) assessment of exercise-related symptoms and signs, (c) unveiling of abnormal cardiopulmonary response, cardiac arrhythmias, coronary insufficiency, or altered haemodynamics, and (d) evaluation of the efficacy of therapeutic interventions. The findings of stress testing may help in the diagnosis, management planning, risk stratification of underlying cardiac conditions, and counselling of patient and family.

Absolute contraindications include active pericarditis and/or myocarditis and severe ventricular outflow obstruction already indicated for surgery. There are groups of cardiac patients who are at higher risk of adverse events and require close medical supervision during stress testing (Box 10.2).

Box 10.2 Cardiac Conditions of Patients at Higher Risk of Adverse Events During Stress Testing

- history suggestive of syncope or myocardial ischaemia during exertion
- cardiomyopathies with heart failure and/or cardiac arrhythmias
- moderate to severe ventricular outflow obstruction
- pulmonary hypertension
- diagnosed long QT syndrome or history of haemodynamically unstable arrhythmias

10.3 Stress Protocols

10.3.1 Exercise Stress

The types of exercise stress used in children include 6-min walk test, exercise testing with ECG monitoring, and cardiopulmonary exercise testing. These yield different parameters and selection depends on patient factors, equipment available, and goal(s) of the stress testing (Table 10.1).

Cardiopulmonary exercise testing can be performed using a treadmill or cycle ergometer. Most exercise laboratories adopt continuous protocols with gradual

Table 10.1 Types of exercise stress testing and their utilization in children

Test	Parameters	Utilization
6-min walk test	Distance	Simple monitoring of exercise capacity in children with chronic heart failure and pulmonary hypertension
	Oxygen saturation	
Exercise testing with ECG monitoring	Exercise time	Assessment of patients with suspected myocardial ischaemia and those with documented or suspected cardiac arrhythmias
	Oxygen saturation	
	Blood pressure	
	Heart rate response	
	ECG changes (myocardial ischaemia, arrhythmias)	
Cardiopulmonary exercise testing	Exercise time	Objective assessment of exercise capacity for planning of management and evaluation of treatment response
	Oxygen saturation	
	Blood pressure	
	Heart rate response	
	ECG changes (myocardial ischaemia, arrhythmias)	
	VO2 max	
	VO2 peak	
	Oxygen pulse	
	Respiratory exchange ratio	
	Ventilatory anaerobic threshold	
	V_E/V_{CO2} slope	
	Spirometric measurements	

Table 10.2 Bruce protocol

Stage	Duration (min)	Speed (miles per hour)	Grade (%)	Metabolic equivalents
1	3	1.7	10	5
2	3	2.5	12	7
3	3	3.4	14	10
4	3	4.2	16	13
5	3	5.0	18	15
6	3	5.5	20	18
7	3	6	22	20

increase in workload. For treadmill testing, the Bruce protocol (an incremental protocol) is the most frequently used protocol for cardiopulmonary exercise testing in children and adolescents (Table 10.2). For cycle ergometry, the pedalling speed is set initially at a rate comfortable for the child followed by gradual increase in the resistance to pedalling (ramp protocol). These exercise protocols can be used for stress echocardiography and stress myocardial perfusion imaging.

10.3.2 Pharmacologic Agents

For patients who are too young or who cannot perform exercise testing, pharmacologic agents are used. Dobutamine infusion is commonly used in stress echocardiography (Chap. 6), while adenosine or dipyridamole is used in stress radionuclide and cardiac magnetic resonance myocardial perfusion scan.

10.4 Interpretation of Exercise Testing Parameters

The maximum workload is estimated from the maximum speed and incline for exercise treadmill testing (Table 10.2) and determined directly from bicycle ergometry settings. Important cardiac and ventilatory parameters are obtained at maximum or peak exercise level (Table 10.3).

Table 10.3 Cardiopulmonary exercise testing parameters

Parameter	Interpretation
VO2 max	Best measure of cardiorespiratory fitness
	Difficult to achieve as exercise until exhaustion is required
	Evidence of near maximal VO2: VO2 plateau, maximum heart rate, maximum respiratory exchange ratio
VO2 peak	The most commonly measured parameter of cardiorespiratory fitness
	Determined by cardiac output and factors affecting oxygen content of arterial and mixed venous blood (e.g. anaemia, peripheral oxygen consumption by skeletal muscle) (based on Fick equation)
	Expressed as % predicted based on prediction equation (based on age, sex, and body size)
Maximum heart rate (HR)	Peak HR = 220 − age
	Reduced in the presence of chronotropic incompetence (e.g. sinus node dysfunction)
Oxygen pulse	VO2/HR = (cardiac output × O2 extraction)/HR = stroke volume × O2 extraction
	Reduced when there is impairment of increase in forward stroke volume with exercise or conditions that decrease oxygen extraction
Oxygen saturation	Worsens during exercise with intracardiac and/or intrapulmonary shunt and pulmonary disease
Blood pressure	Decrease or failure to increase in systolic blood pressure during exercise suggests significant left ventricular dysfunction
Respiratory exchange ratio (RER)	VCO2/VO2
	An indicator of exercise effort (RER ≥1.0 indicates good effort) and the contribution of anaerobic metabolism
Ventilatory anaerobic threshold	The level above which anaerobic metabolism supplements aerobic metabolism
	Shown by an abrupt increase in slope of CO2 production (usually at 40–70% of predicted VO2 peak)
	Interpretation similar to that for VO2 peak
V_E/V_{CO2} slope	Amount of ventilation needed for elimination of CO2 produced
	Based on the linear portion of the VE/VCO2 curve
	An index of gas exchange efficiency and influenced primarily pulmonary flow maldistribution (V/Q mismatch)
	Increased in patients with heart failure and pulmonary hypertension

Part II

Acyanotic Congenital Heart Disease

Left-to-Right Shunts 11

Left-to-right shunts comprise structural abnormalities that allow blood to flow from the systemic (left-sided) to the pulmonary (right-sided) circulation. These include intracardiac defects (atrial septal defect, ventricular septal defect, atrioventricular septal defect) and systemic-to-pulmonary arterial communications (persistent arterial duct, aortopulmonary window).

In these acyanotic congenital heart conditions, the direction of shunting of blood is from the left to the right side of the circulation, as (1) the right ventricular compliance is lower than the left ventricular compliance (for atrial septal defect), (2) the right ventricular pressure is lower than the left ventricular pressure (for ventricular septal defect), and (3) the pressure and resistance of the pulmonary arterial bed is normally lower than that of the systemic arterial bed (for persistent arterial duct and aortopulmonary window).

The haemodynamic consequences of large left-to-right shunts are (1) volume overloading of the left heart (in large ventricular septal defect, persistent arterial duct, and aortopulmonary window), the right heart (in large atrial septal defect) or both sides of the heart (in atrioventricular septal defect), and (2) development of pulmonary arterial hypertension.

11.1 Ventricular Septal Defect

11.1.1 Anatomy

Different types of ventricular septal defects are defined by their location in the ventricular septum (Fig. 11.1), which consists of a small fibrous membranous septum and a larger muscular septum. A perimembranous defect is located in the region of membranous septum, with part of the margin formed by fibrous continuity between the tricuspid and aortic valves. An inlet perimembranous ventricular septal defect

Y.-f. Cheung, *Congenital and Paediatric Acquired Heart Disease in Practice*, https://doi.org/10.1007/978-981-99-2862-0_11

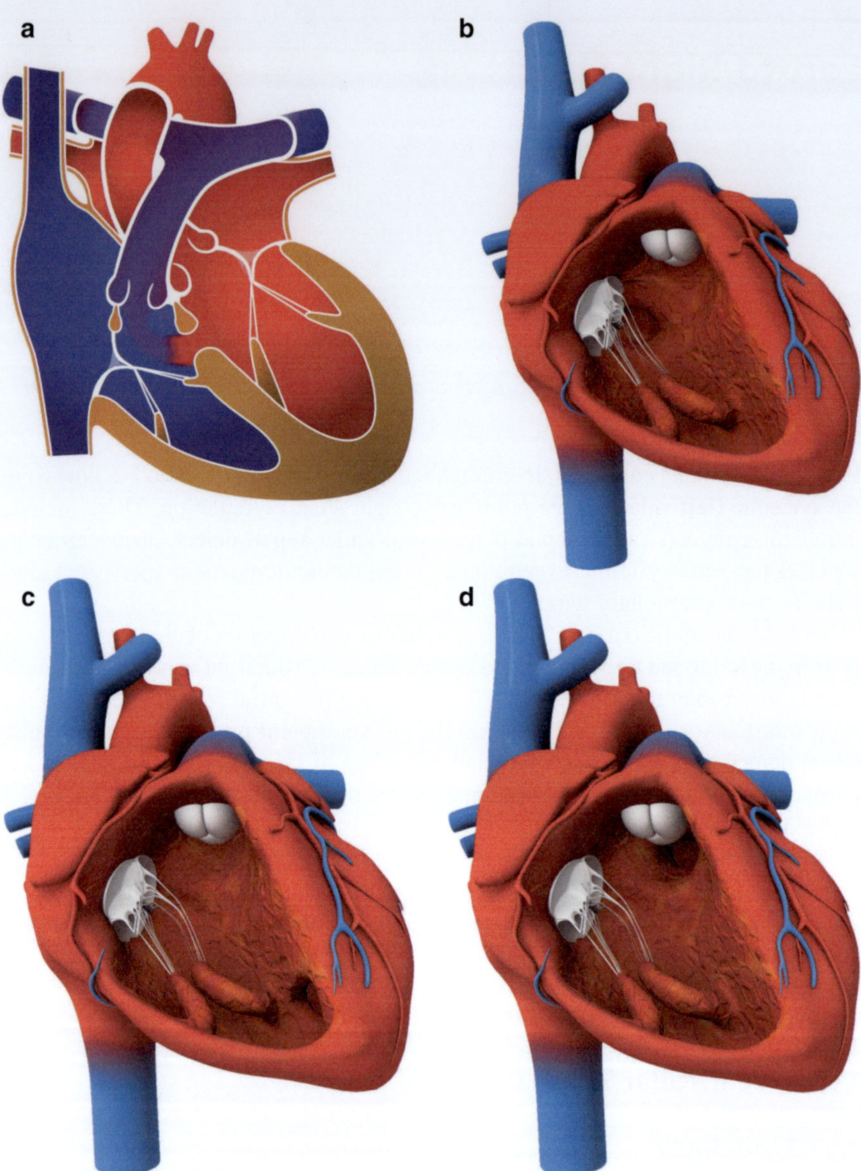

Fig. 11.1 Types of ventricular septal defect. (**a**) Left-to-right shunt through a ventricular septal defect. (**b**) Perimembranous ventricular septal defect. (**c**) Apical muscular ventricular septal defect. (**d**) Subarterial ventricular septal defect

opens into the right ventricular inlet portion, extends along the tricuspid valve, and is mostly covered by its septal leaflet. A muscular defect is bordered entirely by the muscular septum, and a subarterial defect lies just beneath the pulmonary and aortic valves. Coronary cusp prolapse with development of aortic regurgitation and sinus of Valsalva aneurysm are associated commonly with subarterial and outlet muscular defects (right coronary cusp) and less so with perimembranous defects (right and non-coronary cusps).

11.1.2 Pathophysiology

The magnitude of the left-to-right shunt through a ventricular septal defect depends on the size of the defect and pulmonary vascular resistance. At birth when the pulmonary vascular resistance is high, the shunt may appear small. In the first two months after birth, progressive reduction of pulmonary vascular resistance may lead to a gradual increase in left-to-right shunt.

In the presence of a large ventricular septal defect, the pulmonary arterial flow increases, and hence the pulmonary venous return increases and volume overloading of the left atrium and the left ventricle occurs. The right ventricle is, however, not volume overloaded, as it merely functions as a conduit through which blood from the left ventricle enters the pulmonary arterial circulation during systole.

When large left-to-right shunts are allowed to persist, the increase in pulmonary arterial flow causes medial hypertrophy of the pulmonary arterioles and pulmonary arterial hypertension, which in turn leads to pressure overloading of the right ventricle. With further destruction of the pulmonary arterial vasculature, irreversible pulmonary vascular disease (Eisenmenger syndrome) occurs. Significant elevation of pulmonary vascular resistance eventually leads to shunt reversal, with shunting of the deoxygenated blood from the right ventricle to the left ventricle (right-to-left shunt) and systemic hypoxaemia.

11.1.3 Clinical Presentation and Findings

Infants and children with a small ventricular septal defect are asymptomatic and present with incidental finding of a cardiac murmur. Those with a large ventricular septal defect present with symptoms of heart failure at one to two months of age. Signs of small and large ventricular septal defects are shown in Table 11.1.

Improvement of symptoms and signs of heart failure in patients with a large ventricular septal defect may be due to (1) progressive reduction in size or complete closure of the defect (coverage of perimembranous defects by tricuspid valve tissue and muscular defects by myocardial tissue), (2) development of infundibular stenosis (Chap. 12), or (3) increased pulmonary vascular resistance with development of pulmonary vascular disease.

11.1.4 Investigations

CXR: Chest radiograph is normal in children with a small defect and shows pulmonary plethora and cardiomegaly due to left ventricular dilation in patients with a large defect.

Table 11.1 Signs of ventricular septal defect (VSD)

	Small VSD	Large VSD
Signs of heart failure	–	+
Praecordial bulge	–	+
Displaced cardiac apex	–	+
LV impulse	–	+
RV impulse	–	+/–
Loud P2	–	+/–
Murmurs	A soft ejection systolic murmur or a typical pansystolic murmur at the left lower sternal border	A pansystolic murmur at the left lower sternal border, a mid-diastolic murmur at the apex due to increased transmitral flow

ECG: Electrocardiogram is normal in children with a small defect and reveals evidence of left ventricular dilation and right ventricular hypertrophy (when pulmonary hypertension is present) in patients with a large defect.
Echocardiography: Echocardiography confirms the location and size of the defect, permits the quantification of left ventricular dilation and pulmonary arterial pressure (by Doppler evaluation of the transventricular pressure gradient), and assessment of aortic cusp prolapse and aortic regurgitation (Fig. 11.2).

11.1.5 Management Strategy

Spontaneous closure has been estimated to occur in 60–80% of perimembranous and muscular defects, usually before 5 years of age. Subarterial defects do not close. An apparent decrease in the size of subarterial defects is related to prolapse of the right coronary cusp.

Infants and children with a small defect do not require treatment. For infants with heart failure due to moderate-to-large sized ventricular septal defects, medical treatment with diuretics and angiotensin-converting enzyme inhibitors should be started while monitoring for spontaneous partial or complete closure in patients with perimembranous or muscular defects.

Surgical closure of ventricular septal defects, performed usually before six months of age, is indicated in infants with poor medical control of heart failure, failure to thrive, pulmonary hypertension, and recurrent episodes of chest infection. In infants with multiple muscular ventricular septal defects (Swiss cheese defects), initial palliation with placement of a pulmonary arterial band, for better control of heart failure symptoms and growth, is followed later by surgical or transcatheter closure of the defects.

Surgical repair of the defect is also indicated in asymptomatic older children with subarterial, outlet muscular, or perimembranous defects complicated by coronary cusp prolapse and aortic regurgitation (Box 11.1) and in older relatively

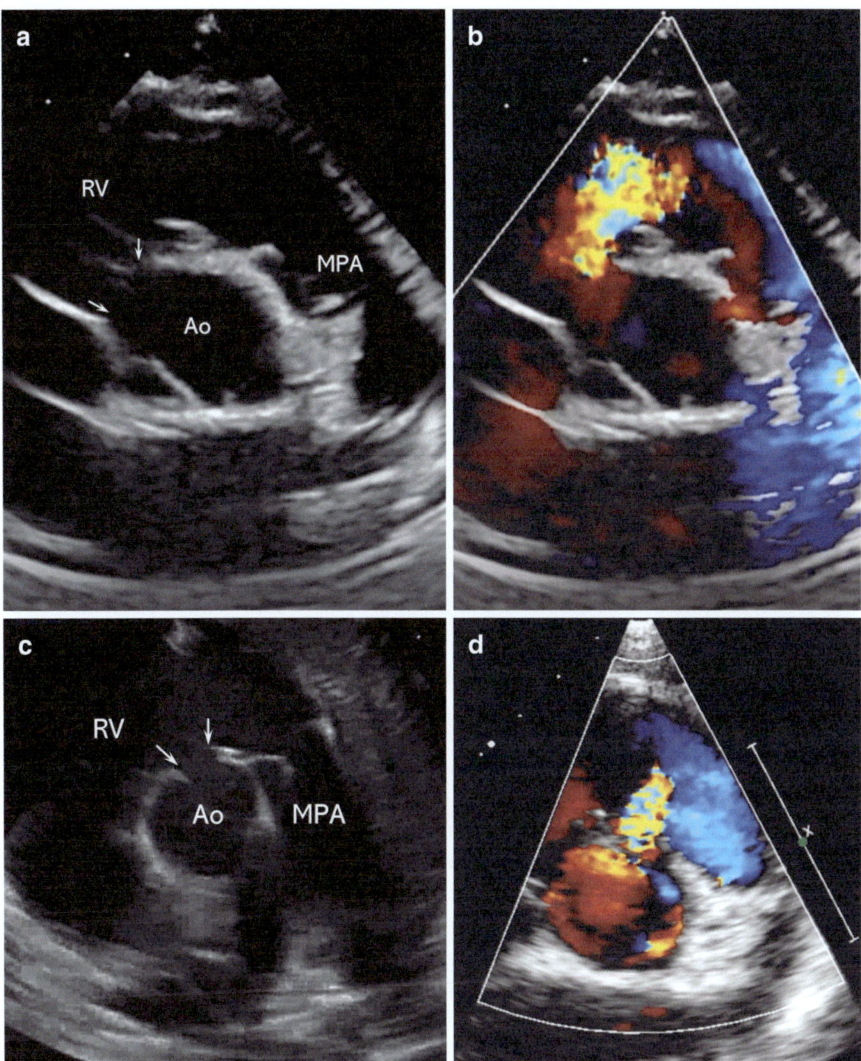

Fig. 11.2 Echocardiographic assessment of ventricular septal defect. (**a**) 2D and (**b**) colour Doppler echocardiographic findings of perimembranous ventricular septal defect (arrows) (**c**) 2D and (**d**) colour Doppler echocardiographic findings of subarterial ventricular septal defect (arrows) (*Ao* aorta, *MPA* main pulmonary artery, *RV* right ventricle)

asymptomatic children with any types of defects causing persistent volume overloading of the left ventricle.

Transcatheter device closure of muscular defects by percutaneous or hybrid perventricular approach may be feasible. In selected patients with perimembranous ventricular septal defects covered partially by tricuspid valve aneurysmal tissue, percutaneous transcatheter device closure can also be contemplated.

Box 11.1 Indications for Surgical Closure of Ventricular Septal Defect with Aortic Regurgitation in Asymptomatic Older Children

- Moderate degree of aortic regurgitation
- Moderate or severe right coronary cusp prolapse in subarterial or outlet muscular ventricular septal defect with any degree of aortic regurgitation
- Moderate or severe right and non-coronary cusp prolapse in perimembranous ventricular septal defect with mild to severe degree of aortic regurgitation
- Unclear indication of closing perimembranous ventricular septal defect with moderate to severe prolapse of the right and/or non-coronary cusp but only trivial degree of aortic regurgitation

11.1.6 Postoperative Considerations

The postoperatively course is usually uncomplicated. Potential complications include low cardiac output syndrome, pulmonary congestion, pulmonary hypertensive crisis, complete heart block, and junctional ectopic tachycardia. Early intensive care management includes fluid restriction, low-dose intravenous milrinone infusion, and diuretics. Extubation is usually possible within the first 24 h of surgery.

11.1.7 Long-Term Monitoring

Long-term outcomes are good in the majority of patients after surgical repair of ventricular septal defects. Increasing follow-up data into adulthood suggest, however, possible occurrence of impaired exercise capacity, right ventricular dysfunction, and cardiac arrhythmias. In patients even after repair of subarterial defects, monitoring for progression of aortic regurgitation and sinus of Valsalva aneurysm, which may rupture during adulthood, is required.

11.2 Atrial Septal Defect

11.2.1 Anatomy

Three types of defects occur in the atrial septum (Fig. 11.3): (1) Secundum atrial septal defect is the most common type and is regarded as the true defect of the atrial septum. It is located in the flap valve that covers the oval fossa. (2) Primum atrial septal defect represents the persistence of the embryonic ostium primum and is considered an incomplete form of complete atrioventricular defect with failure of septation of the atrioventricular junction. It occurs at the lower part of the atrial septum and lies between the free margin of the true atrial septum and orifice of the atrioventricular valves. It is associated with cleft of the left atrioventricular (mitral)

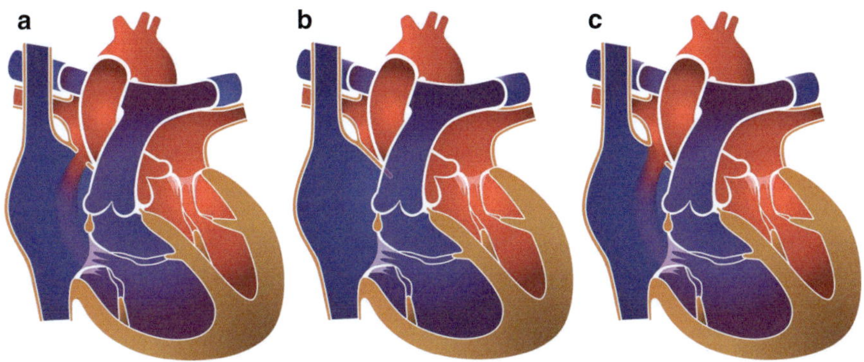

Fig. 11.3 Types of atrial septal defect. (**a**) Secundum atrial septal defect. (**b**) Primum atrial septal defect. (**c**) Sinus venosus atrial septal defect

valve and mitral insufficiency. The primum defect is discussed in greater details in the next section on complete atrioventricular septal defect. (3) Sinus venosus defect is usually found at the entrance of the superior caval vein and occasionally at the mouth of the inferior caval vein. It is associated with partial anomalous drainage of the right pulmonary veins, which usually empty into the right atrium or less commonly (in 10–15% of patients) into the superior caval vein.

Coronary sinus defect is a rare cause of interatrial left-to-right shunting, although this is not usually regarded as a defect of the atrial septum. Rather, this is a defect between the coronary sinus and the left atrium, also referred to as 'unroofing' of the coronary sinus. As the coronary sinus drains into the right atrium, this defect constitutes a left-to-right interatrial shunt.

11.2.2 Pathophysiology

Blood flows from the left atrium to the right atrium through the atrial septal defect throughout the cardiac cycle. The magnitude depends on the size of the defect and relative compliance of the right and left ventricles. After birth, as the pulmonary vascular resistance drops, right ventricular mass decreases and the right ventricle becomes more distensible with promotion of the left-to-right interatrial shunt. A large left-to-right shunt at the atrial level leads to volume overloading of the right heart. Atrial septal defect is the only left-to-right shunt that leads to isolated volume overloading of the right heart.

Unlike other left-to-right shunts, even large left-to-right shunts at the atrial level do not usually result in significant elevation of pulmonary arterial pressure and pulmonary vascular resistance in children. While it remains true that persistent increase in pulmonary arterial flow in the setting of a large atrial septal defect causes medial hypertrophy of the pulmonary arterioles, destruction of the pulmonary arterial vasculature, and irreversible pulmonary vascular disease, development of Eisenmenger syndrome with reversal of atrial shunt flow may not be a uniform response even in adults.

11.2.3 Clinical Presentation and Findings

In contrast to other left-to-right shunts, atrial septal defect is seldom associated with heart failure or pulmonary hypertension in children and adolescents. Rarely, a large atrial septal defect is the cause of heart failure in young infants. Usually, the haemodynamic consequences of a large defect manifest in adult patients at their fourth to fifth decades, who present with symptoms of heart failure due to chronic right ventricular volume overload, atrial arrhythmias due to chronic atrial stretching, and pulmonary hypertension. Signs of small and large atrial septal defects are shown in Table 11.2.

11.2.4 Investigations

CXR: Chest radiograph is normal in children with a small defect and shows an increase in convexity of the right cardiac border due to right atrial dilation, uptilting of the cardiac apex related to right ventricular dilation, and a prominent pulmonary knob in patients with a large atrial septal defect.

ECG: Electrocardiogram is normal in children with a small defect and reveals evidence of right axis deviation, and right atrial and right ventricular dilation in those with a large defect. With volume overloading of the right ventricle, an incomplete right bundle branch block (rsR′) pattern in lead V1 is commonly observed. Whereas the QRS axis is deviated to the right in secundum atrial septal defect, a superior QRS axis (left axis deviation) is characteristic of primum atrial septal defect.

Echocardiography: Echocardiography defines the type, size, and margins of the defect and permits the quantification of right atrial and right ventricular dilation and estimation of pulmonary arterial pressure (by Doppler evaluation of the tricuspid regurgitant jet when present) (Fig. 11.4).

Table 11.2 Signs of atrial septal defect (ASD)

	Small ASD	Large ASD
Signs of heart failure	–	Usually –
Praecordial bulge	–	+
RV impulse	–	+
Wide and fixed splitting of S2	+/–	+
Murmurs	Absent or a soft ejection systolic murmur at the left upper sternal border (pulmonary flow murmur)	A soft pulmonary flow murmur and a mid-diastolic murmur at the left lower sternal border due to increased transtricuspid flow

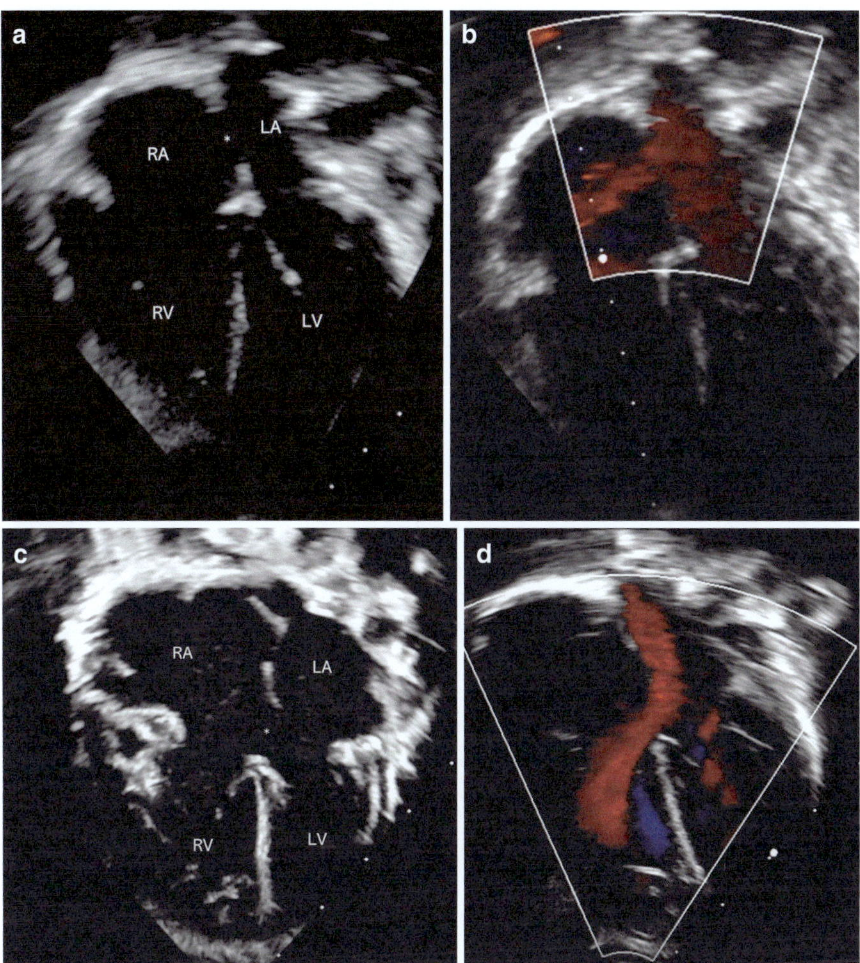

Fig. 11.4 Echocardiographic assessment of atrial septal defect. (**a**) 2D and (**b**) colour Doppler echocardiographic findings of secundum atrial septal defect (asterisk). (**c**) 2D and (**d**) colour Doppler echocardiographic findings of primum septal defect (asterisk) (*LA* left atrium, *LV* left ventricle, *RA* right atrium, *RV* right ventricle)

11.2.5 Management Strategy

Spontaneous closure of secundum atrial septal defects has been reported to vary from 3% to 67%, with the highest incidence being reported in infants during the first year of life. For defects less than 8 mm in size, the rate of spontaneous closure has been reported to exceed 80%.

Infants and children with a small secundum atrial defect do not require treatment. Indications for closure of moderate-to-large sized atrial septal defects include symptomatic heart failure in infants (which is rare) and, in asymptomatic children, evidence of right heart dilation (as assessed by echocardiography). In asymptomatic patients, closure of moderate-to-large sized atrial septal defects is usually not performed in early childhood given the lack of symptoms and possibility of spontaneous closure of the defects. Surgical or transcatheter interventions closure are usually performed in indicated patients at about 5 years of age.

Surgical repair of secundum defects involves either direct suture or patch closure. Transcatheter device closure with secundum atrial septal defects with adequate septal rims is usually performed when the asymptomatic patient reaches a body weight of about 20 kg to facilitate the procedure (Fig. 11.5).

For sinus venosus defects, patch closure of the defect with redirection of the anomalous pulmonary veins into the left atrium is required. Anomalous drainage of the right pulmonary veins to the superior caval vein is repaired by the Warden procedure, which involves division of the superior caval vein, with anastomosis of the cephalic superior caval vein to the right atrial appendage and tunnelling of the caudal superior caval vein to the left atrium. Advantages of this procedure include avoidance of sinus node dysfunction and pulmonary and systemic venous obstruction. In selected adult patients, successful deployment of a covered stent to simultaneously close the sinus venous defect and to redirect the anomalous pulmonary venous drainage to the left atrium behind the covered stent has been reported. Surgical management of primum atrial septal defect is discussed in the next section.

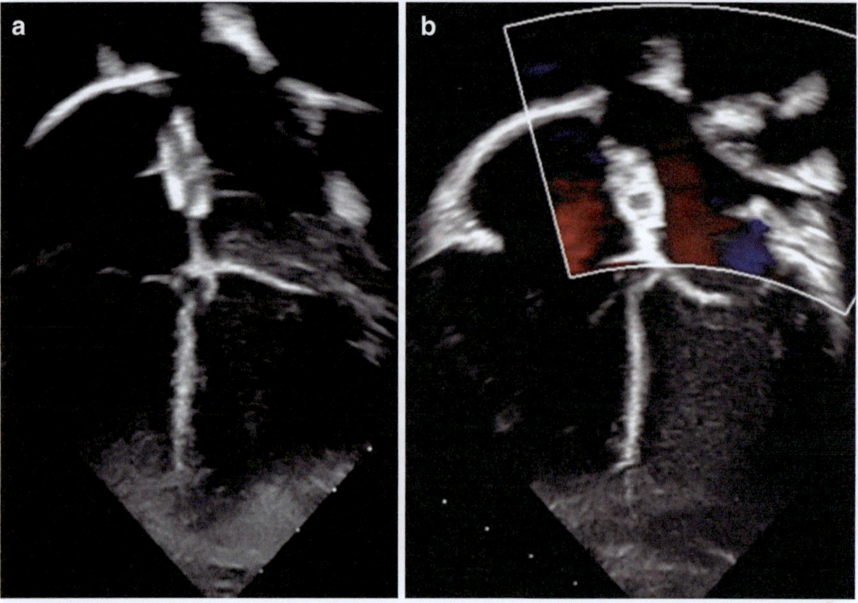

Fig. 11.5 Device occlusion of atrial septal defect. (**a**) 2D and (**b**) colour Doppler echocardiographic demonstration of complete occlusion of a secundum atrial septal defect by an Amplatzer septal occluder

11.2.6 Postoperative Considerations

The postoperative course is usually uncomplicated. Occasional complications immediately after surgical closure of atrial septal defects include sinus node dysfunction, atrial arrhythmia, left ventricular diastolic dysfunction (usually in older patients), and obstruction of superior caval vein and right pulmonary veins (after creation of a baffle for the repair of anomalous drainage of the right pulmonary veins to the superior caval vein).

11.2.7 Considerations After Device Closure of Atrial Septal Defects

Potential complications include embolization of device, atrial arrhythmias, and device erosion (with an estimated absolute risk of erosion of 0.04–0.3% after implantation of an Amplatzer septal occluder). Aspirin is given for six months after device closure to allow for completion of endothelialization.

11.2.8 Long-Term Monitoring

Long-term outcomes are good in most of the patients after surgical repair and transcatheter occlusion of atrial septal defects. There is occasional occurrence of sinus node dysfunction and supraventricular tachyarrhythmias after surgery. Cardiac erosion with development of pericardial effusion and fistula formation (e.g. between the aorta and the right atrium) due to mechanical trauma (especially with the use of an over-sized device) may occur, albeit rarely, after device implantation.

11.3 Atrioventricular Septal Defect

11.3.1 Anatomy

Atrioventricular septal defect, a common congenital cardiac malformation in children with Down syndrome (Chap. 62), comprises cardiac lesions that have deficient atrioventricular septation and an oval common atrioventricular junction (Fig. 11.6a).

11.3.2 Atrioventricular Junction

In atrioventricular septal defect, the atrioventricular valve that guards the common junction comprises five leaflets, namely the superior bridging leaflet, inferior bridging leaflet, left mural leaflet, right anterosuperior leaflet, and right mural leaflet (Fig. 11.6b). The space between the superior and inferior bridging leaflets

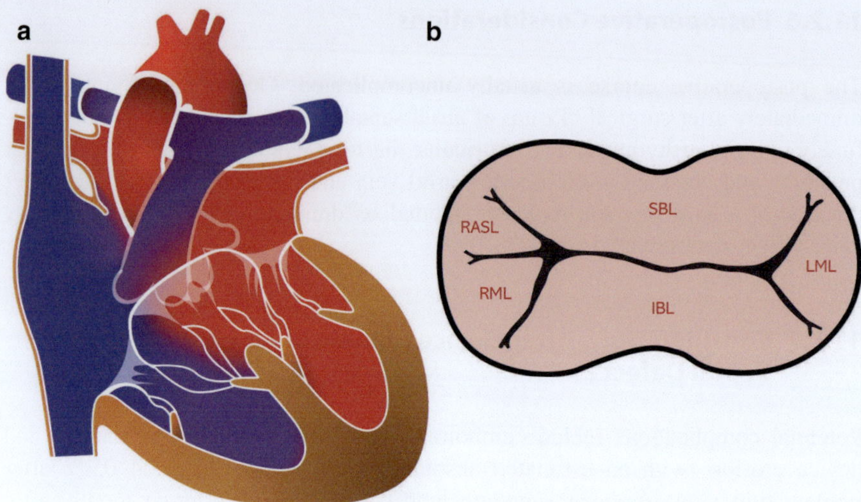

Fig. 11.6 Atrioventricular septal defect. (**a**) Complete atrioventricular septal defect. (**b**) Common atrioventricular valve (*IBL* inferior bridging leaflet, *LML* left mural leaflet, *RASL* right anterosuperior leaflet, *RML* right mural leaflet, *SBL* superior bridging leaflet)

Table 11.3 Rastelli classification

Type	Description
Type A	The most common type, found frequently in Down syndrome, in which the superior bridging leaflet is committed to the left ventricle with chordal attachments to the crest of the ventricular septum
Type B	The least common type, in which the superior bridging leaflet extends into the right ventricle
Type C	Found in combination with other cardiac defects (e.g. tetralogy of Fallot, transposition of the great arteries, heterotaxy syndromes), in which the superior bridging leaflet is large and free floating (with no chordal attachment to the ventricular septum)

constitutes the zone of apposition, commonly referred to as the 'cleft', which may be the site of left atrioventricular valvar regurgitation.

The abnormal atrioventricular valve is usually incompetent. Progressive thickening and prolapse of the valve leaflets further worsen the degree of atrioventricular valvar regurgitation. The Rastelli classification describes the morphology of the atrioventricular valve based on the morphology of the superior bridging leaflet and the chordal insertions (Table 11.3).

In complete atrioventricular septal defect, there are a primum component (an inter-atrial communication between the inferior margin of the true septum and atrial surface of the common atrioventricular valve and junction) and a ventricular component (an inter-ventricular communication between the crest of the ventricular septum and ventricular surface of the common atrioventricular valve and junction). Rarely, the superior and inferior bridging leaflets may be fused to the free margin of the true atrial septum with only a ventricular component (which may be mistaken as a perimembranous inlet ventricular septal defect).

Division of the common atrioventricular junction into a right and a left orifice by valvar tissues joining the two bridging leaflets occurs in a minority of patients. In these patients, the bridging leaflets may be fused to the crest of the ventricular septum and result in a primum atrial septal defect (also referred to as partial atrioventricular septal defect). Incomplete fusion of the bridging leaflets to the ventricular septum, on the other hand, leads to a primum atrial septal defect with an inlet ventricular septal defect. In patients with a primum atrial septal defect, the left atrioventricular (mitral) valve is almost always abnormal with a 'cleft' and varying degrees of left atrioventricular valvar regurgitation.

11.3.2.1 Balance of the Ventricles

Balanced atrioventricular septal defect with right and left ventricles of similar sizes is present in the majority of patients. However, in some patients, the common atrioventricular junction is committed either more to the right ventricle to cause right ventricular dominance or more to the left ventricle to cause left ventricular dominance. In most of these patients, right ventricular dominance is the cause of an unbalanced atrioventricular septal defect. When there is significant hypoplasia of either of the ventricles, biventricular repair is not feasible.

11.3.2.2 Left Ventricular Outflow Tract

The so-called 'goose neck deformity' of the left ventricular outflow tract is characteristic of complete atrioventricular septal defect. This is due to anterosuperior displacement of the aortic valve by the common atrioventricular valve, with the consequence of lengthening of the outlet dimension (apex to aorta) relative to the inlet dimension (atrioventricular valve to apex) and elongating the left ventricular outflow tract. There is usually no obstruction to this elongated outflow. However, several anatomic substrates may contribute to left ventricular outflow obstruction in atrioventricular septal defect: (1) tight binding of superior bridging leaflet to the crest of ventricular septum (especially in partial atrioventricular septal defect), (2) accessory papillary muscle, (3) subaortic membrane, and (4) associated coarctation of the aorta.

11.3.2.3 Associations with Other Cardiac Defects

Associated cardiac defects include tetralogy of Fallot, transposition of the great arteries, secundum atrial septum defect, coarctation of the aorta (although this combination is distinctly uncommon in Down syndrome), and heterotaxy syndrome (in particular right atrial isomerism).

11.3.3 Pathophysiology

The haemodynamic consequences of complete atrioventricular septal defect are:

1. Volume overloading of the right heart due to the left-to-right shunt through the primum atrial septal defect and right atrioventricular valvar regurgitation,
2. Volume overloading of the left heart due to left-to-right shunt through the ventricular septal defect and left atrioventricular valvar regurgitation,

3. Pulmonary hypertension, especially in the presence of a large ventricular component and in children with Down syndrome who commonly have hypoventilation due to upper airway obstruction, and
4. Pressure overloading of the right ventricle due to pulmonary hypertension.

In primum atrial septal defect with or without an inlet ventricular septal defect (usually small in size), the haemodynamic consequences are those of a large atrial septal defect. However, the presence of significant left atrioventricular valvar regurgitation through the cleft would lead to left atrial and left ventricular dilation. In some of these patients, left ventricular-to-right atrial shunting occurs and aggravates the volume overloading of the right heart.

11.3.4 Clinical Presentation and Findings

Infants with a complete atrioventricular septal defect present with symptoms of heart failure at one to two months of age, or even earlier when severe left atrioventricular valvar regurgitation is present. Patients with Down syndrome often, however, remain asymptomatic during infancy due to the persistently increased pulmonary vascular resistance with no postnatal decrease. The physical findings are those of atrial and ventricular septal defects (Table 11.4).

Patients with a primum atrial septal defect with or without an inlet ventricular septal defect may remain relatively asymptomatic and present with incidental cardiac findings of an atrial or ventricular septal defect with or without signs of mitral regurgitation.

Table 11.4 Signs of complete atrioventricular septal defect

Signs	Origins
Signs of heart failure Praecordial bulge Displaced cardiac apex and LV impulse RV impulse	 Cardiomegaly LV volume overload RV volume (± pressure) overload
Wide and fixed splitting of S2 Increased P2	Signifies the atrial component Signifies the presence of pulmonary hypertension
A pansystolic murmur at the left lower sternal border and/or apex	Related to the flow across the ventricular septal defect or right atrioventricular valvar regurgitation and/or left atrioventricular valvar regurgitation
A mid-diastolic flow murmur at the left lower sternal border and/or apex	Related to increased-diastolic flow across the right and/or left atrioventricular valve

11.3.5 Investigations

CXR: In complete atrioventricular septal defect, the degree of cardiomegaly and pulmonary plethora in the chest radiograph is proportional to the magnitude of the left-to-right shunt and the severity of atrioventricular valvar regurgitation. The atrial left-to-right shunt causes enlargement of the right atrium and right ventricle, while the ventricular left-to-right shunt results in enlargement of the left atrium and left ventricle. Enlargement of the left atrium and left ventricle may also be related to significant left atrioventricular valvar regurgitation. The chest radiographic findings of a primum atrial septal defect include an increase in convexity of the right cardiac border due to right atrial dilation, uptilting of the cardiac apex related to right ventricular dilation, and a prominent pulmonary knob.

ECG: In complete atrioventricular septal defect, electrocardiogram reveals a superior QRS axis and, in the presence of large atrial and ventricular components, evidence of right and left ventricular dilation. In primum atrial septal defect, electrocardiogram reveals a superior QRS axis (left axis deviation), and right atrial and right ventricular dilation.

Echocardiography: Echocardiography enables the diagnosis of the type of atrioventricular septal defect and associate cardiac lesions, permits the assessment of the size of the atrial and ventricular components, relative size of the two ventricles, morphology of the atrioventricular valve, and provides an estimation of the severity of atrioventricular valvar regurgitation and left ventricular outflow obstruction (Fig. 11.7). The en face view of the atrioventricular valve obtained by three-dimensional echocardiography may facilitate surgical planning.

Cardiac catheterization: This is usually not indicated. It is performed to assess pulmonary vascular resistance and vascular reactivity in (1) the few patients who

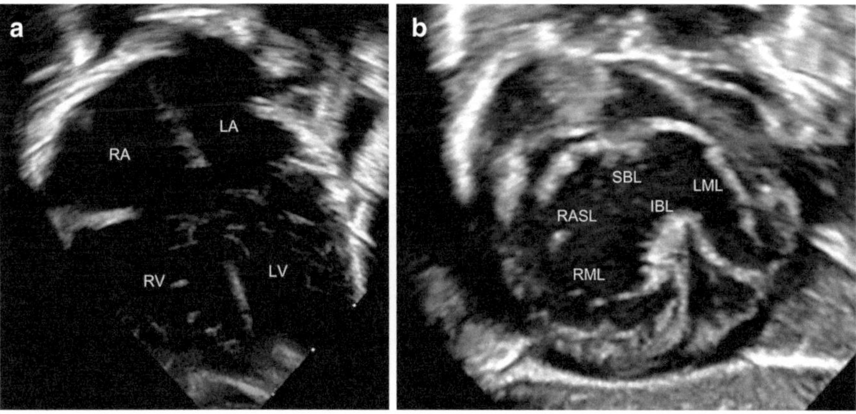

Fig. 11.7 Echocardiographic assessment of atrioventricular septal defect. (**a**) Four-chamber view showing complete atrioventricular septal defect (*LA* left atrium, *LV* left ventricle, *RA* right atrium, *RV* right ventricle). (**b**) Subcostal en face view of the common atrioventricular valve (abbreviations as in Fig. 11.6b)

present late (beyond 12 months of age) and (2) in infants (especially those with Down syndrome) with suspected accelerated development of pulmonary vascular disease (clinical, radiographic and echocardiographic evidence of limited left-to-right shunt and systemic pulmonary hypertension).

11.3.6 Management Strategy

11.3.6.1 Complete Atrioventricular Septal Defect

Medical management: Optimization of nutritional intake is required. Medical therapy with diuretics and systemic vasodilators provides only partial relief of the heart failure symptoms, especially in infants with a large ventricular component and significant left atrioventricular valvar regurgitation.

Surgical intervention for balanced atrioventricular septal defect: Surgical closure of the defect and repair of the atrioventricular valves are required although the timing needs consideration. Valve repair is challenging in neonates and very young infants. On the other hand, if repair is performed beyond 6 months of age, especially in patients with Down syndrome, the risk of developing pulmonary vascular disease is significantly increased.

In infants with relatively well controlled heart failure, elective surgery is usually performed at 3–6 months of age. In infants with refractory heart failure and significant atrioventricular valvar regurgitation, earlier surgical repair at 1–2 months of age may be required, albeit technically more demanding. In very symptomatic neonates, low birth weight infants, and premature babies, pulmonary arterial banding should be considered as an initial palliative intervention.

For the repair of the defect, a single-patch (for closing both the atrial and ventricular components) or a two-patch (an atrial and a ventricular patch) technique in combination with different ways of attaching the bridging leaflets (with or without cutting of the leaflets and attaching either to the patch or crest of ventricular septum) have been used by different surgeons. Closure of the 'cleft' (zone of apposition) of the left atrioventricular valve is usually performed, albeit remains debatable, to reduce the risk of significant postoperative left atrioventricular valvar regurgitation.

Management of unbalanced atrioventricular septal defect: The echocardiographic definition of unbalanced defects is controversial (based on the success of predicting biventricular versus univentricular repair). This may be related to the difficulty of assessing the ventricular size and, more importantly, the predicted change in ventricular size after surgery (removal of right ventricular volume and pressure overload restores septal configuration, increases left ventricular preload, and increases left ventricular size). Several indices have been used in the clinical setting (Table 11.5), although the correlation among these indices has been shown to be poor.

Severe imbalance of the ventricular sizes may require the adoption of a univentricular surgical approach with initial control of the pulmonary flow by pulmonary

Table 11.5 Echocardiographic indices that help to define unbalance

Index	Derivation	Prediction of success or failure of biventricular repair
Atrioventricular valve index	Left atrioventricular valvar area: total atrioventricular valve area ratio (subcostal anterior oblique view)	0.4–0.6 biventricular repair <0.19 univentricular repair 0.19–0.39 heterogenous strategies
Left ventricular inflow index	Width of colour Doppler inflow at its narrowest point into the left ventricle : corresponding left atrioventricular valvar annulus ratio (apical 4-chamber view)	<0.5 is associated with no survival after biventricular repair
Right ventricular/ left ventricular inflow angle	The angle between the hinge points of the right and left atrioventricular valves with the vertex at the crest of the ventricular septum (apical 4-chamber view)	Increasing inflow angle is associated with greater possibility of success for biventricular repair (no cutoff values provided)

arterial banding. Nonetheless, patients with relative right ventricular hypoplasia may still tolerate biventricular repair.

11.3.6.2 Partial Atrioventricular Septal Defect

Elective surgical repair of the primum atrial septal defect with or without significant left atrioventricular valvar regurgitation is usually performed in early childhood to reduce the effect of chronic overloading of the right heart (and of the left heart if there is more than mild degree of mitral regurgitation) and to restore the competence of the left atrioventricular valve. Surgical repair involves patch closure of the primum atrial septal defect and suture of mitral valve cleft together with mitral annuloplasty. An associated inlet ventricular septal defect, which is usually small, is closed by direct suture or with a patch.

11.3.7 Postoperative Considerations

The postoperative course for complete atrioventricular septal defect may be complicated by low cardiac output syndrome, pulmonary hypertensive crisis, complete heart block, and junctional ectopic tachycardia. In patients with low cardiac output syndrome, echocardiographic assessment to define residual left-to-right shunts, severity of left atrioventricular valvar regurgitation and/or stenosis, and ventricular function is important to guide management. On the other hand, patients undergoing repair of a primum atrial septal defect have usually an uncomplicated postoperative course (refer to sections on management after surgery for atrial septal defect and mitral regurgitation).

Initial intensive care management includes fluid restriction, intravenous milrinone infusion, and diuretics. In patients with mildly unbalanced ventricles, increased filling pressure may be necessary because of the restrictive filling of the hypoplastic ventricle. Inhaled nitric oxide therapy is indicated in high-risk patients (high pulmonary vascular resistance preoperatively, Down syndrome) and in patients who develop pulmonary hypertensive crisis.

11.3.8 Long-Term Monitoring

Long-term monitoring is required in patient after repair of complete atrioventricular septal defect for progressive left atrioventricular valvar regurgitation, left ventricular outflow tract obstruction (due to obstruction of the elongated left ventricular outflow by bridging leaflet tissues and/or subaortic membrane), and ventricular dysfunction. Common indications for reoperation include progressive left atrioventricular valvar regurgitation (which may require valvar replacement) and obstruction of the left ventricular outflow tract (which may require subaortic resection, resection of accessory cords and tags, and/or augmentation of the superior bridging leaflet).

11.4 Persistent Arterial Duct

11.4.1 Anatomy

The persistent arterial duct joins the main pulmonary artery at its bifurcation to the descending aorta (Fig. 11.8a). The morphology of the duct varies from a tubular appearance to tapering constriction at either the pulmonary or the aortic end or constrictions at both ends (Fig. 11.8b).

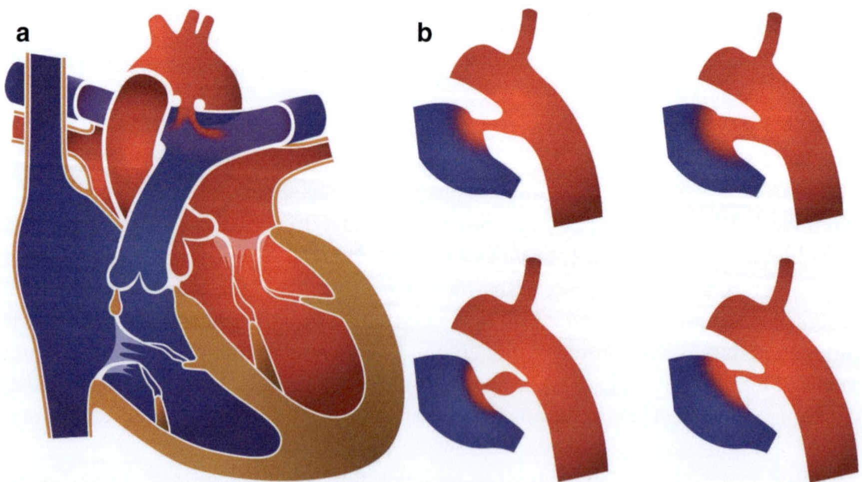

Fig. 11.8 Persistent arterial duct. (**a**) Left-to-right shunt through a persistent arterial duct. (**b**) Different morphologies of persistent arterial ducts

11.4.2 Pathophysiology

Physiologic closure of the arterial duct occurs soon after birth and anatomic occlusion occurs within three months. In preterm infants ≤28 weeks of gestational age, the incidence of persistent arterial duct exceeds 50% although spontaneous closure rates in these infants are high.

When the arterial duct is persistent, blood flows from the descending aorta to the pulmonary arteries to cause a left-to-right shunt. The magnitude of shunt depends on the size of the duct and the relative difference between systemic and pulmonary vascular resistance. As the pulmonary vascular resistance drops progressively in the first two months after birth, shunting through the duct increases. The increase in pulmonary venous return results in volume overloading of the left heart.

High pulmonary flow through a large arterial duct results in pulmonary hypertension. A large persistent arterial duct leads to medial hypertrophy of the pulmonary arterioles, intimal proliferation, and eventual destruction of the arterioles with irreversible pulmonary vascular disease. The resultant increase in pulmonary vascular resistance may result in right-to-left shunting of blood from the pulmonary arteries to the descending aorta through the duct and systemic hypoxaemia (Eisenmenger syndrome). Hence, differential cyanosis with cyanosis of the lower but not the upper extremities and clubbing of only the toes but not the fingers are found in patients with Eisenmenger syndrome due to a large persistent arterial duct.

11.4.3 Clinical Presentation and Findings

Infants and children with a small persistent arterial duct are asymptomatic and present usually with incidental finding of a cardiac murmur. Those with a large persistent arterial duct present with symptoms of heart failure at one to two months of age.

In preterm babies, with improvement of respiratory distress syndrome after surfactant therapy and concomitant decrease in pulmonary vascular resistance, signs of an arterial duct begin to appear few days after birth. They tolerate the left-to-right shunt poorly and develop heart failure earlier due to less effective compensatory mechanisms. In preterm babies, a large left-to-right shunt through a haemodynamically significant duct increases the risk of prolonged ventilation, bronchopulmonary dysplasia, necrotizing enterocolitis, intraventricular haemorrhage, and death.

Signs of small and large persistent arterial ducts are shown in Table 11.6.

11.4.4 Investigations

CXR: Chest radiograph is normal in children with a small duct and shows pulmonary plethora and cardiomegaly due to left ventricular dilation in patients with a large duct.

Table 11.6 Signs of persistent arterial duct (PDA)

	Small PDA	Large PDA
Signs of heart failure	–	+
Bounding pulses	–	+
Praecordial bulge	–	+
Displaced cardiac apex	–	+
LV impulse	–	+
RV impulse	–	+/–
Loud P2	–	+/–
Murmurs	A soft ejection systolic or a continuous murmur at left upper sternal border or left infraclavicular region	A continuous murmur at left upper sternal border or left infraclavicular region (unless with pulmonary vascular disease)

ECG: Electrocardiogram is normal in children with a small duct and reveals evidence of left ventricular dilation and right ventricular hypertrophy (when pulmonary hypertension is present) in patients with a large duct.
Echocardiography: Echocardiography confirms the patency of the duct and enables the quantification of magnitude of left-to-right shunt (by measuring the size of duct and assessment of left atrial and left ventricular dilation), estimation of pulmonary arterial pressure (by Doppler evaluation of the transductal pressure gradient), and diagnosis of isthmus hypoplasia or coarctation of the aorta (Fig. 11.9).

11.4.5 Management Strategy

Transcatheter device closure of duct is the treatment of choice in term infants and children (Fig. 11.10). Closure of ducts associated with a significant left-to-right shunt is indicated for treating the heart failure and eliminating the risk of developing pulmonary vascular disease. Closing small ducts to prevent infective endarteritis, given the low transcatheter procedural risks and complications, is supported by most authorities. However, closing tiny ducts with no audible murmurs (silent ducts) is usually not justified.

In premature babies, there has been a trend toward less aggressive treatment of persistent arterial duct in the last decade. The use of indomethacin as prophylactic treatment fails to confirm a benefit on a composite outcome of survival and neurodevelopment. For symptomatic ducts, supportive treatment includes fluid restriction, diuretics, respiratory support with permissive hypercapnia to limit the left-to-right shunt, and inotropic support. Prostaglandin synthase inhibitors, ibuprofen (oral or intravenous) or indomethacin (intravenous), are the mainstays of medical treatment to close haemodynamically significant ducts in premature babies, although positive effects on long-term outcomes have not been established. Ibuprofen and indomethacin have similar treatment efficacy, while the safety profile

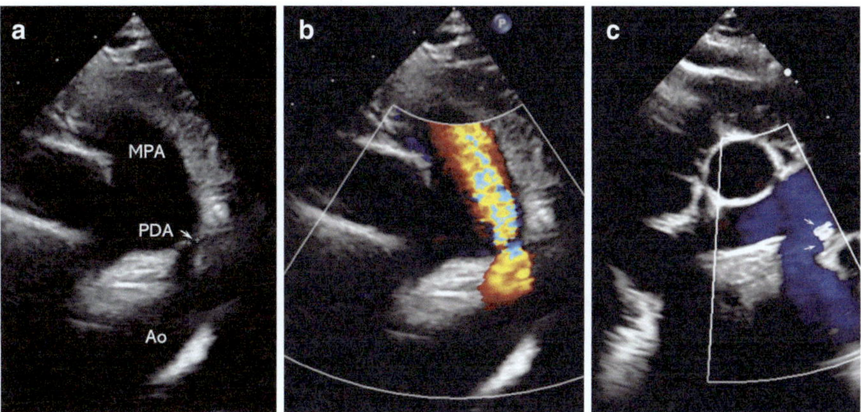

Fig. 11.9 Echocardiographic assessment of persistent arterial duct. (**a**) 2D and (**b**) colour Doppler echocardiographic findings of persistent arterial duct. (**c**) Complete occlusion of the duct by an Amplatzer duct occluder (arrows) (*Ao* aorta, *MPA* main pulmonary artery, *PDA* persistent arterial duct)

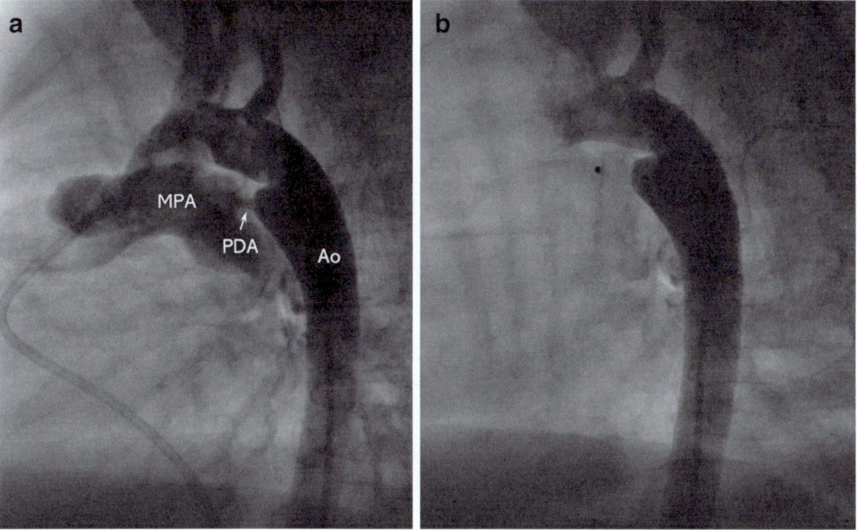

Fig. 11.10 Transcatheter closure of persistent arterial duct. (**a**) Angiographic demonstration of the persistent arterial duct. (**b**) Complete occlusion of the duct by an Amplatzer duct occluder (*Ao* aorta, *MPA* main pulmonary artery, *PDA* persistent arterial duct)

of ibuprofen is superior. Paracetamol (oral or intravenous), thought to act at the peroxidation site of cyclooxygenase, is increasingly used in premature babies in whom ibuprofen and indomethacin are contraindicated or ineffective. The success rate of paracetamol is, however, relatively low.

There are no randomized control trials on pharmacologic closure versus surgical ligation of haemodynamically significant persistent arterial ducts in premature babies. Surgical ligation is performed usually when medical therapy has failed or is contraindicated. Recently, transcatheter closure of the duct in premature babies less than 1000 g has been rendered possible with the introduction of new devices. There are yet no randomized control trials on device closure versus surgical ligation in premature babies and data on long-term outcomes are not available.

11.4.6 Considerations After Surgical Ligation of Ducts in Premature Babies

Potential complications include post ligation cardiac syndrome, injury to the left recurrent laryngeal nerve resulting in left vocal cord dysfunction, incorrect ligation of other vascular structures, chylothorax, development of coarctation of the aorta (especially when isthmus hypoplasia is present).

Post ligation cardiac syndrome with decreased cardiac output is thought to be related to an acute decrease in preload and increase in afterload after ductal ligation. It occurs in up to 50% of premature babies after ductal ligation. Clinical manifestations include hypotension, increased metabolic acidosis, and respiratory failure. Prophylactic intravenous infusion of milrinone may reduce the risk of this complication. This low cardiac output syndrome resolves usually after 24 h. Preliminary data suggest that the incidence of post ligation cardiac syndrome may be lower after transcatheter device closure than surgical ligation of the arterial duct in premature babies.

11.4.7 Considerations After Device Closure of Ducts

Potential complications include embolization of device, haemolysis due to high velocity jet of shunting through a restrictive residual duct, protrusion of device into the main pulmonary artery near to the origin of the left pulmonary artery to cause flow disturbance and stenosis, and protrusion of device into the descending aorta inducing the development of aortic coarctation.

11.5 Aortopulmonary Window

11.5.1 Anatomy

Aortopulmonary window is an abnormal communication, usually large in size, between the proximal aorta and the main pulmonary artery (Fig. 11.11). The presence of separate ascending aorta and main pulmonary trunk distinguishes the condition from truncus arteriosus.

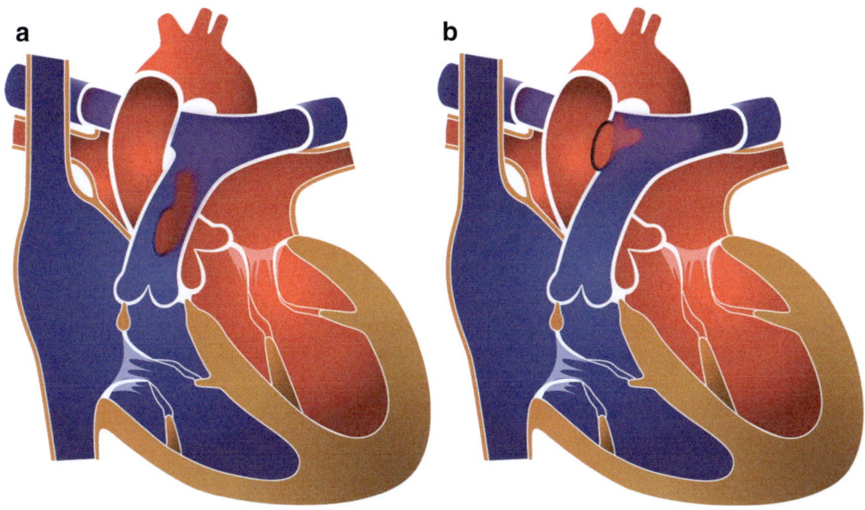

Fig. 11.11 Types of aortopulmonary window. (**a**) Type I (proximal) aortopulmonary window. (**b**) Type II (distal) aortopulmonary window

Table 11.7 Classification of aortopulmonary window

Type	Location	Description
I	Proximal	The commonest type, located just above the sinus of Valsalva with little inferior rim separating the window from the semilunar valves
II	Distal	Located in the uppermost portion of the ascending aorta, where the defect may overlie a portion of the right pulmonary artery, with little superior rim
III	Total	The rarest type, with involvement of most of the ascending aorta (combination of types I and II)
IV	Intermediate	These defects have adequate superior and inferior rims

Four types are recognized based on the classification scheme recommended by the Society of Thoracic Surgeons Congenital Heart Surgery Database Committee (Table 11.7).

Aortopulmonary window can occur in isolation, but in 50–70% of patients, it occurs in association with other cardiac malformations. Common cardiac associations are coarctation of the aorta and interrupted aortic arch (usually type A), while less common ones include ventricular septal defect, atrial septal defect, persistent arterial duct, transposition of the great arteries, and tetralogy of Fallot.

11.5.2 Pathophysiology

The pathophysiology of an aortopulmonary window is similar to that of a large arterial duct, but the magnitude of the left-to-right shunt is even larger as the aortopulmonary window is usually large and unrestrictive. As the pulmonary vascular resistance drops progressively in the first 2 months after birth, the shunting through the aortopulmonary window increases. The increase in pulmonary venous return results in volume overloading of the left heart.

High pulmonary flow through a large aortopulmonary window results in pulmonary hypertension and leads to medial hypertrophy of the pulmonary arterioles, intimal proliferation, and eventual destruction of the arterioles with irreversible pulmonary vascular disease if left unrepaired. The resultant increase in pulmonary vascular resistance may result in right-to-left shunting of blood from the pulmonary arteries to the ascending aorta through the window and systemic hypoxaemia (Eisenmenger syndrome).

11.5.3 Clinical Presentation and Findings

Most of the patients present with symptoms of heart failure at 1–2 months of age as the pulmonary vascular resistance drops. Signs of a large aortopulmonary window are shown in Table 11.8.

11.5.4 Investigations

CXR: Chest radiograph shows pulmonary plethora and cardiomegaly due to left ventricular dilation.
ECG: Electrocardiogram reveals evidence of left ventricular dilation and right ventricular hypertrophy.
Echocardiography: Echocardiography with Doppler colour flow mapping confirms the diagnosis and defines the type of aortopulmonary window (Fig. 11.12). It enables quantification of left-to-right shunt (by measuring the size of window and assessment of left atrial and left ventricular dilation) and pulmonary arterial pressure (by Doppler evaluation of the pressure gradient across the window), and diagnosis of associated cardiac malformations.

Table 11.8 Signs of a large aortopulmonary window

Signs	Origins
Signs of heart failure	Related to large left-to-right shunt
Bounding pulses	Increased pulse pressure due to diastolic runoff to pulmonary artery
Displaced cardiac apex and LV impulse	Volume overloading of left ventricle
RV impulse and loud P2	Pulmonary hypertension
Systolic murmur at the left sternal border	Flow across the window, usually systolic and not continuous due to early onset pulmonary hypertension

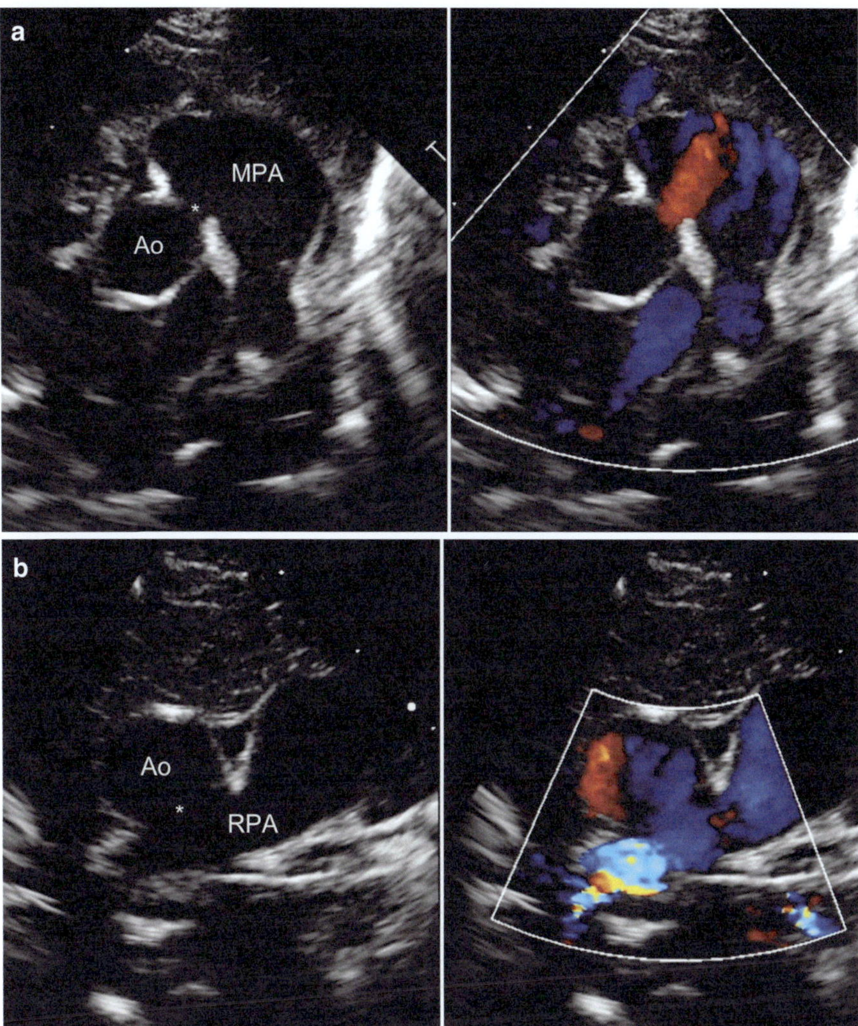

Fig. 11.12 Echocardiographic assessment of aortopulmonary window. (**a**) Proximal aortopulmonary window (asterisk). (**b**) Distal aortopulmonary window with the defect (asterisk) overlying the proximal right pulmonary artery (*Ao* aorta, *MPA* main pulmonary artery, *RPA* right pulmonary artery)

11.5.5 Management Strategy

Medical management: Optimization of nutritional intake is required. Medical therapy with diuretics and systemic vasodilators provides only partial relief of the heart failure symptoms.

Surgical and catheter intervention: Surgical closure of the aortopulmonary window, usually with the use of a patch, is indicated in all patients. Ligation of a small restrictive aortopulmonary window may suffice the purpose. Selected patients, usually those with a small aortopulmonary window with adequate superior and inferior rims, may be suitable candidates for transcatheter device closure.

11.5.6 Postoperative Considerations

The postoperative course is usually smooth for isolated aortopulmonary window, although low cardiac output syndrome and pulmonary hypertensive crisis can occur. These postoperative complications are more common in patients requiring concurrent repair of associated cardiac abnormalities. Initial intensive care management includes fluid restriction, intravenous milrinone infusion, and diuretics. Inhaled nitric oxide therapy is required in high-risk patients (patients presenting late and with evidence of high pulmonary vascular resistance preoperatively) and in patients who develop pulmonary hypertensive crisis.

11.5.7 Long-Term Monitoring

The outcome after surgery for isolated aortopulmonary window is usually excellent. Monitoring for pulmonary arterial stenosis in the long term is required.

Right Ventricular Outflow Obstructive Lesions

12

Right ventricular outflow obstruction is caused by lesions that obstruct blood flow from the right ventricle to the pulmonary arterial circulation. Most commonly, the obstruction is at the level of the pulmonary valve. Less frequently, the obstruction is caused by narrowing of the infundibulum beneath the pulmonary valve or stenosis of the peripheral pulmonary arteries.

12.1 Valvar Pulmonary Stenosis

12.1.1 Anatomy

The pulmonary valve cusps are fused and open incompletely during systole in valvar pulmonary stenosis. The opening is usual central in location (Fig. 12.1). In the most severe form of so-called critical pulmonary stenosis, the cusps are severely fused to leave only a pin-hole opening. Tethering of valve leaflets at the sinotubular junction may cause additional supravalvar stenosis. In children with Noonan syndrome (Chap. 62), the valve cusps are usually dysplastic, thickened and mucoid in appearance. Post-stenotic dilation of the pulmonary trunk occurs as a result of the turbulent blood flow in the main pulmonary artery.

12.1.2 Pathophysiology

The haemodynamic consequence of right ventricular outflow obstruction is pressure overloading of the right ventricle. Severe valvar pulmonary stenosis causes right ventricular hypertrophy. Systolic pressure of the right ventricle may exceed that of the left ventricle. The right ventricular end-diastolic pressure also increases and leads to right atrial hypertension and hypertrophy.

Y.-f. Cheung, *Congenital and Paediatric Acquired Heart Disease in Practice*, https://doi.org/10.1007/978-981-99-2862-0_12

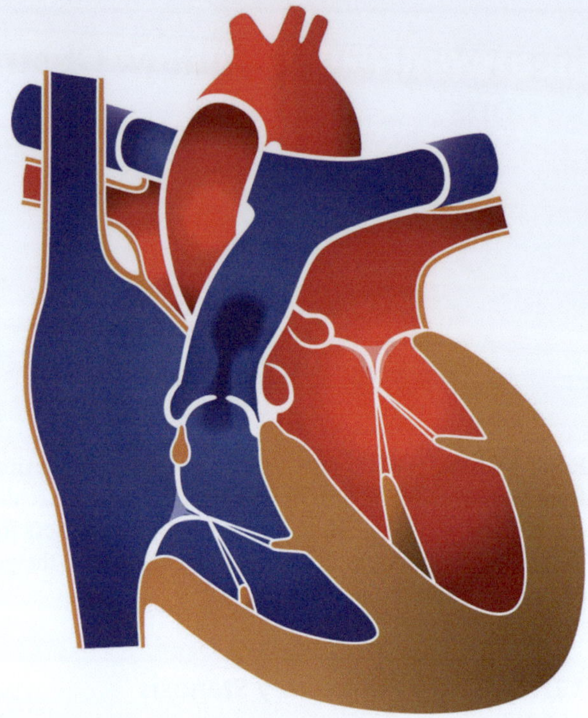

Fig. 12.1 Valvar pulmonary stenosis. Thickening and incomplete opening of the pulmonary valve with turbulent flow in the main pulmonary artery

In the absence of intracardiac defects, most infants and children are usually acyanotic even in the presence of significant right ventricular outflow obstruction as there is no right-to-left shunting of blood. However, in neonates with critical pulmonary stenosis, the elevated right atrial pressure may cause right-to-left shunting of blood through the patent oval foramen to cause cyanosis. In the latter situation, the pulmonary flow is dependent on patency of the arterial duct (duct-dependent pulmonary circulation).

12.1.3 Clinical Presentation and Findings

Infants and children with even moderate to severe valvar pulmonary stenosis are usually asymptomatic and present with cardiac murmurs. Neonates with critical pulmonary stenosis present with cyanosis as explained above. Signs of mild and moderate to severe valvar pulmonary stenosis are shown in Table 12.1.

12.1.4 Investigations

CXR: Chest radiograph shows a prominent pulmonary knob due to post-stenotic dilation of the pulmonary trunk in valvar, but not infundibular or supravalvar, pulmonary stenosis. The heart size and pulmonary vascular markings are usually

Table 12.1 Signs of mild and severe valvar pulmonary stenosis (PS)

	Mild PS	Moderate to severe PS
Cyanosis	–	Usually– (present in critical PS)
RV impulse	–	+
Suprasternal pulsation or thrill	–	+/–
Delayed and soft P2 or a single S2	–	+
Ejection click	+	+
Murmurs	An ejection systolic murmur at the left upper sternal border	An ejection systolic murmur at the left upper sternal border

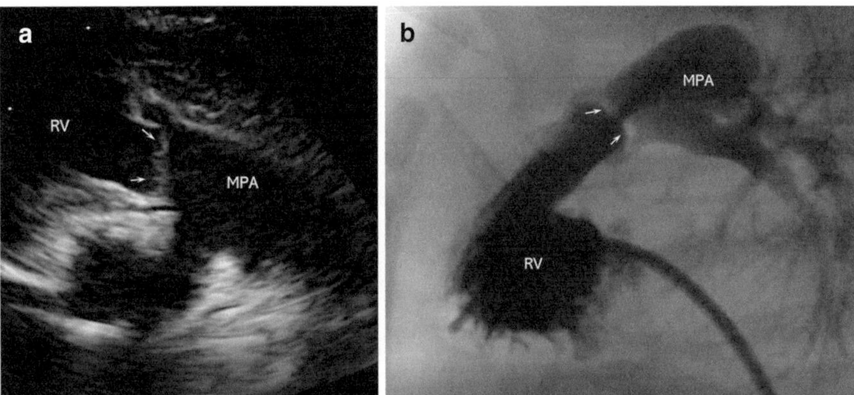

Fig. 12.2 Echocardiographic and angiographic assessment of valvar pulmonary stenosis. (**a**) Echocardiographic and (**b**) angiographic illustration of thickening and doming of the stenotic pulmonary valve (*MPA* main pulmonary artery, *RV* right ventricle)

normal. In neonates with critical pulmonary stenosis, the lung fields may appear oligaemic.

ECG: Electrocardiogram shows right axis deviation, right atrial hypertrophy, and right ventricular hypertrophy.

Echocardiography: Echocardiography confirms the type and level of right ventricular outflow obstruction (Fig. 12.2), enables the assessment of the morphology of the pulmonary valve, supravalvar tethering of the leaflets, right ventricular contractility, and right-to-left shunt of blood through the interatrial communication, and provides an estimation of the peak systolic pressure gradient across the right ventricular outflow tract and right ventricular systolic pressure by Doppler interrogation.

12.1.5 Management Strategy

In neonates with critical pulmonary stenosis, intravenous prostaglandin E infusion is used to maintain ductal patency and systemic oxygenation before intervention.

Transcatheter balloon pulmonary valvoplasty is the treatment of choice. The indications for intervention are (1) critical pulmonary stenosis in neonates, (2) a significant echocardiographically derived peak instantaneous gradient of ≥40 mmHg (based on the 2011 American Heart Association recommendation) (historically >50–60 mmHg) in infants and older children, and (3) clinically significant valvar pulmonary stenosis in the presence of right ventricular dysfunction in infants and older children. Over-sized balloons at about 120% of the diameter of the pulmonary valve annulus are used. Use of balloons larger than then 130–140% of the diameter of the pulmonary valve annulus may increase the risk of significant pulmonary regurgitation.

Surgical valvotomy is reserved for patients with dysplastic pulmonary valves (common in Noonan syndrome) not responding to balloon dilation and for those with hypoplastic pulmonary valve annulus. In the latter group of patients, transannular patch enlargement of the right ventricular outflow tract is required.

12.1.6 Considerations After Transcatheter Balloon Pulmonary Valvoplasty

In neonates with critical pulmonary stenosis, cyanosis may persist in the first few days after balloon valvoplasty due to impaired diastolic filling of the hypertrophic poorly compliant right ventricle with significant right-to-left atrial shunting. Maintenance of prostaglandin E is often required initially but can usually be weaned off in less than 2 weeks after transcatheter intervention.

12.1.7 Long-Term Monitoring

Functional outcomes of the patients are usually good after transcatheter balloon pulmonary valvoplasty or surgical valvotomy and the need for reintervention for residual stenosis is low. However, monitoring for progression of pulmonary regurgitation and right ventricular volume overload is required in the long term.

12.2 Other Levels of Right Ventricular Outflow Obstruction

Obstruction of blood flow from the right ventricle to the pulmonary circulation due to infundibular stenosis (subvalvar pulmonary stenosis) or stenosis of the peripheral pulmonary arteries is less common than that due to valvar pulmonary stenosis (Fig. 12.3).

Signs that help to localize the level of right ventricular outflow obstruction are shown in Table 12.2.

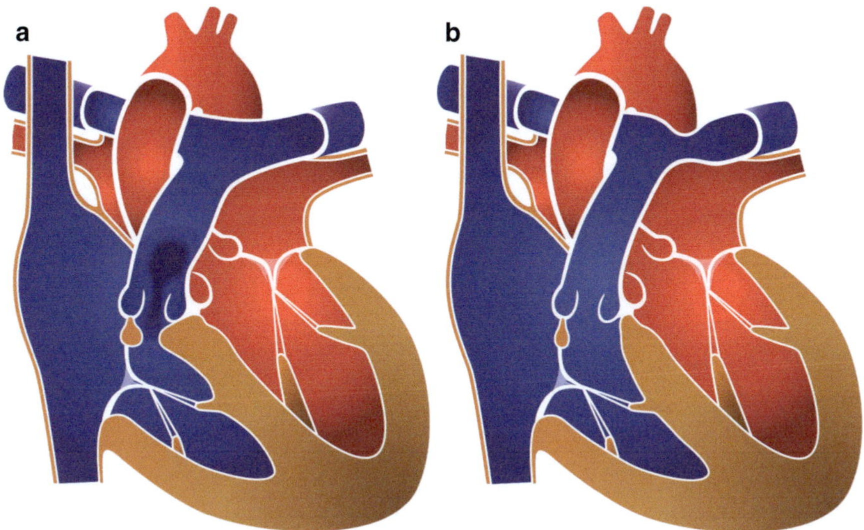

Fig. 12.3 Stenosis at other levels of the right ventricular outflow. (**a**) Subpulmonary (infundibular) pulmonary stenosis. (**b**) Branch pulmonary arterial stenosis

Table 12.2 Signs that help to localize the level of right ventricular outflow obstruction

	Subvalvar stenosis	Valvar stenosis	Pulmonary arterial stenosis
RV impulse	+	+	+
Soft P2	–	+	–
Ejection click	–	+	–
Ejection systolic murmur at left upper sternal border	Louder at left upper, but also audible at left lower sternal border	May radiate to the back and neck (much less obvious than in aortic stenosis)	Radiates to the axilla and the back, but not the neck

Isolated infundibular stenosis with an intact ventricular septum is uncommon. Subvalvar pulmonary stenosis may occur in association with (1) a perimembranous ventricular septal defect with hypertrophy of the septomarginal trabeculation causing a so-called double-chamber right ventricle (the defect may be closed by the hypertrophic myocardium), (2) a subarterial or outlet muscular septal defect with severe prolapse of the right coronary cusp (which may obliterate the shunt through the defect), and (3) severe valvar pulmonary stenosis as part of the right ventricular hypertrophic response. Infundibular resection or repair of the subarterial or outlet muscular ventricular septal defect is required for the relief of significant obstruction.

Peripheral pulmonary arterial stenosis occurs in congenital rubella syndrome, Alagille syndrome (Chap. 62), Williams syndrome (Chap. 62), and tetralogy of Fallot (Chap. 16). The branch pulmonary arteries may also be hypoplastic, which increases right ventricular afterload. Management of peripheral pulmonary arterial stenosis is discussed in the respective chapters.

13 Left Ventricular Outflow Obstructive Lesions

Left ventricular outflow obstruction comprises cardiac lesions that obstruct blood flow from the left ventricle to the systemic circulation. The obstruction may occur at three levels: (1) valvar or near the valvar level (valvar, subvalvar and supravalvar aortic stenosis), (2) arterial level (coarctation of the aorta, interrupted aortic arch, midaortic syndrome), and (3) the ventricular level (hypoplastic left heart syndrome) (Chap. 21).

13.1 Valvar Aortic Stenosis

13.1.1 Anatomy

Obstruction is at the level of the aortic valve, which is thickened and opening incompletely, is the most common cause of left ventricular outflow obstruction (Fig. 13.1). Fusion of the three cusps to form a unicuspid aortic valve with a pin-hole opening is typically found in neonates with critical aortic stenosis. In these neonates, there may be varying degrees of hypoplasia of the left ventricle and other left-sided structures (Chap. 31). In infants and older children with congenital valvar aortic stenosis, a bicuspid aortic valve is most frequently found. The valve can be truly bicuspid or functionally bicuspid due to fusion of commissure. A tricuspid aortic valve, on the other hand, is uncommonly found in congenital valvar aortic stenosis. Regardless of the morphology of the cusps, congenital valvar aortic stenosis is progressive in nature.

Bicuspid aortic valve, the most common cause of congenital valvar aortic stenosis, is also regarded as the most common congenital heart condition given its prevalence of 0.5–2% in the general population. It can occur in association with coarctation of the aorta and interrupted aortic arch. Bicuspid aortic valve is

The original version of the chapter has been revised. A correction to this chapter can be found at https://doi.org/10.1007/978-981-99-2862-0_65

Y.-f. Cheung, *Congenital and Paediatric Acquired Heart Disease in Practice*, https://doi.org/10.1007/978-981-99-2862-0_13

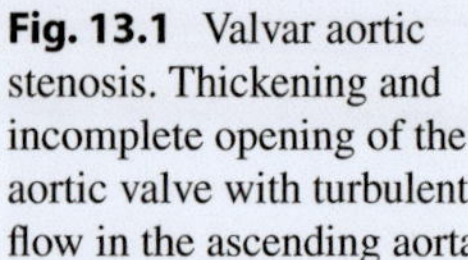

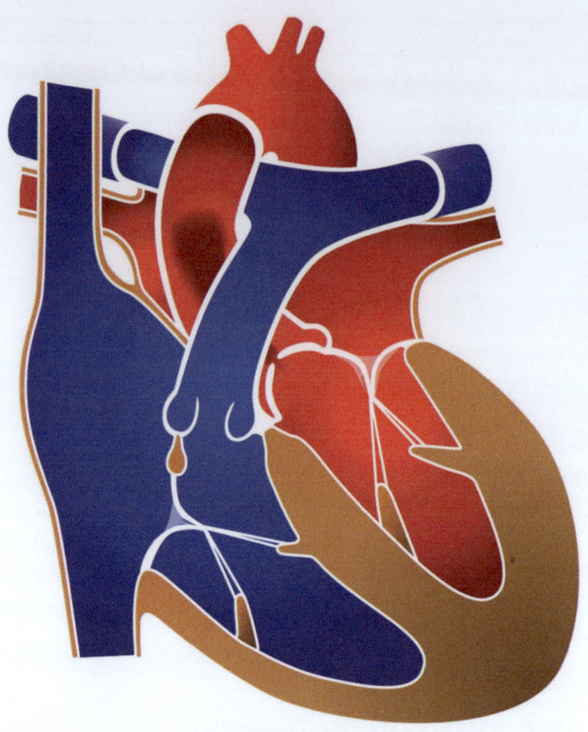

Fig. 13.1 Valvar aortic stenosis. Thickening and incomplete opening of the aortic valve with turbulent flow in the ascending aorta

associated with dilation of the aortic root and ascending aortic aneurysm disproportionate to the degree of aortic stenosis, which suggests an intrinsic developmental abnormality of the aortic wall (bicuspid aortopathy).

13.1.2 Pathophysiology

Valvar aortic stenosis causes pressure overloading and concentric hypertrophy of the left ventricle, although the systolic function of the left ventricle is usually preserved in children. Severe aortic stenosis impairs coronary perfusion (due to elevated left ventricular end-diastolic pressure) that leads to subendocardial ischaemia, increases myocardial oxygen consumption (related to increased left ventricular systolic pressure), and promotes myocardial fibrosis. Progressive dilation of the left ventricle and impairment of left ventricular contractility would eventually occur. Left ventricular systolic function may be severely impaired in some of the neonates with critical aortic stenosis at presentation.

13.1.3 Clinical Presentation and Findings

Neonates with critical aortic stenosis typically present with early-onset heart failure or cardiogenic shock within the first 2 weeks of life when the arterial duct closes. Ductal closure causes systemic hypotension and weak pulses (duct-dependent systemic circulation). A right, instead of a left, ventricular impulse is prominent as the right ventricle supports the systemic circulation via the arterial duct. The cardiac murmur is absent or soft and nonspecific.

Infants and older children with aortic stenosis are usually asymptomatic, even when the stenosis is moderate to severe in degree. Adolescents with severe aortic stenosis may present with exercise intolerance, and on exertion, chest pain, syncope or sudden death.

Signs of valvar aortic stenosis in children are shown in Table 13.1, and signs that help to localize the level of obstruction are highlighted in Table 13.2. It is worthwhile to note that the ejection systolic murmur of aortic stenosis is best audible along the axis of the left ventricular outflow (from the left mid sternal border to the right upper sternal border) with radiation to the carotid arteries.

Table 13.1 Signs of aortic stenosis (AS)

	Mild AS	Severe AS
Weak, slow-rising pulse	–	+
Left ventricular impulse	–	+
Suprasternal pulsation/thrill	–	+
Delayed A2 or a single S2	–	+
Ejection click	+	+
Murmurs	An ejection systolic murmur at left middle and right upper sternal border with radiation to the neck	An ejection systolic murmur at the left middle and right upper sternal border with radiation to the neck

Table 13.2 Signs that help to localize the level of aortic stenosis

	Valvar stenosis	Subvalvar stenosis	Supravalvar stenosis
Associated syndrome	Turner syndrome	–	Williams syndrome
Pulse	–	–	Right upper pulse limb pulse stronger than the left
Ejection click	+	–	–
Murmur of aortic insufficiency	Uncommon	Common	–

13.1.4 Investigations

CXR: Cardiomegaly and increased pulmonary vascular markings due to pulmonary venous congestion are present in neonates with critical aortic stenosis and heart failure. In older children and adolescents, the heart size and pulmonary vascular markings are usually normal. Post-stenotic dilation of the aortic root is usually caused by valvar rather than subvalvar or supravalvar aortic stenosis.

ECG: Electrocardiogram shows right ventricular hypertrophy in neonates with critical aortic stenosis. In infants and older children with moderate to severe valvar aortic stenosis, the electrocardiogram shows left axis deviation and left ventricular hypertrophy.

Echocardiography: Echocardiography defines the type and level of left ventricular outflow obstruction, enables the assessment of the morphology of the aortic valve, aortic root dilation, left ventricular contractility and hypertrophy (Fig. 13.2), and provides an assessment of severity of stenosis by estimating the peak and mean systolic pressure gradients across the stenotic aortic valve by Doppler interrogation (Table 13.3) and derivation of the aortic valve area by the continuity equation (Box 13.1).

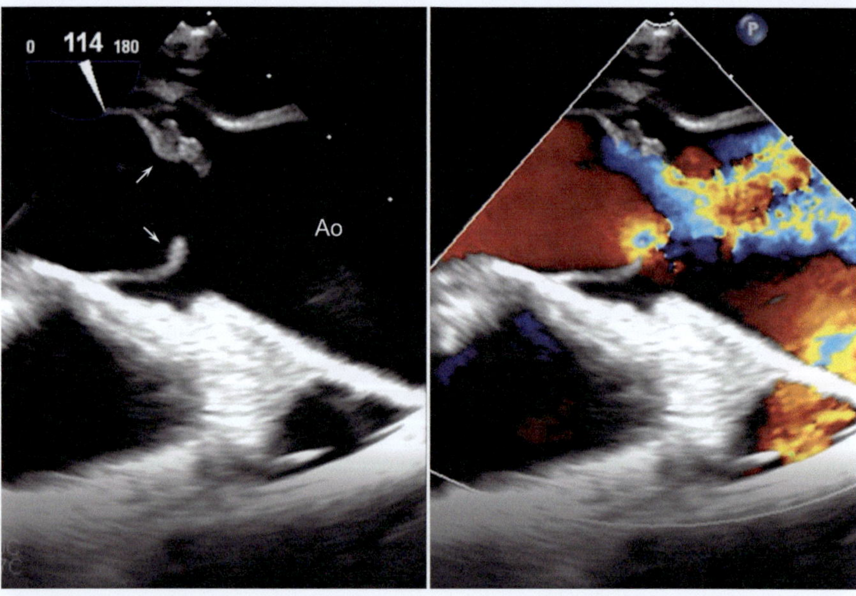

Fig. 13.2 Transesophageal assessment of valvar aortic stenosis. Thickening and doming of the stenotic aortic valve (arrows) (left) with dilation of and high-velocity flow in the ascending aorta (right) (*Ao* aorta)

Table 13.3 Severity of aortic stenosis by Doppler echocardiography

Severity	Jet velocity (m/s)	Peak instantaneous gradient (mmHg)	Mean gradient (mmHg)	Aortic valve area (cm^2)	Indexed aortic valve area (cm/m^2)
Mild	<3	<36	<20	>1.5	>0.85
Moderate	3–4	36–64	20–40	1–1.5	0.6–0.85
Severe	>4	>64	>40	<1.0	<0.6

Adapted with modifications from Baumgartner et al. Eur Heart J Cardiovasc Imaging 2017;18:254–275

Box 13.1 Derivation of Aortic Valve Area by Doppler Echocardiography Using Continuity Equation

The continuity equation is based on the concept that the stroke volume ejected through the left ventricular outflow tract (SV_{lvot}) passes entirely through the stenotic aortic valve (SV_{av})

$$\mathbf{SV_{av} = SV_{lvot}}$$

Flow volume = cross-sectional area ($\pi \times$ diameter^2/4) × Doppler-derived velocity time integral (VTI)

$$\textbf{Aortic valve area} \times \mathbf{VTI_{av}} = \textbf{LVOT area} \times \mathbf{VTI_{lvot}}$$

Hence

$$\textbf{Aortic valve area} = \left(\textbf{LVOT area} \times \mathbf{VTI_{lvot}}\right) / \mathbf{VTI_{av}}$$

The continuity equation can be simplified based on the premise that the shapes of the Doppler-derived velocity curves area are similar between the LVOT and aorta. Hence, the ratio of VTI_{av}: VTI_{lvot} may be similar to the ratio of the maximum velocity (Vmax) across aortic valve: Vmax across LVOT

Simplified continuity equation

$$\textbf{Aortic valve area} = \left(\textbf{LVOT area} \times \mathbf{Vmax_{lvot}}\right) / \mathbf{Vmax_{av}}$$

The following echocardiographic measurements are required for calculation of aortic valve area: (1) pulsed wave Doppler assessment for VTI_{lvot} or $Vmax_{lvot}$, (2) continuous wave Doppler for VTI_{av} or $Vmax_{av}$, and (3) LVOT diameter for calculation of cross-sectional area).

13.1.5 Management Strategy

Initial stabilization and interventions in neonates with critical aortic stenosis: Critically ill neonates with critical aortic stenosis requires immediate stabilization with infusion of prostaglandin E, inotropic support, intubation with ventilatory support, correction of metabolic acidosis, and urgent intervention. While transcatheter balloon aortic valvoplasty is the treatment of choice in many centres, surgical valvotomy with shaving, mobilization, and tricuspidalization of the aortic cusps has gained momentum as the initial intervention of neonates with critical aortic stenosis. Early mortality is comparable between the two interventions (10–15% after balloon aortic valvoplasty versus 5–20% after surgery).

Children and adolescents: In children and adolescents with valvar aortic stenosis, the following aspects of management should be considered: (1) exercise restriction, (2) prevention against infective endocarditis, and (3) timing and choice of initial intervention.

13.1.5.1 Exercise Restriction

Exercise restriction in patients depends on the severity of valvar aortic stenosis (Table 13.4).

13.1.5.2 Prevention Against Bacterial Endocarditis

Valvar aortic stenosis is a risk factor for infective endocarditis. Patients and their parents should be counselled on the importance of good dental and skin hygiene. While antibiotic prophylaxis prior to dental and other procedures are not recommended by the current guidelines (Chap. 49), the views may differ among practitioners.

13.1.5.3 Intervention

Indications for intervention are better defined for symptomatic patients but are less so for asymptomatic children and adolescents (Box 13.2). In asymptomatic patients, other factors including the progression of systolic pressure gradient across the stenotic aortic valve, serial results of exercise testing, and intention of patient to participate in competitive sports should be considered.

For initial intervention, transcatheter balloon aortic valvoplasty for isolated valvar aortic stenosis is the intervention of choice in many centres. A balloon size at 80–100% of the diameter of the aortic valve annulus is used. Stabilization techniques during balloon inflation include rapid right ventricular pacing, intravenous boluses of adenosine, use of extra-stiff guidewires, and use of long sheaths and long balloons. Proponents of surgical valvotomy as the primary intervention have provided data to suggest better durability of the procedure and lower prevalence of

Table 13.4 Exercise restriction (based on 2015 AHA/ACC Scientific Statement)

Severity	Recommendations
Mild	No exercise restriction if the maximal exercise response is normal
Moderate	Can participate in low and moderate static or low and moderate dynamic competitive sports if exercise tolerance testing is normal to the level of the activity
Severe	No participation in competitive sports even if asymptomatic

aortic regurgitation. Primary surgical repair of the aortic valve is usually performed in patients with associated cardiac lesions that require surgical interventions at the same time and in those with significant aortic regurgitation.

Box 13.2 Indications for Intervention of Valvar Aortic Stenosis in Children and Adolescents

Symptomatic patients

- angina, syncope, exertional dyspnoea, heart failure
- evidence of left ventricular systolic dysfunction

Asymptomatic patients (as yet no consensus agreement)

- abnormal exercise stress testing response (anginal symptom, ST and T wave changes, progressive worsening of exercise capacity)
- Doppler-derived mean gradient >60 mmHg
- catheterization-derived peak-to-peak gradient of ≥50 mmHg between the left ventricle and aorta
- patients wanting to participate in competitive sports and female patients contemplating pregnancy with catheterization-derived peak-to-peak gradient of ≥40 mmHg

13.1.6 Considerations After Transcatheter Balloon Aortic Valvoplasty

Damage to the femoral artery and thrombotic complications are rarely seen in the current era. For low birthweight babies with critical aortic stenosis, carotid artery cutdown facilitates transcatheter intervention and primary repair of the artery after intervention reduces the risk of arterial complications.

13.1.7 Postoperative Considerations

In neonates undergoing surgical aortic valvotomy, left ventricular diastolic dysfunction may be present and requires judicious fluid administration, low dose intravenous milrinone support, esmolol infusion to slow down the heart rate for better ventricular filling (proposed by some groups but data are limited in this regard), and the use of higher positive end expiratory ventilatory pressure. In older children and adolescents, the hypertrophic left ventricle may appear 'hypercontractile' and requires judicious fluid administration and use of inotropes, control of systemic blood pressure, and reduction of afterload.

13.1.8 Long-Term Monitoring

Congenital valvar aortic stenosis runs a progressive course in all patients both before and after transcatheter or surgical interventions. Reinterventions for restenosis and/or progressive aortic regurgitation are commonly required. Meta-analysis of reported studies suggests that freedom from reintervention is worse after balloon valvoplasty than surgical valvotomy (46% versus 73% at 10-year follow up). In patients with a bicuspid aortic valve, follow up for progressive dilation of the aortic root and development of ascending aortic aneurysm and dissection is required.

Replacement of the dysfunctional aortic valve may eventually be required at an older age. Options include (1) prosthetic mechanical valve replacement, (2) Ross procedure (or Ross-Konno procedure if the aortic annulus is hypoplastic), and (3) the recently described Ozaki procedure (Box. 13.3).

Box 13.3 Replacement of Dysfunctional Aortic Valve

Valve replacement

- bioprosthetic valve not an option in children due to early degeneration
- mechanical prosthesis has no growth potential and requires anticoagulation

Ross or Ross-Konno procedure

- Ross procedure (pulmonary autograft): replacement of the aortic valve with the patient's own pulmonary valve, the pulmonary valve being replaced by a pulmonary homograft or other valved conduit
- Ross-Konno procedure: combination of the Ross procedure with incision of the ventricular septum at the outflow and resecting obstructive fibrous or muscular tissue (Konno procedure)
- long-term issues include neoaortic root dilation and regurgitation and the need to replace pulmonary homograft or valved conduit

Ozaki procedure

- complete removal of aortic valve leaflets with recreation of new leaflets using autologous or bovine pericardium
- limited experience in paediatric patients

13.2 Subvalvar Aortic Stenosis

Subvalvar aortic stenosis comprises lesions that cause fixed or dynamic obstruction of the left ventricular outflow beneath the level of the aortic valve.

13.2.1 Anatomy

Fixed subvalvar stenosis is most commonly caused by a discrete fibrous membrane or a fibro-muscular ridge. Rarely, diffuse tunnel-like obstruction of the outflow is cause by the hypertrophic myocardium together with a hypoplastic aortic annulus. Associated cardiac malformations include ventricular septal defect, atrioventricular septal defect, coarctation or interruption of the aorta, and Shone complex. Other causes of fixed left ventricular outflow obstruction include accessory mitral valvar tissue, abnormal insertion of mitral papillary muscle, and cardiac tumours.

Dynamic left ventricular outflow obstruction is usually caused by hypertrophic obstructive cardiomyopathy and associated systolic anterior motion of the mitral valve (Chap. 44).

13.2.2 Pathophysiology

Subvalvar aortic stenosis, when severe, causes pressure overloading and hypertrophy of the left ventricle. Subaortic stenosis progresses over time and may be rapid during childhood in some of the patients. It has been proposed that turbulent flow and shear stress promote the progressive fibrotic narrowing of the left ventricular outflow.

Damage to the aortic valve leaflets and interference of the motion of the leaflets by the high velocity turbulent jet of blood flow predispose to development of progressive aortic regurgitation.

13.2.3 Clinical Presentation and Findings

Infants and children with subvalvar aortic stenosis are usually asymptomatic, even when the stenosis is moderate to severe in degree, and present usually with incidental finding of a cardiac murmur. The signs are those of left ventricular outflow obstruction (Table 13.2).

The absence of an ejection systolic click distinguishes the condition from valvar aortic stenosis. The presence of a double apical impulse suggests hypertrophic obstructive cardiomyopathy. Performance of Valsalva manoeuvre decreases murmur intensity in fixed subvalvar aortic stenosis and increases murmur intensity in hypertrophic obstructive cardiomyopathy. The presence of an early diastolic murmur at the left lower sternal border suggests development of aortic regurgitation.

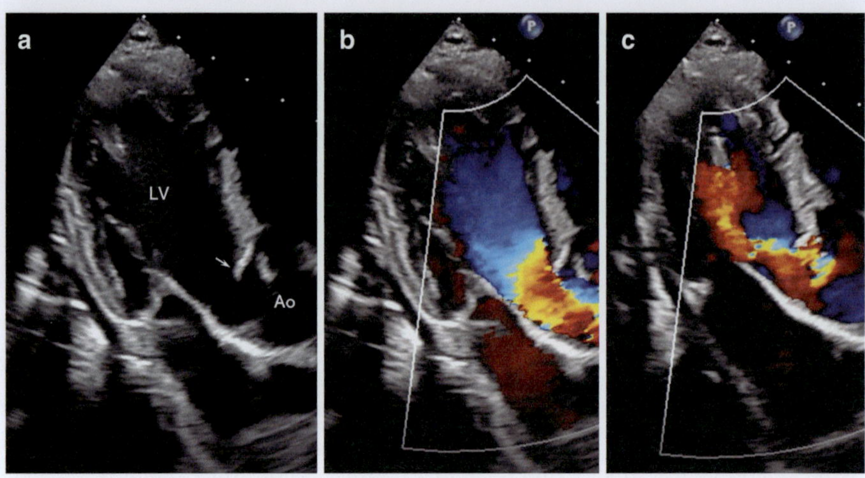

Fig. 13.3 Echocardiographic assessment of subaortic stenosis. (**a**) 2D echocardiographic demonstration of a subaortic membrane (arrow) (**b**) Colour flow mapping showing the origin of flow turbulence originates from the subaortic region (**c**) Mild degree of aortic regurgitation is evident (*Ao* aorta, *LV* left ventricle)

13.2.4 Investigations

CXR: The chest radiograph is usually normal.
ECG: Electrocardiogram may be normal or show left axis deviation and left ventricular hypertrophy.
Echocardiography: Echocardiography defines the type and cause of subvalvar aortic stenosis and enables the assessment of morphology, motion, and competence of the aortic valve, evaluation of left ventricular contractility and hypertrophy, and quantification of severity of subvalvar aortic stenosis by estimating the peak and mean pressure gradients across the stenosis by Doppler interrogation (Fig. 13.3). Three-dimensional echocardiography provides additional information to facilitate surgical planning.
Cardiac catheterization: This is usually not required and reserved for the few patients who require exact documentation of the peak gradient across the left ventricular outflow tract before surgery is contemplated.

13.2.5 Management Strategy

Monitoring: Regular annual or biannual (if there is concern of rapid progression) echocardiography for monitoring of the progression of subvalvar aortic stenosis and development of aortic regurgitation is necessary.
Indications for intervention: Indications for intervention are better defined for symptomatic patients (Box 13.4). There is, however, no consensus agreement on the indications for asymptomatic patients.

Factors that may influence the decision to perform surgery to relieve the outflow obstruction include (1) the progressive nature of subaortic valvar stenosis, (2) relatively high rate of recurrence after surgery and the need for reintervention (about 10–20% reintervention rate after resection of a discrete fibrous membrane), (3) risk of development of aortic regurgitation, which may persist even after surgery, and (4) the intention of patients to participate in competitive sports and the planning of pregnancy.

Box 13.4 Indications for Intervention of Isolated Subvalvar Aortic Stenosis

Symptomatic patients

- angina, syncope, exertional dyspnoea
- evidence of left ventricular systolic dysfunction

Asymptomatic patients (as yet no consensus agreement)

- Doppler-derived peak instantaneous gradient ≥50–60 mmHg
- Doppler-derived mean gradient ≥30–40 mmHg
- progressive worsening of aortic regurgitation
- presence of left ventricular hypertrophy (left ventricular mass index z score > 2)
- indications and optimal timing of surgery in patients with no aortic regurgitation or left ventricular hypertrophy are controversial

Surgery: Surgical correction can vary from simple resection of the subaortic membrane to circumferential excision of the fibromuscular ridge with or without septal myomectomy. For diffuse tunnel-like obstruction of the outflow, modified Konno procedure (removal of the obstructive tissue, resection of subaortic interventricular septum with creation of a ventricular septal defect, and closure of the defect with a patch) is performed. If the aortic annulus is also hypoplastic in addition to the diffuse subaortic obstruction, the Ross-Konno operation is required.

13.2.6 Postoperative Considerations

The postoperative course in usually smooth. Potential complications related to extensive septal myomectomy include complete heart block and inadvertent creation of a ventricular septal defect. In patients with hypertrophic left ventricles, the postoperative hypercontractile state and diastolic dysfunction require judicious fluid administration just adequate to maintain normal haemodynamics, judicious use of inotropes, esmolol infusion to slow down the heart rate for better ventricular filling (proposed by some groups but data are limited in this regard), control of blood pressure, and reduction of afterload.

13.2.7 Long-Term Monitoring

Recurrence of subaortic narrowing is relatively common after surgery for subvalvar aortic stenosis and reintervention is required in 10–20% of patients. Risk factors include early age at diagnosis and initial surgery, a short distance between the subaortic membrane and aortic valve, extension of the membrane to involve the aortic valve, and a high peak Doppler-derived Doppler gradient of ≥60 mmHg. Aortic regurgitation may progress despite relief of the subaortic stenosis and needs regular monitoring.

13.3 Supravalvar Aortic Stenosis

Congenital supravalvar aortic stenosis is the least common form of left ventricular outflow tract obstruction. It is regarded as a form of arteriopathy with disruption of elastin due to haploinsufficiency of the elastin gene *ELN*. Haploinsufficiency of *ELN* occurs in (1) William syndrome (William-Beuren syndrome) (Chap. 62), a de novo contiguous gene deletion syndrome with heterozygous microdeletion on chromosome 7q11.23 that includes *ELN*, (2) an autosomal dominant familial form of supravalvar aortic stenosis with point mutation in *ELN*, and (3) a non-familial sporadic form.

13.3.1 Anatomy

Two forms of supravalvar aortic stenosis in terms of morphology are recognized: (1) an hourglass-narrowing of the ascending aorta with proximity to the sinotubular junction, which occurs in most of the patients, and (2) more diffuse narrowing of the ascending aorta with possible extension to the aortic arch (Fig. 13.4). Histologically, the arterial media is thickened with disorganization of elastin fibres, increased collagen deposition, and hypertrophy of vascular smooth muscle cells.

Associated cardiovascular abnormalities include (1) coronary arterial stenosis due to ostial narrowing, adhesion of the thickened aortic valvar leaflets to the sinotubular junction, or diffuse coronary arterial stenosis, (2) supravalvar pulmonary stenosis and branch pulmonary arterial stenosis that usually improves with time, (3) coarctation of the aorta and midaortic syndrome (4) stenoses of the origins of carotid, renal, iliac, and other peripheral arteries, and (v) mitral valve prolapse.

13.3.2 Pathophysiology

The pathophysiology of supravalvar aortic stenosis is similar to that of valvar and subvalvar aortic stenosis, which is characterized by pressure overloading and hypertrophy of the left ventricle.

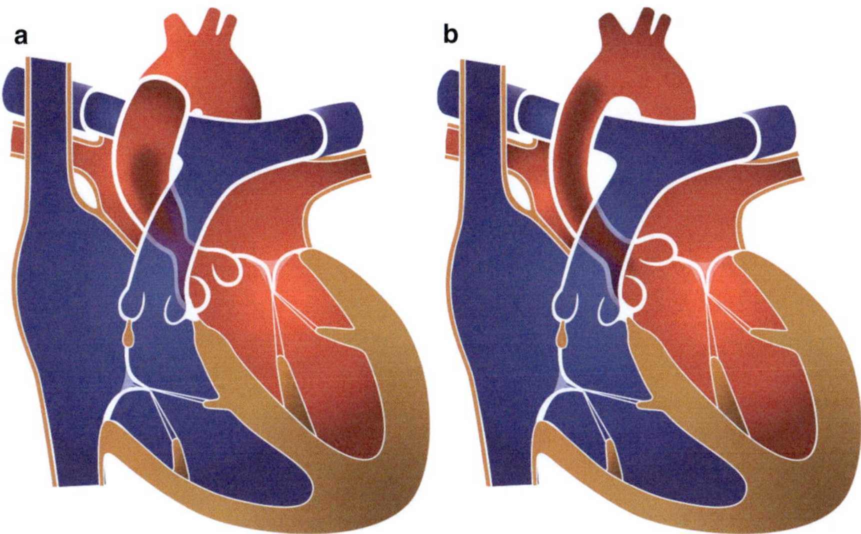

Fig. 13.4 Supravalvar aortic stenosis. (**a**) Hourglass-narrowing of ascending aorta (**b**) Diffuse narrowing of the ascending aorta

Systemic hypertension, commonly found in patients with William syndrome, further increases the left ventricular afterload. Hypertension may be related to renal arterial stenosis and/or mid aortic syndrome. Even in the absence of these associated conditions, disruption of elastin per se increases arterial stiffness to cause hypertension. In supravalvar aortic stenosis, the blood pressure is higher, and the pulse is stronger in the right than the left upper limb. This is explainable by the Coanda effect (the tendency of a jet of fluid emerging from an orifice to follow an adjacent surface). Hence, the high velocity jet of blood stream emerging from the supravalvar region has the tendency to flow along the right side of the aortic wall with transfer of kinetic energy of flow to the right innominate artery, from which the right subclavian arises.

Coronary arterial flow may be compromised as a result of coronary ostial stenosis, adhesion of the thickened aortic valvar leaflets to the sinotubular junction, diffuse coronary arterial stenosis, and premature atherosclerosis due to exposure of the coronary arteries to high perfusion pressure proximal to the site of supravalvar narrowing. Increased risk of sudden death in supravalvar aortic stenosis may be related to impairment of coronary perfusion.

13.3.3 Clinical Presentation and Findings

Infants and children with non-syndromic subvalvar aortic stenosis are usually asymptomatic and present with a cardiac murmur. Patients with William syndrome may be diagnosed based on the dysmorphic facies (Chap. 62). The signs are those of left ventricular outflow obstruction (Table 13.2). The absence of an ejection systolic click distinguishes the condition from valvar aortic stenosis. Differential upper limb pulse volume, stronger on the right than the left arm (Coanda effect) and unequal carotid arterial pulsation (due to differential stenosis of the origins of the right and left carotid arteries) suggest supravalvar origin of aortic stenosis.

13.3.4 Investigations

CXR: The chest radiograph is usually normal.
ECG: Electrocardiogram may be normal or show left axis deviation and left ventricular hypertrophy. The presence of ST and T wave changes suggests associated coronary arterial ischaemia.
Echocardiography: Echocardiography defines the morphology (hourglass narrowing versus diffuse narrowing of ascending aorta) of the supravalvar stenosis, enables the assessment of thickening and motion of the aortic valve leaflets, coronary arterial flow and evidence of ostial stenosis, and provides an estimation of the severity of supravalvar aortic stenosis (the peak and mean pressure gradients) by Doppler interrogation. Further imaging should aim to assess for associated diffuse hypoplasia of the ascending aorta, aortic arch, and abdominal aorta (mid aortic syndrome), and supravalvar and branch pulmonary arterial stenosis.
CT and CMR: These provide information on arteriopathy involving different parts of the arterial tree (including the abdominal aorta and renal arteries) (Fig. 13.5) and ostial stenosis of the coronary arteries.
Genetic evaluation: Genetic testing for 7q11.23 microdeletion and mutation of *ELN* is required (Chap. 62).

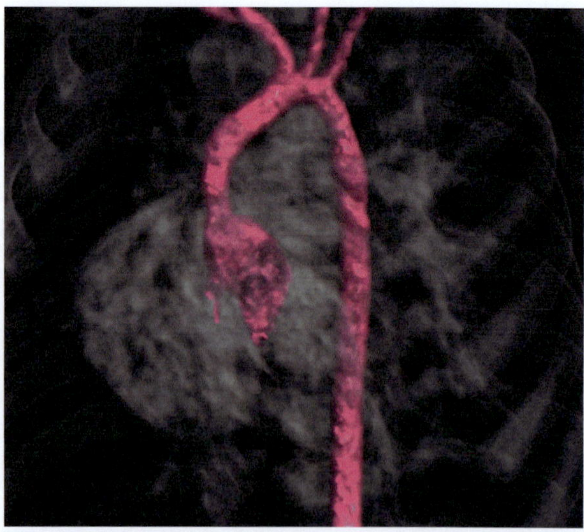

Fig. 13.5 Supravalvar aortic stenosis. Computed tomography showing diffuse narrowing of the ascending aorta and aortic arch in a child with William syndrome

13.3.5 Management Strategy

Monitoring: Regular annual or biannual (if there is concern of rapid progression) echocardiography for monitoring of progression of supravalvar aortic stenosis and evidence of coronary ischaemia is necessary.
Indications for intervention: Indications for intervention are better defined for symptomatic patients (Box 13.5). Similar to valvar and subvalvar aortic stenosis, consensus agreement on the indications for asymptomatic patients with supravalvar aortic stenosis is lacking.

Box 13.5 Indications for Intervention of Supravalvar Aortic Stenosis

Symptomatic patients
- angina, syncope, exertional dyspnoea
- evidence of resting or inducible myocardial ischaemia
- evidence of left ventricular systolic dysfunction

Asymptomatic patients (as yet no consensus agreement)
- Doppler-derived peak instantaneous gradient >60 mmHg
- Doppler-derived mean gradient >40 mmHg
- Catheterization-derived peak-to-peak gradient >40–50 mmHg

Surgical intervention: Patients with significant supravalvar aortic stenosis are at high risk of myocardial ischaemia and cardiovascular collapse during induction of general anaesthesia. Coronary perfusion must be maintained by ensuring an adequate preload and taking precautions to avoid hypotension, lowering of systemic vascular resistance, and tachycardia.

For discrete hourglass narrowing of the ascending aorta, different techniques including single patch enlargement, inverted bifurcated patch technique, and three-patch aortoplasty have been described. More extensive patch aortoplasty or resection of the stenotic segment with insertion of an autograft may be required for repairing the diffuse form of supravalvar aortic stenosis. Experience on transcatheter intervention (balloon dilation and stent implantation) is limited and surgical repair remains the treatment of choice. Branch pulmonary arterial stenosis can be managed, if indicated, by balloon angioplasty or surgery.

13.3.6 Postoperative Considerations

Important aspects of postoperative monitoring include coronary insufficiency and systolic and diastolic dysfunction of the hypertrophic left ventricle. Judicious fluid administration just adequate to maintain normal haemodynamics and cautious use of inotropes and diuretics are necessary. Systemic vasoconstrictors may be required to maintain diastolic coronary perfusion.

13.3.7 Long-Term Monitoring

Long-term monitoring for recurrent supravalvar aortic stenosis after surgery, progressive stenosis of other arteries, systemic hypertension, and aortic valvar disease is required. Reintervention is required in about 10–20% of patients. Risk factors include diffuse form of supravalvar aortic stenosis and associated aortic valvar disease.

13.4 Coarctation of the Aorta

13.4.1 Anatomy

Coarctation of the aorta is usually a discrete narrowing of the aorta opposite to the site of insertion of the arterial duct. The shelf that protrudes into the lumen of the aorta represents ductal tissue that encircles the isthmus (the segment between the arterial duct and origin of the left subclavian artery) (Fig. 13.6). Less commonly, the segment of narrowing may be long and tortuous. There may be varying degrees of hypoplasia of the aortic arch. Associated cardiac lesions include ventricular septal

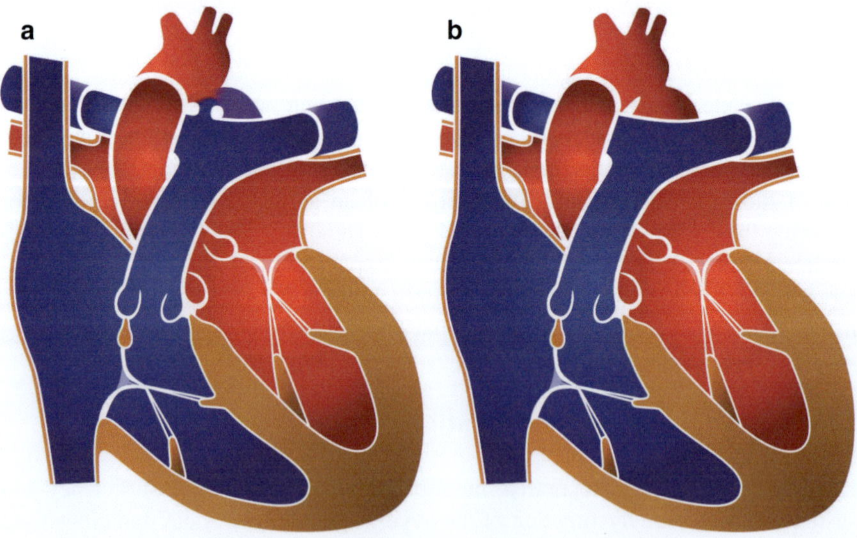

Fig. 13.6 Coarctation of the aorta. (**a**) Severe coarctation of the aorta in the newborn with duct-dependent systemic circulation (**b**) Non-duct-dependent coarctation of the aorta

defect, bicuspid aortic valve, aortopulmonary window, Taussig-Bing anomaly (double-outlet right ventricle with subpulmonary ventricular septal defect), and aberrant origin of the right subclavian artery from the descending aorta distal to the site of coarctation. Coarctation of the aorta may also occur in the setting of a right-sided aortic arch.

13.4.2 Pathophysiology

In neonates with severe coarctation, adequate perfusion of the descending aorta and its branches depends on patency of the arterial duct (duct-dependent systemic circulation). In the early neonatal period, the right ventricle is the dominant ventricle that supplies blood to the descending aorta by way of the persistent arterial duct. The consequences of closure of the arterial duct are an acute increase in pressure load causing left ventricular failure and jeopardized descending aortic perfusion resulting in bowel ischaemia, renal failure, and metabolic acidosis. Metabolic acidosis worsens left ventricular contraction further. Early-onset heart failure therefore occurs in neonates with severe coarctation.

In infants, children, and adolescents with non-duct-dependent coarctation of the aorta, the left ventricle supplies blood to the descending aorta. Pressure overload results in compensatory left ventricular hypertrophy. In older children and adolescents, a collateral circulation by way of the branches of the right and left subclavian arteries and the internal thoracic (mammary) artery, with enlargement of the intercostal arteries (which cause rib notching), may develop to augment blood flow to the descending aorta. Permanent alteration of arterial structure and mechanics proximal to the site of coarctation results in arterial stiffening and persistence of systolic hypertension despite repair of the coarctation.

13.4.3 Clinical Presentation and Findings

Neonates with severe coarctation of the aorta present with early-onset heart failure and even in a collapsed state within the first 2 weeks of life. Ductal closure causes weak or absent lower limb pulses and oliguria due to poor renal perfusion. In the presence of aberrant origin of the right subclavian artery from the descending aorta, the right upper limb is also weak. The cardiac murmur is either absent or soft and nonspecific.

Neonates with mild coarctation of the aorta and mild hypoplasia of the aortic arch or isthmus are asymptomatic with no abnormal physical signs. Presentations include suspicious fetal echocardiographic findings of a small aortic arch or mild arch narrowing and postnatal detection of a cardiac murmur that prompts echocardiographic assessment. There are situations in which prediction of progression of these conditions to severe coarctation of the aorta may be difficult (discussed later in the section).

Table 13.5 Signs of coarctation of the aorta

	Neonates (duct-dependent)	Older children and adolescents
Weak lower limb pulses	+	+
Abnormal cardiac impulse	Right ventricular impulse	Left ventricular impulse
Murmurs	Inaudible or a soft ejection systolic murmur at the left upper sternal border	An ejection systolic murmur at the left upper sternal border, radiating to the left interscapular area at the back
		In older children with a well-developed collateral circulation, soft continuous murmurs may be audible throughout the chest

Infants and older children with coarctation of the aorta are usually asymptomatic, even when the narrowing is moderate to severe. A common presentation is incidental finding of a cardiac murmur or systemic hypertension of the upper limb proximal to the site of coarctation. Clinical findings of significant coarctation of the aorta are shown in Table 13.5.

13.4.4 Investigations

CXR: Cardiomegaly and increased pulmonary vascular markings due to pulmonary venous congestion are present in neonates with severe coarctation of the aorta. In older children and adolescents, the heart size and pulmonary vascular markings are usually normal. In the latter group of patients, rib notching due to erosion of the inferior surfaces of the ribs by the well-developed collateral circulation may be seen. Additionally, the cardinal 'figure 3 sign', caused by indentation at the site of coarctation with pre- and post-stenotic aortic dilation, may be found.

ECG: Electrocardiogram shows right ventricular hypertrophy in neonates with severe aortic stenosis as the right ventricle is the dominant ventricle supporting the descending aortic flow by way of the arterial duct. In infants and older children with significant aortic coarctation, the electrocardiogram shows left axis deviation and left ventricular hypertrophy.

Echocardiography: Echocardiography defines the site and severity of coarctation (Fig. 13.7a, b), and enables the assessment of the arch dimension, patency and size of the arterial duct (right-to-left shunting from the pulmonary artery to the descending aorta during systole), associated cardiac lesions, and left ventricular contractility, and provides an estimation of peak systolic pressure gradient across the site of coarctation by Doppler interrogation. The diastolic tail of the Doppler flow pattern is characteristic (Fig. 13.7d). In the presence of a large arterial duct supplying blood flow to the descending aorta in neonates with severe coarctation, the pressure gradient can be grossly underestimated.

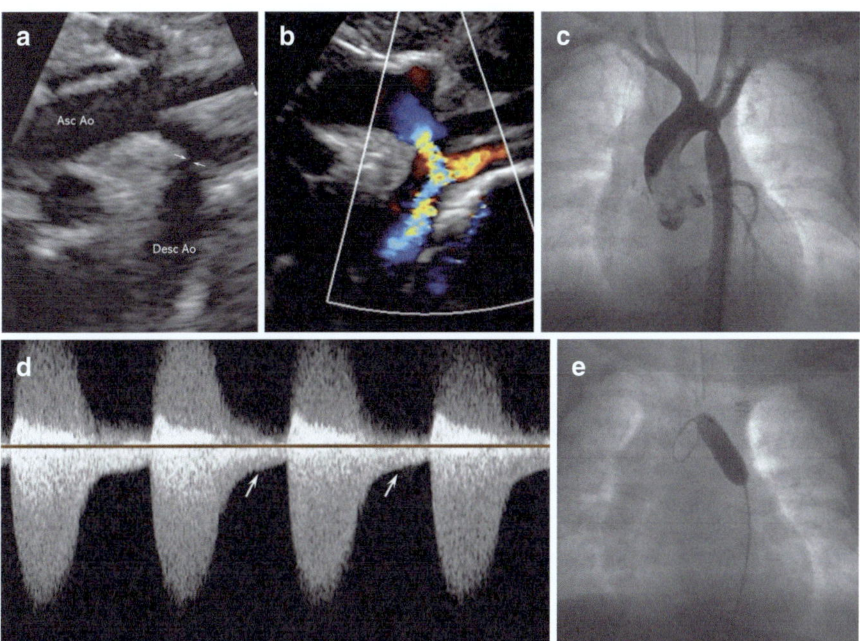

Fig. 13.7 Imaging and transcatheter intervention of coarctation of the aorta. (**a**) Suprasternal view demonstrating severe coarctation of the aorta (arrows) (**b**) Doppler colour flow mapping and (**c**) angiographic demonstration of aortic recoarctation after previous surgical repair (**d**) Characteristic diastolic tail (arrows) in the continuous wave Doppler pattern (**e**) Balloon angioplasty for recoarctation of the aorta (*Asc Ao* ascending aorta, *Desc Ao* descending aorta)

CT: Computed tomography angiography may be useful when the arch anatomy and aortic sidedness is unclear on echocardiographic assessment of critically ill neonates at presentation. In older children and adolescents, it assists in the planning and evaluation of the outcomes of stenting of aortic coarctation.

CMR: In older children and adolescents, cardiac magnetic resonance provides information on the morphology of the aortic arch and coarctation, flow gradient across the coarctation or recoarctation site, collateral flow, and left ventricular systolic function. In patients after stent implantation, artifact may be present, however.

13.4.5 Management Strategy

Initial stabilization: Critically ill neonates with severe coarctation of the aorta requires immediate stabilization with infusion of prostaglandin E, inotropic support, intubation with ventilatory support, and correction of metabolic acidosis.

Neonatal surgical intervention: Early surgical repair is commonly performed by resection of the stenotic segment with extended end-to-end anastomosis (sliding of

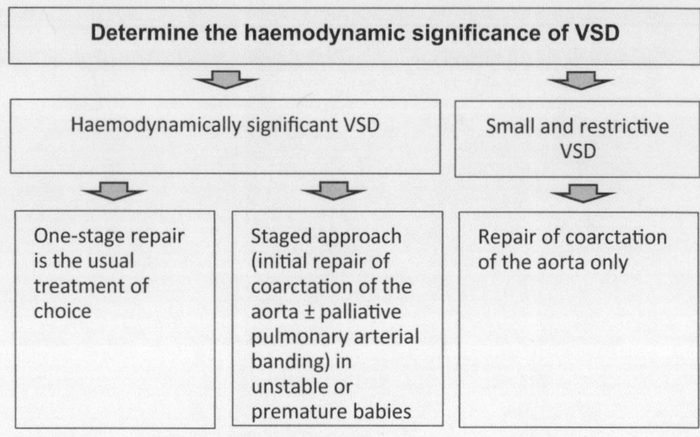

Fig. 13.8 Management of ventricular septal defect with coarctation of the aorta. *VSD* ventricular septal defect

the incised distal aorta to the extended incision made of the underside of the aortic arch). Less commonly, the subclavian artery is ligated and mobilized for repair of coarctation (subclavian flap aortoplasty).

For neonates with severe coarctation of the aorta and an associated ventricular septal defect, approaches vary dependent of the size of the defect and clinical condition of the patient (Fig. 13.8).

Neonatal catheter intervention: Transcatheter balloon angioplasty in neonates and infants is associated with increased risk of complications (femoral artery injury, aortic aneurysm) and a high rate of recoarctation (about 80% for neonatal intervention). Hence, surgical repair of native coarctation of the aorta is usually the treatment of choice.

Neonatal watchful waiting approach: For neonates with suspected mild coarctation of the aorta and/or hypoplasia of the aortic arch or isthmus, there are situations in which prediction of progression to severe coarctation of the aorta may be difficult. A 'watchful waiting' management approach can be adopted in these situations (Fig. 13.9).

Intervention beyond the neonatal period: Beyond the neonatal period, transcatheter balloon angioplasty is indicated in older infants and children with a resting systolic pressure gradient across the narrowed segment >20 mmHg and in those with a gradient <20 mmHg (due to extensive collaterals or left ventricular dysfunction) but with severe coarctation demonstrable by imaging. Balloon angioplasty is the intervention of choice for recurrent coarctation after previous surgical repair (Fig 13.7e).

In adolescents and young adults, stent implantation has increasingly been adopted as the primary approach for native and recurrent coarctation of the aorta (Fig. 13.10). Bare metal stents and covered stents, the latter being used in selected patients at risk of aortic wall injury, have been used with good immediate relief of the pressure gradient across the site of (re)coarctation.

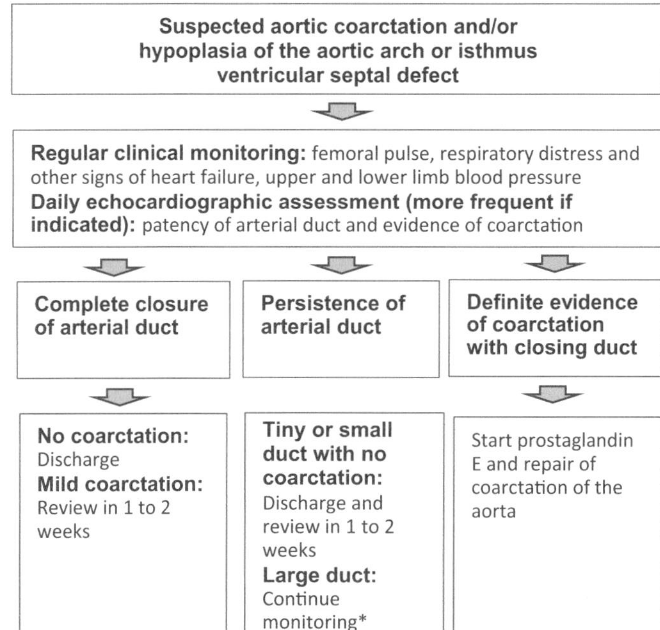

Fig. 13.9 'Watchful waiting' approach to managing neonates with suspected coarctation of the aorta and/or hypoplasia of the aorta arch or isthmus. *If ligation of the large arterial duct is required for the management of heart failure, intraoperative assessment for aortic coarctation is required after ductal ligation. Repair of the significant aortic coarctation unmasked after ligation of the arterial duct should be performed in the same setting

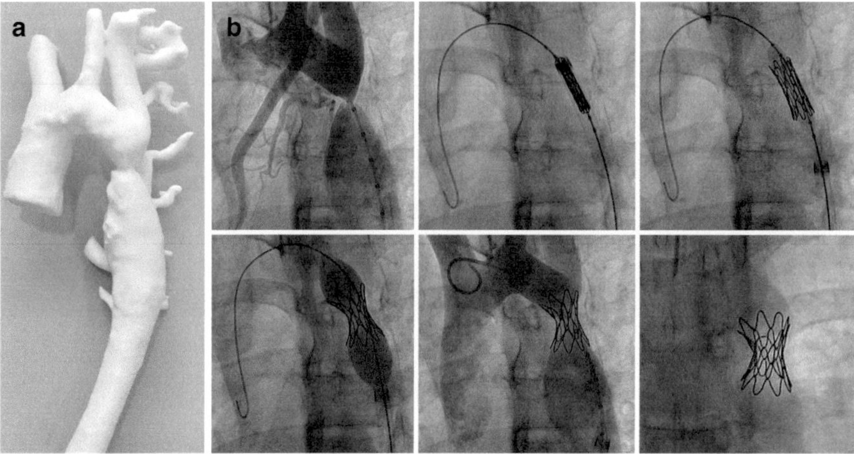

Fig. 13.10 Stenting of coarctation of the aorta. (**a**) 3D printing based on CT findings for planning of aortic stenting (**b**) Stenting of native aortic coarctation in an adolescent

13.4.6 Postoperative Considerations

Potential complications after surgical repair of coarctation of the aorta include low cardiac output syndrome (especially in those with poor left ventricular function preoperatively), paradoxical hypertension, postcoarctectomy syndrome, spinal cord ischaemia, injury to the phrenic nerve and recurrent laryngeal nerve, Horner syndrome, and chylothorax.

Paradoxical hypertension occurs immediately after surgery as a result of reduced stretching of the baroreceptors in the aortic arch and carotid arteries. This may increase the risk of bleeding from the suture lines and postcoarctectomy syndrome. Management includes adequate analgesia and sedation and the use of alpha- and beta-receptor blockers and systemic vasodilators.

Postcoarctectomy syndrome, uncommon in neonates, occurs usually at 2–3 days after surgery. It is probably related to exposure of the distal arterial bed to postoperative increase in perfusion pressure, which results in arterial spasm and ischaemia. Clinical manifestations include abdominal pain, abdominal distension with ileus, and bowel ischaemia. Management includes fasting, nasogastric decompression, and the use of beta-receptor blockers and angiotensin-converting enzyme inhibitor (as renin level is increased after surgery).

Neurological complications include spinal cord ischaemia and injury to the phrenic nerve and recurrent laryngeal nerve. Complete recovery of phrenic nerve and recurrent laryngeal nerve palsy occurs in almost all of the patients. The risk of spinal cord ischaemia is higher in older patients with poor collateral development. Minimizing the time of aortic clamping and the use of partial bypass may reduce the risk.

13.4.7 Considerations After Transcatheter Interventions

Important complications to be monitored after transcatheter interventions for coarctation of the aorta are those related to femoral arterial cannulation (bleeding, thrombosis, and impairment of lower limb perfusion) and systemic hypertension. When distal perfusion of the lower limb is impaired, intravenous heparin infusion, Doppler evaluation of arterial flow to the lower limbs, and consultation with vascular surgeons are required.

13.4.8 Long-Term Monitoring

Patients after intervention of coarctation of the aorta require monitoring of complications including systemic hypertension, recoarctation of the aorta, and aortic aneurysm formation. In patients with a bicuspid aortic valve, progressive aortic stenosis may occur on follow up and require further intervention. These complications chronically increase left ventricular afterload and impair left ventricular diastolic function.

Systemic hypertension is reported to occur in up to about 50% of patients despite satisfactory repair of aortic coarctation. Persistence of systemic hypertension has been hypothesized to be related to permanent structural and functional alteration of the arterial bed proximal to the site of coarctation and an unfavourable shape and flow dynamics of the aortic arch. This may contribute to the higher risk of premature coronary artery disease found in patients after repair of coarctation the aorta.

Aortic aneurysm at the coarctation site may occur after patch repair, balloon angioplasty, and stent implantation. Intracranial aneurysms have been reported in occur with a higher incidence in adults with coarctation of the aorta compared with the general population, although similar data have not been reported in paediatric patients. The need for routine imaging to assess intracranial aneurysms in children and adults with coarctation of the aorta remains controversial.

13.5 Interrupted Aortic Arch

13.5.1 Anatomy

The aortic arch may be interrupted at one of the three locations: (1) distal to the left subclavian artery (type A), (2) between the left common carotid and left subclavian arteries (type B), and (3) between the innominate and the left common carotid arteries (type C) (Fig. 13.11). Type B interruption is the commonest type (75%) of interruption and is associated with DiGeorge syndrome, while type A interruption accounts for most of remaining 25% of interruption and type C is extremely rare. Interrupted aortic arch may also occur in the setting of a right-sided aortic arch. Ventricular septal defect is a frequent association, and, in this setting, posterior deviation of the muscular outlet septum may cause severe left ventricular outflow obstruction. Other associated cardiac lesions are similar to those of coarctation of the aorta.

13.5.2 Pathophysiology

Perfusion of the descending aorta and its branches depends entirely on blood flow through the arterial duct in interrupted aortic arch (duct-dependent systemic circulation). The right ventricle is hence the dominant ventricle that supplies blood to the descending aorta by way of the persistent arterial duct. With closure of the arterial duct, distal perfusion is compromised with development of renal failure, acidosis, and shock. Early-onset heart failure is characteristic of aortic interruption.

13.5.3 Clinical Presentation and Findings

Neonates with interrupted aortic arch usually present with early-onset heart failure or circulatory collapse within the first 2 weeks of life (Table 13.6). The femoral pulses become weak or absent with closure of the arterial duct. Poor renal perfusion results in oliguria. The auscultatory findings are non-specific and unhelpful.

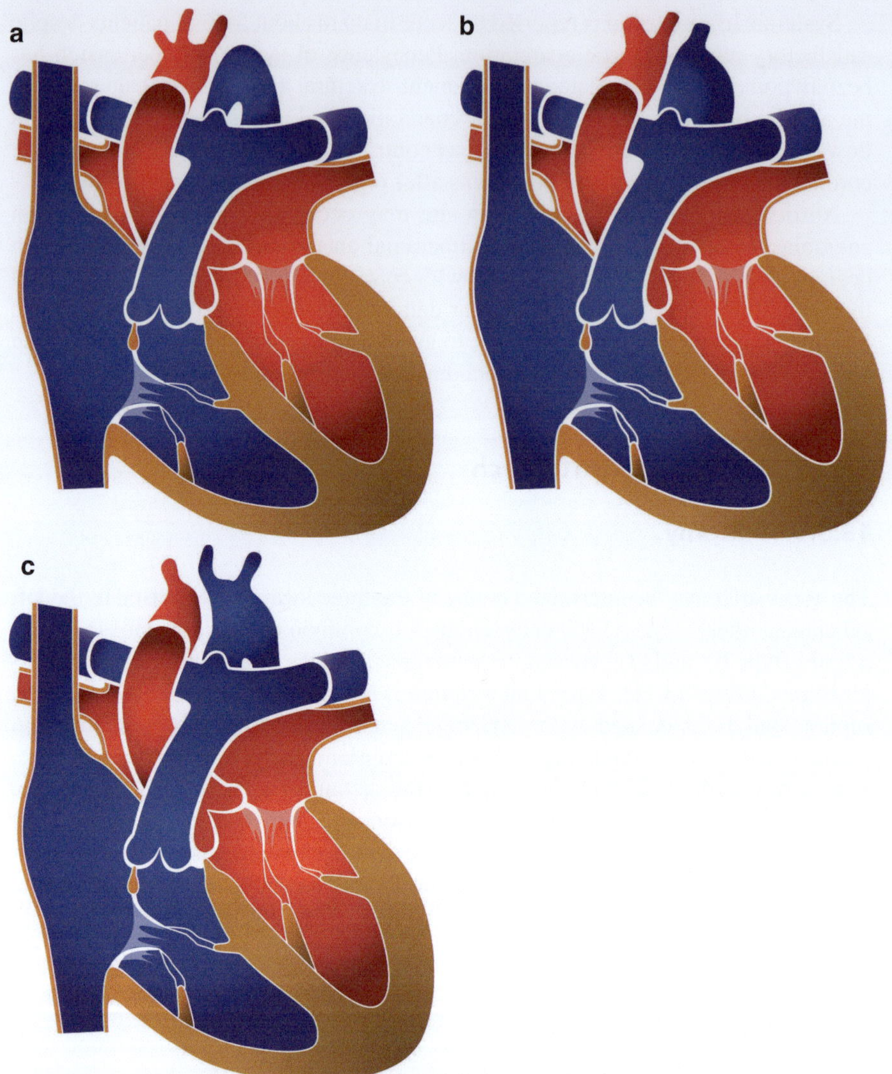

Fig. 13.11 Types of Interrupted aortic arch. (**a**) Type A (**b**) Type B (**c**) Type C

Table 13.6 Signs of interrupted aortic arch

Signs	Origins
Signs of heart failure	
Weak femoral pulses	Type A: Equally strong upper limb pulses
	Type B: Weak left upper limb pulse as well
	Type C: Weak left upper limb pulse and left carotid pulse as well
	(note that the lower limb pulses may not be weak in the presence of a large arterial duct)
Differential cyanosis	Oxygen saturation in the right upper extremity is higher than that in the lower extremities

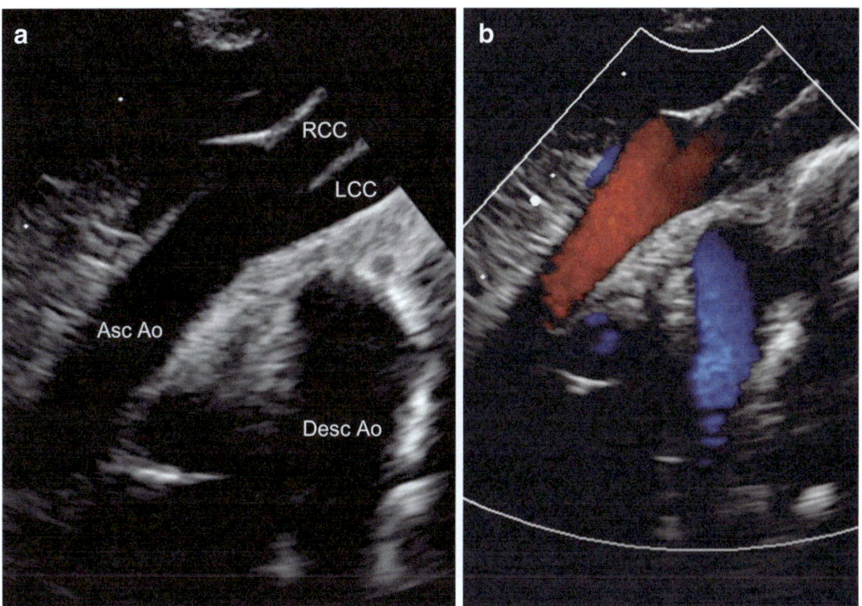

Fig. 13.12 Echocardiographic assessment of interrupted aortic arch. (**a**) 2D and (**b**) colour Doppler echocardiographic findings of type B interrupted bovine aortic arch (*Asc Ao* ascending aorta, *Desc Ao* descending aorta, *LCC* left common carotid artery, *RCC* right common carotid artery)

13.5.4 Investigations

CXR: Cardiomegaly and increased pulmonary vascular markings due to pulmonary venous congestion are present. The absence of thymus, a feature of DiGeorge syndrome, suggests type B interruption.

ECG: Electrocardiogram shows right ventricular hypertrophy as the right ventricle is the dominant ventricle supporting the descending aortic flow by way of the arterial duct.

Echocardiography: Echocardiography defines the site of interruption (Fig. 13.12), and enables the assessment of the arch dimension, patency and size of the arterial

duct (right-to-left shunting from the pulmonary artery to the descending aorta during systole), associated cardiac lesions, and left ventricular contractility.
CT: Computed tomography angiography may be useful when the arch anatomy and aortic sidedness is unclear on echocardiographic assessment of critically ill neonates at presentation.
Genetic evaluation: Genetic testing for 22q11.2 microdeletion and assessment for associated features of DiGeorge syndrome (Chap. 62) is required especially in patients with type B interruption and absence of thymus in the chest radiograph.

13.5.5 Management Strategy

Initial stabilization: Critically ill neonates with aortic interruption requires immediate stabilization with infusion of prostaglandin E, inotropic support, intubation with ventilatory support, and correction of metabolic acidosis.
Surgical intervention: Surgical repair is performed by end-to-end or end-to-side anastomosis. In the presence of significant left ventricular outflow obstruction in association of a ventricular septal defect and normal-sized left ventricle, surgical options include (1) Yasui procedure (reconstruction of aortic arch by Norwood-type operation or Damus-Kaye-Stansel procedure with repair of the interrupted arch, redirection of left ventricular outflow through the ventricular septal defect, and establishment of right ventricle-to-pulmonary arterial continuity using a valved conduit), and (2) Ross-Konno procedure (discussed in the section on valvar aortic stenosis in this Chapter).

13.5.6 Postoperative Considerations and Long-Term Monitoring

Potential complications after surgical repair of interrupted aorta and issues requiring long-term monitoring are those after repair of coarctation of the aorta. An issue more commonly encountered after repair of interrupted aortic arch but not coarctation of the aorta is development of subaortic stenosis due to discrete subaortic membrane, fibromuscular ridge, or posterior deviation of ventricular septum despite repair of the associated ventricular septal defect.

13.6 Midaortic Syndrome

13.6.1 Anatomy

Midaortic syndrome is a rare condition characterized by segmental or diffuse narrowing of the abdominal aorta with varying involvement of renal and splanchnic arterial branches. While the cause in most of the patients is unknown, midaortic syndrome can occur in association with genetic, inflammatory, and infective conditions (Table 13.7).

Table 13.7 Causes of midaortic syndrome

Causes
Idiopathic
Association with genetic disorders
Neurofibromatosis type I (von Recklinghausen disease)
Alagille syndrome
William syndrome
Tuberous sclerosis
Inflammatory or infective causes
Takayasu arteritis
Congenital infection syndrome (especially congenital rubella infection)

Narrowing of the abdominal aorta may be segmental and located at the suprarenal (above the coeliac or superior mesenteric artery), inter-renal (at or above the renal arteries, but below the superior mesenteric artery), or infrarenal (below the renal arteries) aorta or diffuse in nature. Involvement of renal arteries may be unilateral or bilateral. For the splanchnic arteries, stenosis of the superior mesenteric and coeliac arteries is more common than that of the inferior mesenteric artery. Histologically, intimal thickening and fibrous proliferation of the media without inflammation are seen in idiopathic cases.

13.6.2 Pathophysiology

Abdominal aortic obstruction increases the afterload to the left ventricle and causes left ventricular hypertrophy. Activation of the renin–angiotensin system secondary to reduced renal blood flow worsens the systemic hypertension, which would eventually lead to left ventricular dysfunction. The limitation of blood flow to the lower limbs and the intestine can lead respectively to intermittent claudication and abdominal angina.

13.6.3 Clinical Presentation and Findings

Children with midaortic syndrome present with incidental finding of severe systemic hypertension, headache, and even encephalopathy. Intermittent claudication and abdominal angina as the presenting complaints are uncommon.

Physical signs include strong upper limb pulses (but not in patients with Takayasu arteritis in which one or both upper pulses may be absent), weak or absent femoral pulses, left ventricular impulse, and abdominal bruit. Signs of heart failure indicate left ventricular dysfunction. The findings of upper limb hypertension and absent femoral pulses in the absence of echocardiographic finding of coarctation of the aorta should prompt the suspicion of and further investigations for midaortic syndrome.

In patients with genetic syndromes, dysmorphic facies (Alagille syndrome, William syndrome) and cutaneous lesions (neurofibromatosis type I, tuberous

Table 13.8 The EULAR/PRINTO/PRES criteria for childhood Takayasu arteritis

Criterion	Definition
Angiographic abnormality (mandatory criterion)	Angiography (conventional, computed tomography, or magnetic resonance imaging) of the aorta or its main branches and pulmonary arteries showing aneurysm/dilation, narrowing, occlusion or thickened arterial wall not due to fibromuscular dysplasia, or similar causes; changes usually focal or segmental
Pulse deficit or claudication	Lost/decreased/unequal peripheral artery pulse(s)
	Claudication: Focal muscle pain induced by physical activity
Blood pressure discrepancy	Discrepancy of four limb systolic blood pressure > 10 mmHg difference in any limb
Bruits	Audible murmurs or palpable thrills over large arteries
Hypertension	Systolic/diastolic blood pressure greater than 95th percentile for height
Acute phase reactants	Erythrocyte sedimentation rate > 20 mm per first hour or C-reactive protein of any value above normal (according to the local laboratory)

Adapted from Ozen et al. Ann Rheum Dis 2010;69:798–806

sclerosis) are present. In patient with congenital rubella infection, cataract, deafness, and splenomegaly may be found.

For diagnosis of Takayasu arteritis in children, the European League Against Rheumatism (EULAR), the Pediatric Rheumatology European Society (PRES) and by the Pediatric Rheumatology International Trials Organization (PRINTO) criteria is adopted (Table 13.8). The presence of angiographic abnormalities in the aorta or its main branches and pulmonary arteries (mandatory criterion) with at least one of the five other features fulfil the diagnosis of Takayasu arteritis in children.

13.6.4 Investigations

Echocardiography: Echocardiography shows left ventricular hypertrophy and hypoplastic abdominal aorta with turbulent flow and absence of coarctation of the aorta in idiopathic midaortic syndrome. Additional echocardiographic findings may include cardiac tumours (tuberous sclerosis) and other sites of arterial stenoses (William syndrome, Alagille syndrome, and Takayasu arteritis).

Cardiac catheterization: Angiography with haemodynamic assessment by cardiac catheterization has been the standard in diagnosing patients with midaortic syndrome and associated arterial abnormalities. Increasingly, computed tomography and magnetic resonance angiography are used for noninvasive imaging of these abnormalities.

CT and MR angiography: These modalities delineate the entire arterial tree for assessment of the extent of disease and surgical planning (Fig. 13.13).

Assessment of renovascular hypertension: Investigations include Doppler assessment for renal arterial stenosis, renal ultrasound, measurement of plasma renin activity, and renal function test.

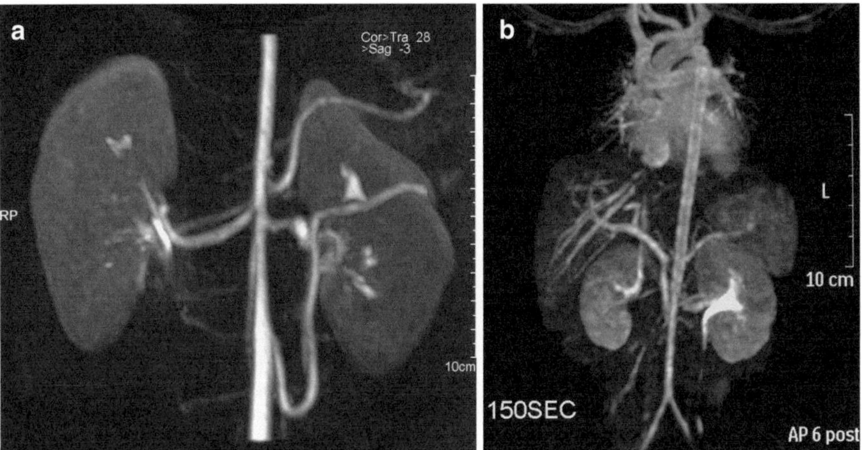

Fig. 13.13 Midaortic syndrome. (**a**) Long-segment stenosis of the abdominal aorta above the level of the inferior mesenteric artery branching (**b**) Long-segment narrowing the distal abdominal aorta between the renal arteries and the iliac arteries

Measurement of inflammatory markers: Increased erythrocyte sedimentation rate or C reactive protein suggests an inflammatory cause of midaortic syndrome.
Genetic evaluation: Depending on the associated clinical features, further genetic evaluation may be indicated.

13.6.5 Management Strategy

Medical management: Medical therapy aims at optimizing the control of hypertension, which may be difficult to manage. Often, the use of multiple antihypertensive medications is required. The use of angiotensin-converting enzyme inhibitors and angiotensin II receptor blockers requires caution. Close monitoring for possible deterioration of renal function is necessary. Medical treatment represents the mainstay of treatment in patients deemed not suitable (e.g. complex lesions, young age) for endovascular or surgical intervention. For patients with Takayasu arteritis, the mainstay of therapy is systemic glucocorticoids in conjunction with glucocorticoid-sparing agent (e.g. methotrexate, azathioprine) and/or anti-tumour necrosis factor-alpha agents (e.g. infliximab).
Endovascular interventions: Balloon angioplasty and stenting have been performed in children with poorly controlled blood pressure. These procedures are generally regarded as palliative as the rate of restenosis is high but may postpone the timing of surgery.
Surgical interventions: The timing and indications of surgery are individualized and based on the age and body size of patient, severity of symptoms (hypertension, intermittent claudication, and abdominal angina), risk of renal compromise (due to

severe stenosis of the renal artery), response to antihypertensive treatment, and complexity of the arterial lesions.

Surgery involves aorto-aortic bypass grafting with or without revascularization of the renal and splanchnic artery. For severe renal artery stenosis with renovascular hypertension, aorta-renal bypass (with a prosthetic graft or autologous grafts) and auto-renal transplantation are possible options. If renal revascularization is not possible, nephrectomy may be required.

13.6.6 Long-Term Monitoring

Monitoring of blood pressure and continuous use of antihypertensive medications even after interventions are necessary. Restenosis and the lack of growth of the prosthetic graft in children inevitably requires replacement and further interventions in the long term.

14 Left-Sided Inflow Obstructive Lesions

Obstruction of the left ventricular inflow is rare in children. It may occur at the level of the mitral valvar apparatus or, less commonly, proximal to the mitral valvar orifice. Cortriatriatum, a fibromuscular partition within the left atrium, may restrict flow from the proximal to the distal left atrial compartment and limit left ventricular inflow. The consequences common to significant left ventricular inflow obstruction due to different causes are pulmonary venous obstruction, pulmonary hypertension, right ventricular dysfunction, and reduced systemic cardiac output.

14.1 Mitral Stenosis

Mitral stenosis can be congenital or acquired due to rheumatic heart disease (Chap. 48). Congenital mitral stenosis is a rare condition, which can occur in isolation or, more commonly, in association with varying degrees of left ventricular hypoplasia (Chap. 21) and left ventricular outflow obstruction (Chap. 31).

14.1.1 Anatomy

Congenital mitral stenosis is contributed by heterogeneous structural abnormalities that may occur at one or more levels of the mitral inflow: supravalvar level, leaflets, chordae tendineae, and papillary muscles (Fig. 14.1).

Different classification systems have been proposed to describe congenital mitral valvar lesions. The Carpentier classification proposed in 1976, based on functional analysis of leaflet mobility, is a commonly utilized classification (Table 14.1). A haemodynamic and anatomic classification was proposed by the Congenital Heart Surgery Nomenclature and Database Project in 2000 (Table 14.2).

Y.-f. Cheung, *Congenital and Paediatric Acquired Heart Disease in Practice*, https://doi.org/10.1007/978-981-99-2862-0_14

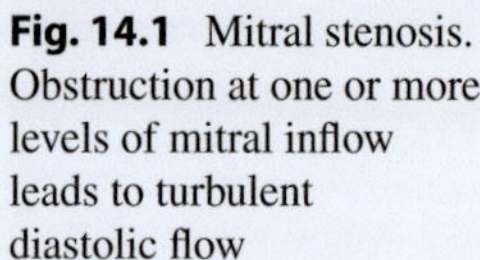

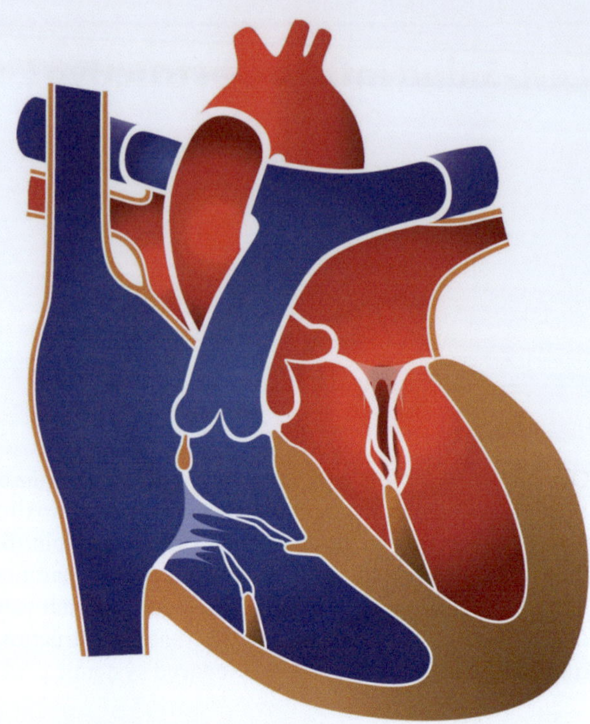

Fig. 14.1 Mitral stenosis. Obstruction at one or more levels of mitral inflow leads to turbulent diastolic flow

Table 14.1 Carpentier classification of congenital mitral valvar lesions

Type	Leaflet mobility	Functional correlation
I	Normal leaflet motion	Valvar regurgitation due to annular dilation of cleft leaflet
II	Leaflet prolapse	Valvar regurgitation due to chordal elongation or agenesis or papillary muscle elongation
III	Restricted leaflet motion	Mitral stenosis ± regurgitation due to commissural fusion of thickening or shortening of subvalvar apparatus

Each type can be subdivided in A (normal papillary muscle) or B (abnormal papillary muscle: parachute mitral valve, hammock mitral valve, or papillary muscle hypoplasia)

Table 14.2 Congenital Heart Surgery Nomenclature and Database Project classification of congenital mitral valvar lesions

Type	Description
1	Supravalvar
2	Valvar (a) Annular defects (b) Leaflet defects
3	Subvalvar (a) Abnormalities of the chordae tendineae (b) Defects of papillary muscles
4	Mixed lesions

Each anatomic type is considered in the context of the haemodynamics: mitral stenosis, mitral regurgitation, or mixed

Certain distinct pathological entities (e.g. parachute and hammock mitral valves) have been described, although they probably belong to part of a continuous spectrum. Supravalvar mitral ring, although commonly regarded as congenital mitral valvar anomaly, is probably acquired in relation to mitral inflow obstructive lesion.

14.1.1.1 Parachute Mitral Valve

Abnormalities of the papillary muscle cause the so-called parachute mitral valve. Absence or severe hypoplasia of one of the papillary muscles results in the insertion of all chordae tendineae into one papillary muscle to form a parachute-like appearance. This is often associated with abnormalities of other components of the mitral valvar apparatus to cause mitral stenosis with or without mitral regurgitation. Parachute mitral valve constitutes also one of the components of Shone complex (Chap. 31).

14.1.1.2 Hammock Mitral Valve

Hammock mitral valve describes the appearance of the mitral valvar apparatus when viewed from the left atrial aspect. The intermixing of chordae tendineae with the abnormally enlarged papillary muscle causes this appearance and results in mitral stenosis and/or mitral regurgitation.

14.1.1.3 Supravalvar Mitral Ring

The supravalvar mitral ring is attached to the mitral valvar annulus and is commonly associated with stenotic lesions of the mitral valve. This ring is believed to be an acquired lesion secondary to turbulent flow across a stenotic mitral valve and worsens mitral inflow obstruction.

14.1.2 Pathophysiology

Mitral stenosis results in a diastolic pressure gradient between the left atrium and left ventricle. Pressures in the left atrium, pulmonary veins, and pulmonary capillaries are increased. Hence, the consequences of severe mitral stenosis include pulmonary oedema, reflex pulmonary arterial vasoconstriction, pulmonary hypertension, and right ventricular dysfunction.

14.1.3 Clinical Presentation and Findings

Congenial mitral stenosis is often diagnosed when the patients are assessed for associated cardiac abnormalities. Infants with severe congenital mitral stenosis present with shortness of breath, poor feeding and failure to thrive. Older children are usually asymptomatic, although they may complain of shortness of breath after strenuous exertion. Rarely, palpitations due to atrial arrhythmias may occur. The physical signs are shown in Table 14.3.

Table 14.3 Signs of mitral stenosis

	Mild mitral stenosis	Severe mitral stenosis
Weak pulses	–	+
RV impulse	–	+
Soft S1	±	+
Increased P2	–	+
Opening snap	–	±
Murmur	A soft, low-frequency mid-diastolic murmur at the apex	A low-frequency mid-diastolic murmur at the apex

14.1.4 Investigations

CXR: Dilation of the left atrium and pulmonary venous congestion are evident in the presence of moderate to severe mitral stenosis.
ECG: Electrocardiogram may show bifid P waves (P-mitrale), and, with pulmonary hypertension, right axis deviation and right ventricular hypertrophy.
Echocardiography: Detailed echocardiographic assessment is required for evaluation of associated cardiac malformations and all components of the mitral valvar apparatus: supravalvar region, annulus, leaflets and commissures, chordae tendineae, and papillary muscles. Three-dimensional echocardiographic imaging provides unique en face views to visualize the abnormal mitral valvar apparatus. Two-dimensional imaging and Doppler flow mapping further allow the assessment of the severity of mitral stenosis (Fig. 14.2). The available cutoff values for the mean transmitral gradient and valve area are derived from adults. In children, there is no standardized approach for quantitative echocardiographic assessment of mitral stenosis, but in general, the same four aspects as shown in Box 14.1 are evaluated.
Cardiac catheterization: This is usually not required for initial diagnosis. In patients considered for mitral valvar interventions, diagnostic catheterization enables an accurate assessment of the transmitral pressure gradient (by simultaneous measurement of the pulmonary arterial wedge pressure or left atrial pressure and left ventricular end-diastolic pressure), pulmonary arterial pressure, and pulmonary vascular resistance. Transcatheter intervention with transseptal puncture and balloon mitral valvoplasty can be performed in the same setting.

Box 14.1 Echocardiographic Evidence of Moderate to Severe Mitral Stenosis in Adults

- Dilation of the left atrium
- Mitral valve area (2D planimetry) $\leq 1.5\ \text{cm}^2$
- Mean transmitral gradient ≥ 5 mmHg
- Moderate to severe pulmonary hypertension

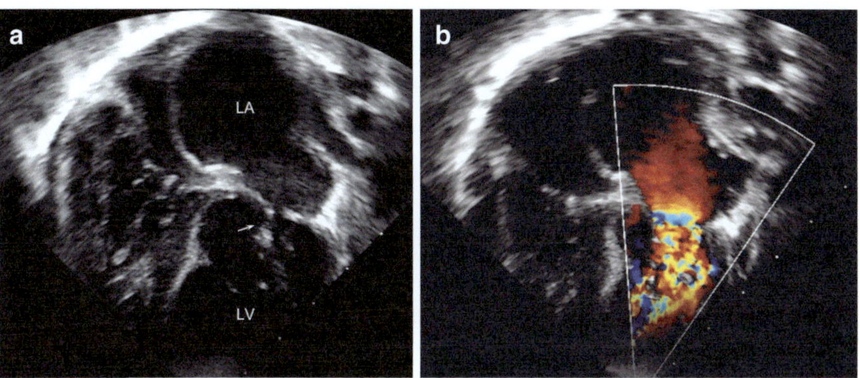

Fig. 14.2 Echocardiographic assessment of mitral stenosis. (**a**) Thickening of the mitral valve leaflets (arrow) and dilation of the left atrium in congenital mitral valve stenosis (**b**) Colour Doppler flow mapping showing high-velocity flow across the mitral valve during diastole (*LA* left atrium, *LV* left ventricle)

14.1.5 Management Strategy

In symptomatic infants, diuretics may provide partial symptomatic relief. Mitral valvar intervention is indicated in symptomatic children with evidence of moderate to severe mitral stenosis. The indications are, however, less well defined in asymptomatic patients. Nonetheless, parameters as shown in Box 14.1, development of atrial arrhythmias, and clear definition of the abnormal mitral valvar substrates provide the basis for planning transcatheter or surgical intervention.

Depending on the size of patients, nature of substrate causing mitral stenosis, and associated cardiac malformations, options include percutaneous balloon mitral valvoplasty, surgical mitral valvoplasty, resection of supravalvar ring, and mitral valvar replacement.

Two issues of importance related to mitral valve replacement in young infants are (a) the need for supra-annular implantation, which allows a larger prosthesis and reduces the risk of heart block and subaortic stenosis, and (b) the difficulties in adjusting warfarin dosage and anticoagulation monitoring. Recent reports on the use the stented bovine jugular vein graft (Melody valve) as a surgical implant in the mitral position in infants are encouraging.

14.2 Cortriatriatum

14.2.1 Anatomy

The term 'cortriatriatum' refers to a heart with three atria. However, this condition in essence has only two atria and is characterized by division of usually the left atrium or rarely the right atrium by a fibromuscular partition. Partition of the left

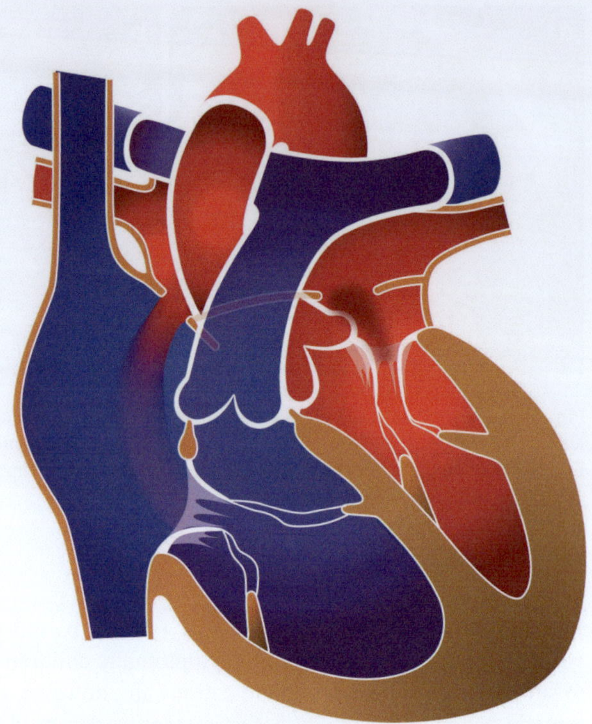

Fig. 14.3 Cortriatriatum. Partition of the left atrium with an atrial septal defect between the proximal chamber and the right atrium

atrium into a proximal compartment (pulmonary venous compartment) that connects to the pulmonary veins and a distal compartment (vestibular compartment) that communicates with the mitral valvar orifice by the partition (Fig. 14.3) is the only important type of cortriatriatum of clinical relevance seen in children and is discussed in this section. The communication between the proximal and distal compartments is usually small and obstructs blood flow from the proximal into the distal compartment. The atrial septum may be intact or harbours an atrial septal defect. The atrial septal defect, if present, is usually a secundum defect located between the proximal chamber and the right atrium.

14.2.2 Pathophysiology

The pathophysiology depends on whether the communication between the proximal and distal compartments is restrictive or not and whether there is an associated atrial septal defect. Pulmonary venous obstruction is most severe in the presence of a restrictive communication and an intact atrial septum. A restrictive communication aggravates the left-to-right interatrial shunt in the presence of a secundum atrial septal defect, which allows blood to drain from the proximal chamber to the right atrium. The obstructive pulmonary venous flow causes pulmonary venous hypertension, pulmonary oedema, reflex pulmonary arteriolar constriction, and secondary pulmonary arterial hypertension. Muscularization of the pulmonary venules and arterioles further contribute further to the increase in pulmonary vascular resistance.

14.2.3 Clinical Presentation and Findings

Patients with a non-restrictive communication between the proximal and distal compartments and an atrial septal defect, which is uncommon, may present with an asymptomatic heart murmur. Typically, infants present with shortness of breath due to pulmonary venous congestion (a restrictive communication between the proximal and distal compartments) and increased left-to-right atrial shunt (when an atrial septal defect is present). The signs are those of pulmonary venous obstruction and pulmonary hypertension (Table 14.4).

14.2.4 Investigations

CXR: The presence of radiographic evidence of pulmonary venous congestion suggests a restrictive communication between the proximal and distal compartments. Cardiomegaly due to right atrial and right ventricular dilation may be present in patients with a large atrial septal defect.

ECG: The electrocardiogram shows right ventricular hypertrophy.

Echocardiography: Echocardiographic assessment confirms the diagnosis by showing a partition within the left atrium and demonstrates associated atrial septal defect (Fig. 14.4). The degree of restrictive flow through the partition and severity of pulmonary hypertension can be assessed by Doppler echocardiography.

Table 14.4 Signs of cortriatriatum with a restrictive communication between proximal and distal compartments

Signs	Origins
Respiratory distress	Pulmonary venous congestion
Right ventricular impulse	Right ventricular pressure overload due to pulmonary hypertension
Increased P2	Pulmonary hypertension
An ejection systolic murmur at the left upper sternal border	High pulmonary flow in the presence of a large atrial septal defect with blood draining from the proximal left atrial chamber to the right atrium

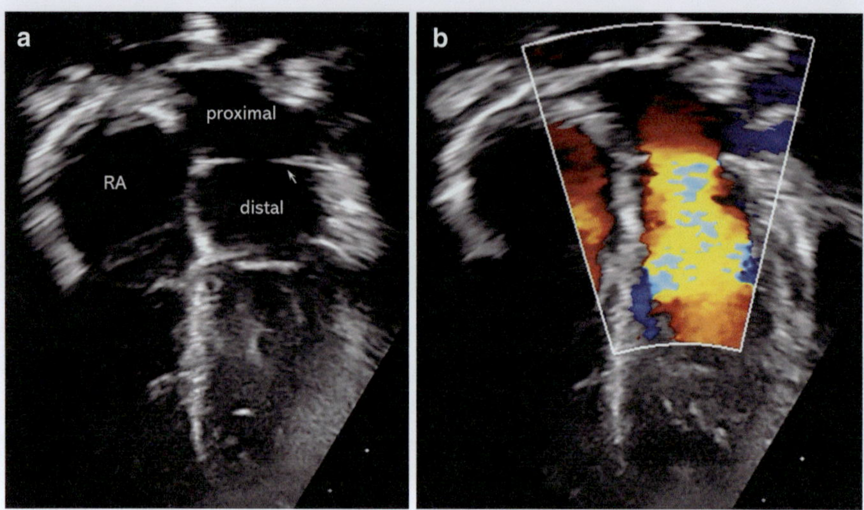

Fig. 14.4 Echocardiographic assessment of cortriatriatum. (**a**) Echocardiographic demonstration of fibromuscular partitioning of the left atrium in a proximal and a distal chamber (**b**) Colour Doppler flow mapping reveals turbulent flow originating at the level of the fibromuscular partition (Abbreviation: *RA* right atrium)

14.2.5 Management Strategy

Surgical resection of the partition and closure of the atrial septal defect, if present, is the definitive treatment. Postoperative management of pulmonary hypertensive crisis may be a challenge.

14.2.6 Postoperative Considerations

Important postoperative complications are similar to those after repair of obstructed total anomalous pulmonary venous connection (Chap. 37). These include pulmonary hypertensive crisis, low cardiac output syndrome, and supraventricular tachyarrhythmias.

Chronic pulmonary venous obstruction results in muscularization of the pulmonary arterioles and venules. Increased reactivity of the pulmonary vasculature predisposes to development of pulmonary hypertensive crisis postoperatively. In situations when pulmonary hypertension and hypertensive crisis appear refractory to treatment, accelerated pulmonary vascular disease and lymphangiectasia have to be considered.

Chronic volume unloading of the left ventricle preoperatively reduces its compliance. Judicious fluid replacement after surgery is necessary to avoid significant increase in left atrial pressure (which can lead to pulmonary oedema and aggravate pulmonary hypertension). Afterload reduction may be beneficial.

Left- and Right-Sided Valvar Regurgitation

15

Valvar regurgitation in children is usually secondary to acquired valvar abnormalities or associated heart conditions rather than due to congenital valvar abnormalities. Regurgitation of the left-sided valves (mitral and aortic valves) causes volume overloading of the left ventricle, while regurgitation of the right-sided valves (tricuspid and pulmonary valves) results in volume overloading of the right ventricle.

15.1 Aortic Regurgitation

15.1.1 Aetiology

Isolated aortic regurgitation is uncommon in childhood. Congenital aortic valvar abnormalities (Chap. 13) may cause stenosis or insufficiency. In children, aortic regurgitation is often found in association with other congenital cardiac malformations or acquired disorders (Table 15.1).

Table 15.1 Causes of aortic regurgitation in children

Nature of lesion	Cardiac condition
Congenital valvar abnormalities	Bicuspid aortic valvar degeneration Truncal valvar dysfunction
Damage of the valvar cusp(s)	Infective endocarditis Rheumatic heart disease Turbulent flow related to subaortic stenosis
Dilation of aortic annulus	Marfan syndrome Loeys-Dietz syndrome Ehlers-Danlos syndromes Neoaortic dilation (post arterial switch operation and Ross procedure)
Prolapse of the coronary cusp(s)	Subarterial, outlet muscular, and perimembranous ventricular septal defects

Y.-f. Cheung, *Congenital and Paediatric Acquired Heart Disease in Practice*,
https://doi.org/10.1007/978-981-99-2862-0_15

15.1.2 Pathophysiology

In chronic moderate to severe aortic insufficiency, a significant volume of blood regurgitates from the aorta into the left ventricle during diastole and results in volume overloading of the left ventricle.

The left ventricle initially adapts by (a) eccentric hypertrophy to normalize the left ventricular volume-to-mass ratio and wall stress (law of Laplace) and (b) increasing the force of contraction to maintain ejection fraction in response to the increased preload (Frank-Starling mechanism). Late decompensation of the left ventricle with systolic failure and diastolic dysfunction (related to myocardial hypertrophy and fibrosis) may be seen, albeit uncommon, in children.

Acute onset of severe aortic regurgitation (e.g. due to damage of the aortic valve in infective endocarditis) can, however, lead to rapid decompensation as there is no time for compensatory response of the left ventricle to develop. The pathophysiologic consequences are low effective cardiac output, hypotension, and pulmonary oedema.

15.1.3 Clinical Presentation and Findings

Most children with aortic insufficiency are relatively asymptomatic. Those with chronic severe aortic regurgitation may have shortness of breath on exertion or symptoms of frank heart failure.

The characteristic physical signs are large volume or collapsing pulses, signs of left ventricular volume overload, and a blowing early diastolic murmur (Table 15.2). In severe aortic insufficiency, a mid-diastolic rumbling murmur at the apex (Austin Flint murmur) due to interference of mitral valve opening by the regurgitating blood stream may be audible.

15.1.4 Investigations

CXR: Cardiomegaly occurs in the presence of moderate to severe degree of aortic insufficiency due to left ventricular dilation. In addition, the aortic knuckle may be prominent due to dilation of the ascending aorta.

Table 15.2 Signs of aortic regurgitation

	Mild aortic regurgitation	Severe aortic regurgitation
Bounding pulses	–	+
Displacement of cardiac apex	–	+
Left ventricular impulse	–	+
Murmur	A short early diastolic murmur at the left mid sternal border	A long early diastolic murmur at the left mid sternal border, Austin Flint murmur

ECG: The electrocardiogram shows left ventricular dilation and hypertrophy.

Echocardiography: Echocardiography demonstrates the aortic valve pathologies, shows aortic root dilation, and enables semi-quantitative assessment of the severity of aortic regurgitation (Box 15.1) (Fig. 15.1).

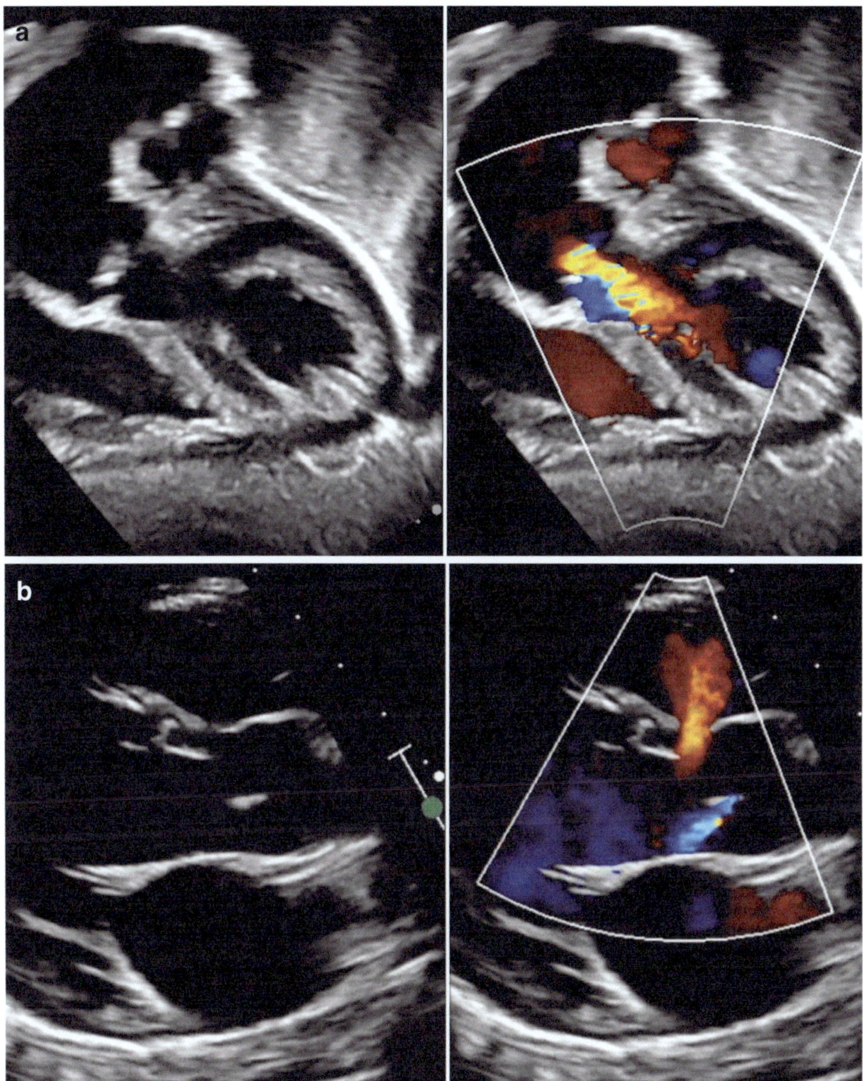

Fig. 15.1 Echocardiographic assessment of aortic regurgitation. (**a**) Trivial degree of aortic regurgitation (blue mosaic colour jet in the right panel) due to prolapse of the right coronary cusp (left panel) in the presence of a subarterial ventricular septal defect (**b**) Moderate degree of truncal valve regurgitation (mosaic colour jet in the right panel) persists despite repair of truncus arteriosus in an infant

Box 15.1 Echocardiographic Evidence of Moderate to Severe Aortic Regurgitation

- Dilation of the left ventricle
- Large regurgitant colour jet width in the left ventricular outflow tract
- Increased regurgitant colour jet width/left ventricular outflow tract width ratio (≥25%)
- Dense aortic regurgitant jet as assessed by continuous wave Doppler echocardiography
- Obvious diastolic flow reversal in the descending aorta as assessed by pulsed Doppler echocardiography

15.1.5 Management Strategy

Afterload reduction with systemic vasodilators (angiotensin-converting enzyme inhibitor is usually used, other options include hydralazine and nifedipine) may benefit asymptomatic children with moderate to severe aortic insufficiency, symptomatic children, and in those with systemic hypertension in addition with aortic regurgitation.

Aortic valve surgery is indicated in symptomatic children and in those with evidence of impaired or deteriorating left ventricular function (Box 15.2). The indications are, however, less well defined in asymptomatic patients. Unlike in adults, left ventricular dimensions have not been incorporated in the management guidelines of aortic regurgitation in children.

Box 15.2 Indications for Intervention of Aortic Regurgitation

- Angina, syncope, exertional dyspnoea, heart failure
- Evidence of left ventricular systolic dysfunction
- Progressive worsening of left ventricular function and/or size in asymptomatic patients
- Progressive worsening of exercise capacity in asymptomatic patients

The choice between repair and replacement the aortic valve depends on the following factors: (a) patient factor (age, body size, exercise participation, preference on the use of anticoagulants), (b) underlying aetiology (prolapse through a ventricular septal defect, infective damage, connective tissue disease), (c) anatomic factors (size of aortic and pulmonary annulus, subaortic stenosis, concomitant aortic root dilation), and (d) centre experience on valve repair versus prosthetic valve replacement, Ross procedure, and Ozaki procedure (Chap. 13).

15.2 Mitral Regurgitation

15.2.1 Aetiology

Congenital mitral regurgitation is uncommon and may be related to cleft of the mitral valve leaflet. Often in children, mitral regurgitation is found in association with other congenital cardiac malformations, connective tissue disorders, or acquired disorders (Table 15.3).

Dysplastic mitral valve can be associated with mitral regurgitation and/or mitral stenosis. A cleft in the mitral valve is usually an isolated lesion that involves the anterior mitral valvar leaflet (rarely the posterior leaflet is involved). Mitral valve prolapse, which may be congenital or acquired occurs when the mitral valve leaflets extend above the plane of the atrioventricular junction during ventricular systole. In most cases, it is primary in nature, but it may also be associated with papillary muscle dysfunction and connective tissue abnormalities. In children with mitral valve prolapse, the associated mitral insufficiency when present is usually mild in degree.

15.2.2 Pathophysiology

In the presence of moderate-to-severe degree of mitral regurgitation, a significant volume of blood regurgitates into the left atrium during systole, resulting in left atrial dilation and increasing the risk of atrial arrhythmias. The combined pulmonary venous return and regurgitant volume leads to volume overloading of the left ventricle. Contraction of the left ventricle is, however, usually preserved until a late stage when left ventricular decompensation occurs with impaired contraction, pulmonary venous congestion, and pulmonary hypertension.

Table 15.3 Causes of mitral regurgitation in children

Nature of lesion	Cardiac condition
Congenital valvar abnormalities	Dysplastic mitral valve Cleft mitral valve Mitral valve prolapse (may also be acquired)
Damage to the valve leaflets	Infective endocarditis Rheumatic heart disease
Papillary muscle dysfunction	Kawasaki disease Anomalous origin of the left coronary artery from the pulmonary artery
Connective tissue disease	Marfan syndrome Loeys-Dietz syndrome Ehlers-Danlos syndromes
Lysosomal storage disease	Mucopolysaccharidosis
Functional regurgitation (stretching of the mitral annulus due to left ventricular dilation)	Left-to-right shunts Myocarditis Dilated cardiomyopathy

Table 15.4 Signs of mitral regurgitation

	Mild mitral regurgitation	Severe mitral regurgitation
Displaced cardiac apex	–	+
Left ventricular impulse	–	+
Mid-systolic click	When mitral valve prolapse is present	When mitral valve prolapse is present
Murmur	A soft pansystolic murmur at the apex ± radiation to left axilla	A loud pansystolic murmur at the apex with radiation to the left axilla, a diastolic flow murmur at the apex

15.2.3 Clinical Presentation and Findings

Most children with mitral regurgitation are relatively asymptomatic. Those with severe regurgitation may have shortness of breath on exertion and reduced exercise tolerance. Palpitations may suggest the complication of atrial arrhythmias. In patients with mitral valve prolapse, ill-defined chest pain, fatigue, and palpitations are common symptoms.

The physical signs of significant mitral regurgitation are those of left ventricular volume overloading and a pansystolic murmur at the cardiac apex with radiation to the left axilla (Table 15.4). The presence of a mid-systolic click and a late systolic murmur suggest mitral valve prolapse.

15.2.4 Investigations

CXR: Cardiomegaly occurs in the presence of moderate to severe mitral regurgitation due to enlargement of the left atrium and the left ventricle. The pulmonary vascular markings may be prominent because of pulmonary venous congestion secondary to increased left atrial pressure.

ECG: The electrocardiogram shows left atrial and left ventricular dilation.

Echocardiography: Echocardiography demonstrates the mitral valve pathologies (Fig. 15.2), enables the assessment the causes of functional mitral regurgitation, and allows semi-quantitative assessment of the severity of mitral regurgitation (Box 15.3).

Box 15.3 Echocardiographic Evidence of Moderate to Severe Mitral Regurgitation

- Dilation of the left atrium and left ventricle
- Large regurgitant colour jet area (the area of an eccentric colour jet may appear small even with moderate to severe mitral regurgitation)
- Dense mitral regurgitant jet as assessed by continuous wave Doppler echocardiography

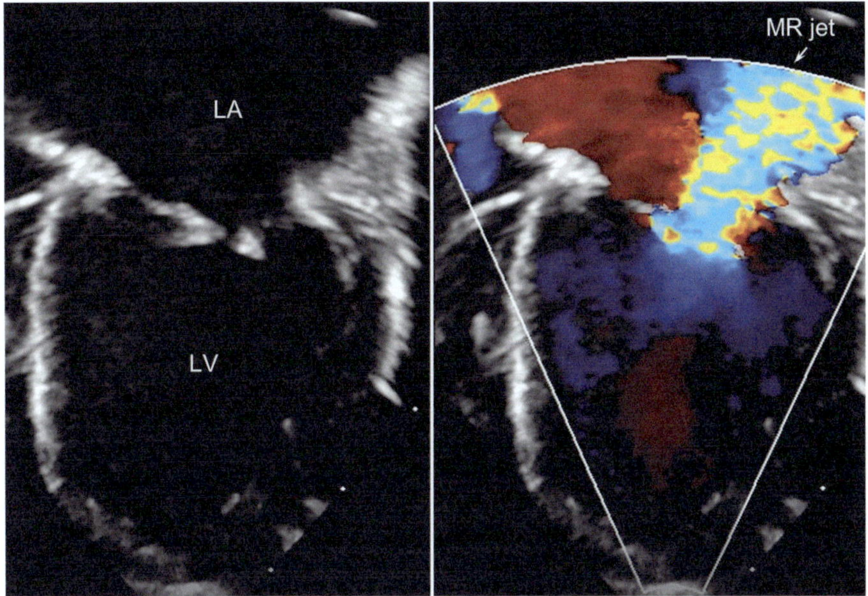

Fig. 15.2 Echocardiographic assessment of dysplastic mitral valve with mitral regurgitation. Thickening with incomplete coaptation of the mitral valve (left panel) with Doppler colour flow mapping showing severe degree of mitral regurgitation (Abbreviations: LA, left atrium, LV, left ventricle, MR, mitral regurgitation)

15.2.5 Management Strategy

Afterload reduction with systemic vasodilators and diuretics are useful in the management of children with moderate to severe mitral insufficiency. Mitral valve repair and annuloplasty is indicated in symptomatic children not responsive to medical therapy and in those with impaired or deteriorating left ventricular function. Mitral valve replacement is usually considered after failed attempts of repair.

15.3 Pulmonary Regurgitation

15.3.1 Aetiology

Isolated pulmonary regurgitation is uncommon in childhood. The detection of trivial degree of pulmonary regurgitation by Doppler colour flow mapping is usually regarded as a physiologic phenomenon. In children and adolescents, pulmonary regurgitation is usually seen after surgery or transcatheter intervention to relieve right ventricular outflow obstruction (Table 15.5).

Table 15.5 Causes of pulmonary regurgitation in children

Nature of lesion	Cardiac condition
Congenital valvar abnormalities	Tetralogy of Fallot with absent pulmonary valve syndrome
Damage to the pulmonary valve	Post repair of tetralogy of Fallot with transannular patch Post balloon valvoplasty for pulmonary stenosis Post transcatheter perforation and balloon valvoplasty for pulmonary valve atresia with intact ventricular septum
Dysfunction of valved conduit (usually with concomitant stenosis, which is the predominant abnormality)	Post repair of pulmonary atresia with ventricular septal defect Post repair of truncus arteriosus Ross procedure Rastelli operation

15.3.2 Pathophysiology

In chronic moderate to severe pulmonary regurgitation, a significant volume of blood regurgitates from the pulmonary artery into the right ventricle during diastole, and results in volume overloading of the right ventricle. Progressive increase in right ventricular end-diastolic volume is followed by an increase in right ventricular end-systolic volume as the right ventricular systolic function worsens. Stretching of the tricuspid annulus leads to functional tricuspid regurgitation, which in turn further aggravates volume loading of the right ventricle.

The adaptive response of the right ventricle depends on severity and chronicity of the pulmonary regurgitation, restrictive physiology of the right ventricle (Chap. 27), dilation and dysfunction of the right ventricular outflow tract, and impedance of the pulmonary vasculature. Increased pulmonary vascular impedance in the presence of branch pulmonary arterial stenosis and left ventricular dysfunction worsens the severity of pulmonary regurgitation. Transannular patch repair of tetralogy of Fallot leads to aneurysmal dilation, akinesia, and dysfunction of the right ventricular outflow, all of which aggravate the severity of pulmonary regurgitation.

Chronic dilation of the right ventricle increases inhomogeneity of activation and slows conduction velocity. This mechano-electrical interaction may create re-entry circuits that predispose to development of ventricular tachycardia and sudden death, which are well documented in patients with severe pulmonary regurgitation after repair of tetralogy Fallot. Furthermore, right ventricular dilation may impair left ventricular function through adverse ventricular-ventricular interaction (Chap. 28).

15.3.3 Clinical Presentation and Findings

Most children with pulmonary regurgitation are asymptomatic. Adolescents with chronic severe pulmonary regurgitation may have exercise intolerance and, infrequently, palpitations related to atrial and/or ventricular arrhythmias. Symptoms and signs of right heart failure due to systolic right ventricular dysfunction (shortness of breath, exercise intolerance, increased jugular venous pressure, hepatomegaly, peripheral oedema) are rare in children.

Table 15.6 Signs of moderate to severe pulmonary regurgitation

Signs	Origins
Right ventricular impulse	Right ventricular volume overloading
Single S2	Soft and absent P2
An ejection systolic murmur and an early diastolic murmur at the left sternal border	The systolic murmur can be related to increased right ventricular stroke volume and/or concomitant residual pulmonary stenosis

Physical signs of moderate to severe pulmonary regurgitation in children and adolescents are those of right ventricular volume overloading and a diastolic regurgitant murmur at the left sternal border (Table 15.6).

15.3.4 Investigations

CXR: Cardiomegaly occurs in the presence of moderate to severe pulmonary regurgitation due to enlargement of the right ventricle.
ECG: The electrocardiogram shows right ventricular dilation. The presence of right bundle branch block pattern in patients after repair of Fallot may mask the evidence of right ventricular dilation or hypertrophy. Increased QRS duration reflects right ventricular dilation, and in adults with repaired tetralogy of Fallot, a QRS duration ≥180 ms is predictive of ventricular tachycardia and sudden death.
Echocardiography: Echocardiography enables the assessment of the right ventricular outflow tract and allows semi-quantitative assessment of the severity of pulmonary regurgitation (Box 15.4) (Fig. 15.3) and concomitant pulmonary stenosis.
CMR: Cardiac magnetic resonance is the gold standard for the determination of the ventricular volumes and ejection fraction. For assessing the pathophysiologic consequence of pulmonary regurgitation and timing of intervention, the following data obtained by magnetic resonance imaging are useful: right ventricular systolic and diastolic volumes, right and left ventricular ejection fraction, pulmonary regurgitant fraction, late gadolinium enhancement (myocardial fibrosis), and residual cardiac lesions (e.g. residual ventricular septal defect, branch pulmonary arterial stenosis).

Box 15.4 Echocardiographic Evidence of Severe Pulmonary Regurgitation

- Dilation of the right ventricle
- Large regurgitant colour jet width in the right ventricular outflow tract
- Increased regurgitant colour jet width/right ventricular outflow tract width ratio (>50%)
- Dense pulmonary regurgitant jet as assessed by continuous wave Doppler echocardiography
- Diastolic flow reversal in the branch pulmonary arteries
- Pressure half-time <100 ms (but inaccurate in the presence of restrictive right ventricular physiology and increased right ventricular diastolic pressure)

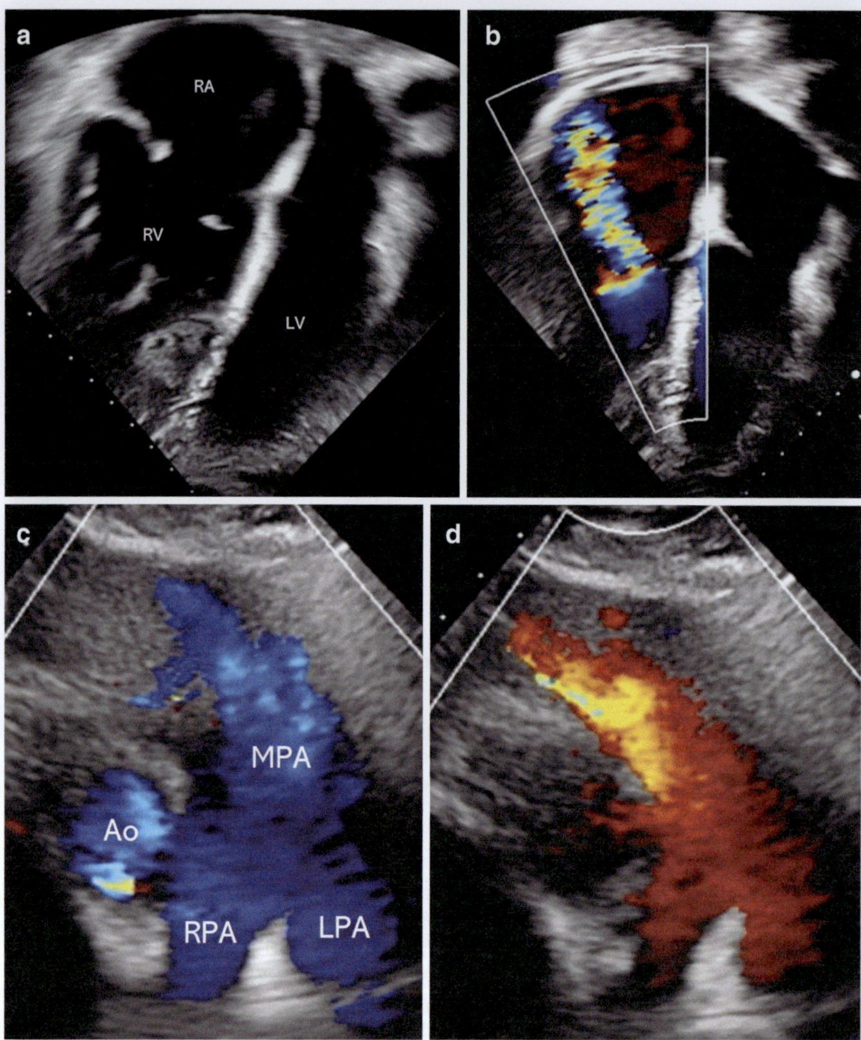

Fig. 15.3 Echocardiographic assessment of pulmonary regurgitation. (**a**) Volume overloading of the right ventricle due to severe pulmonary regurgitation (**b**) Functional tricuspid regurgitation related to right ventricular dilation (**c**) Doppler colour flow mapping shows low-velocity antegrade pulmonary flow during systole and (**d**) severe pulmonary regurgitation with diastolic flow reversal in the branch pulmonary arteries (Abbreviations: *Ao* aorta, *LPA* left pulmonary artery, *LV* left ventricle, *MPA* main pulmonary artery, *RA* right atrium, *RPA* right pulmonary artery, *RV* right ventricle)

15.3.5 Management Strategy

The usefulness of angiotensin-converting enzyme inhibitor in the management of pulmonary regurgitation is unclear. It has not been shown to reduce pulmonary regurgitation or right ventricular size in patients with repaired tetralogy of Fallot. In patients with branch pulmonary arterial stenosis, relief of the obstruction by balloon angioplasty or stenting may reduce pulmonary regurgitation.

The optimal timing of pulmonary valve replacement, in particular in patients with repaired tetralogy of Fallot, remains to be a focus of discussion. Implanting the valve too early predicts the need for early multiple subsequent reinterventions, while implanting it too late may confer the risk of passing the threshold for recovery of right ventricular function.

Implantation of the pulmonary valve, surgical or transcatheter, is indicated in symptomatic patients with shortness of breath and exercise intolerance. The indications are, however, less well defined in asymptomatic patients. In asymptomatic patients, the right ventricular volumes and function, severity of right-sided valvar regurgitation and exercise stress testing parameters should be considered when deciding on the timing of pulmonary valve replacement. Guidelines for surgical pulmonary valve replacement in asymptomatic patients with pulmonary regurgitation after repair of tetralogy of Fallot from the American Heart Association (AHA), European Society of Cardiology (ESC), and Canadian Cardiovascular Society (CCS) are shown in Table 15.7. There are no specific recommendations for transcatheter pulmonary valve replacement, which targets at a wider spectrum of patients who have not only predominantly pulmonary regurgitation, but also pulmonary outflow obstructive lesions and mixed obstructive and regurgitant lesions.

Other factors to consider when determining the timing and indications of pulmonary valve implantation include the degree of left ventricular dysfunction and the presence of residual cardiac lesions that might require concurrent surgical interventions (e.g. obstruction or aneurysmal dilation of the right ventricular outflow tract, branch pulmonary arterial stenosis, aortic root dilation and aortic regurgitation).

Table 15.7 Guidelines for surgical pulmonary valve replacement in asymptomatic patients

Criteria	AHA 2018	ESC 2020	CCS 2009
RV end-diastolic volume	≥160 ml/m^2 or RVEDV ≥2 × LVEDV	≥160 ml/m^2	>170 ml/m^2
RV end-systolic volume	≥80 ml/m^2	≥80 ml/m^2	Not specified
RV or LV systolic function	Mild on moderate RV or LV systolic dysfunction	Progressive RV dysfunction	≥ moderate RV dysfunction
RV hypertension due to outflow obstruction	RVSP ≥2/3 systemic pressure	>80 mmHg	RV systolic pressure ≥2/3 systemic pressure
Pulmonary regurgitation	Moderate or severe	Severe	Free
Tricuspid regurgitation	≥ moderate	≥ moderate	Important
Arrhythmias	Sustained tachyarrhythmias	Not specified	Atrial or ventricular tachycardia
Cardiopulmonary exercise testing	Decreased	Decreased	Not specified

Abbreviations: *EDV* end-diastolic volume, *LV* left ventricular, *RV* right ventricular, *RVSP* right ventricular systolic pressure

15.4 Tricuspid Regurgitation

15.4.1 Aetiology

Isolated congenital tricuspid regurgitation due to dysplasia of the tricuspid valve is uncommon. In children, tricuspid regurgitation is often found in association with other congenital cardiac malformations or acquired disorders (Table 15.8).

Tricuspid valvar dysplasia can occur in the absence of Ebstein malformation (Chap. 22). In this condition, the hinge points of the leaflets are normal at the atrioventricular junction. The leaflets may be thickened but are completely delaminated from the right ventricular myocardium. The right ventricular myocardium in tricuspid valvar dysplasia, unlike in Ebstein malformation, is usually normal.

15.4.2 Pathophysiology

In the presence of moderate-to-severe degree of tricuspid regurgitation, a significant volume of blood regurgitates into the right atrium during systole, resulting in right atrial dilation and increasing the risk of atrial arrhythmias. Increased right atrial pressure leads to central venous hypertension and liver congestion. The combined systemic venous return and regurgitant volume leads to volume overloading of the right ventricle. Contraction of the right ventricle is usually preserved in childhood and only rarely would right ventricular decompensation occur with impaired contraction and worsening of systemic venous congestion.

Table 15.8 Causes of tricuspid regurgitation in children

Nature of lesion	Cardiac condition
Congenital valvar abnormalities	Dysplastic tricuspid valve Ebstein malformation Pulmonary atresia with intact ventricular septum Complete atrioventricular septal defect
Damage to the valve leaflets	Infective endocarditis Post congenital heart surgery or transcatheter interventions
Connective tissue disease	Marfan syndrome Loeys-Dietz syndrome Ehlers-Danlos syndromes
Lysosomal storage disease	Mucopolysaccharidosis
Functional regurgitation (stretching of the tricuspid annulus due to right ventricular dilation)	Severe pulmonary regurgitation in repaired tetralogy of Fallot Atrial septal defect Pulmonary hypertension Systemic right ventricular dysfunction (tricuspid valve being the systemic atrioventricular valve)

Table 15.9 Signs of moderate to severe tricuspid regurgitation

Signs	Origins
Right ventricular impulse	Right ventricular volume overloading
Abnormal S2	Single S2 in repair tetralogy of Fallot or pulmonary atresia with intact ventricular septum, loud P2 suggests pulmonary hypertension
A pansystolic murmur at the left lower sternal border	The characteristic murmur of tricuspid regurgitation
Increased jugular venous pressure	Presence of 'cv wave' with attenuation of the x descent (Chap. 53)
Hepatomegaly and pulsatile liver	Liver congestion with transmission of atrial contraction and right ventricular systolic pressure wave to the liver

15.4.3 Clinical Presentation and Findings

Most children with tricuspid regurgitation are asymptomatic. Those with severe regurgitation may have symptoms of heart failure.

The physical signs of moderate to severe tricuspid regurgitation are those of right ventricular volume overloading and a pansystolic murmur at the left lower sternal border (Table 15.9).

15.4.4 Investigations

CXR: Cardiomegaly occurs in the presence of moderate to severe tricuspid regurgitation due to enlargement of the right atrium and the right ventricle.
ECG: The electrocardiogram shows right atrial and right ventricular dilation.
Echocardiography: Echocardiography demonstrates the tricuspid valve pathologies, enables the assessment the causes of functional tricuspid regurgitation (Fig. 15.4), and allows semi-quantitative assessment of the severity of tricuspid regurgitation (Box 15.5).

Box 15.5 Echocardiographic Evidence of Moderate to Severe Tricuspid Regurgitation

- Dilation of the right atrium and right ventricle
- Large regurgitant colour jet area
- Dense tricuspid regurgitant jet as assessed by continuous wave Doppler echocardiography
- Dilation of inferior caval vein
- Systolic flow reversal in hepatic veins

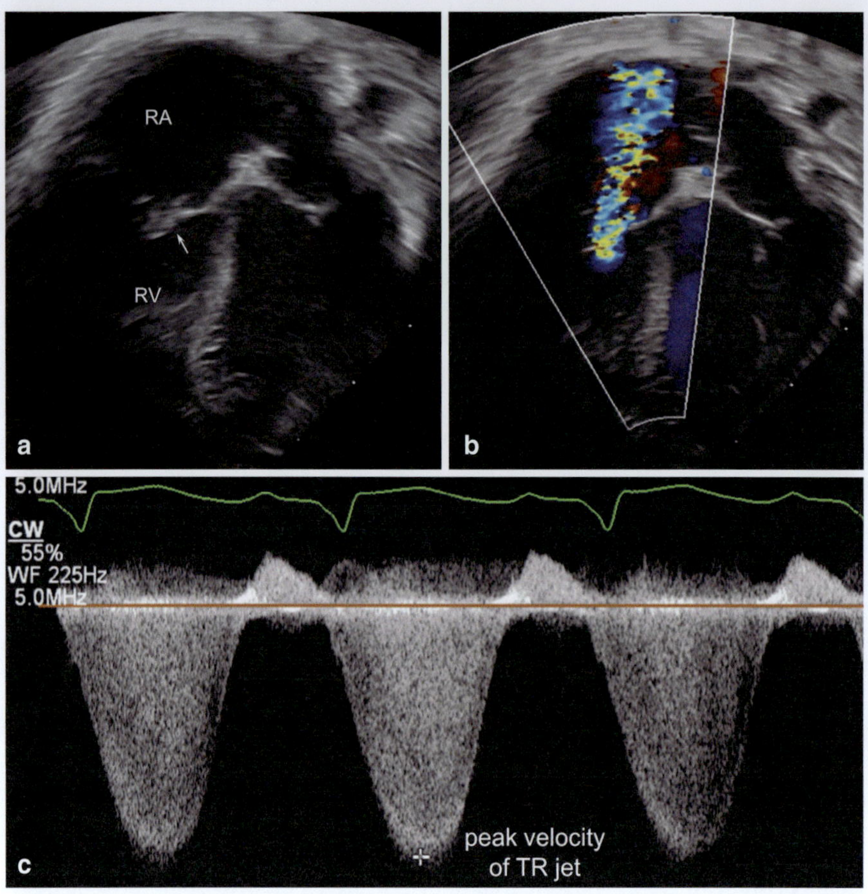

Fig. 15.4 Echocardiographic assessment of tricuspid regurgitation. (**a**) 2D echocardiography shows thickening of the tricuspid valve leaflets (arrow) in congenital dysplastic tricuspid valve (**b**) Doppler colour flow mapping demonstrates moderate tricuspid regurgitation (**c**) The dense tricuspid regurgitant jet as assessed by continuous wave Doppler echocardiography suggests at least moderate tricuspid regurgitation (Abbreviations: *RA* right atrium, *RV* right ventricle, *TR* tricuspid regurgitation)

15.4.5 Management Strategy

Diuretics may benefit patients with significant systemic venous congestion. Surgical intervention for tricuspid regurgitation is indicated in symptomatic patients. Functional tricuspid regurgitation related to severe pulmonary regurgitation in repaired tetralogy of Fallot and large atrial septal defects generally improve with management of the underlying conditions and reduction of right ventricular volume load and may not require tricuspid valvar intervention.

Part III

Cyanotic Congenital Heart Disease

16 Right Ventricular Outflow Obstructive Lesions with Right-to-Left Shunt

Cyanotic congenital heart lesions associated with right ventricular outflow obstruction is characterized by reduced blood flow to the pulmonary circulation and right-to-left shunting of blood at either the ventricular level (tetralogy of Fallot, pulmonary atresia with ventricular septal defect) or the atrial level (pulmonary atresia with intact ventricular septum).

Right-to-left shunting of blood refers to the flow of deoxygenated blood in the right-sided circulation to the systemic circulation, thereby causing arterial hypoxaemia and cyanosis clinically. Congestive heart failure is not a feature of cyanotic heart lesions with right ventricular outflow obstruction as the pulmonary flow is diminished and ventricular volume overloading is absent.

16.1 Tetralogy of Fallot

Tetralogy of Fallot is the most common cyanotic congenital heart disease. The detailed description in 1888 by Dr. Étienne-Arthur Louis Fallot, a French professor of hygiene and legal medicine, of the components of this common cause of 'la maladie bleu' (the blue disease) has led to the eponymous condition of tetralogy of Fallot.

16.1.1 Anatomy

Tetralogy of Fallot comprises four components: obstruction of the right ventricular outflow tract, right ventricular hypertrophy, a large ventricular septal defect, and an aorta that overrides the ventricular septum (Fig. 16.1).

The narrowest part of the right ventricular outflow tract is usually at the subpulmonary infundibulum, which is between the anterior-superiorly deviated outlet septum and the septoparietal trabeculations. Other levels of right ventricular outflow obstruction are frequently present and include valvar and supravalvar pulmonary

Y.-f. Cheung, *Congenital and Paediatric Acquired Heart Disease in Practice*, https://doi.org/10.1007/978-981-99-2862-0_16

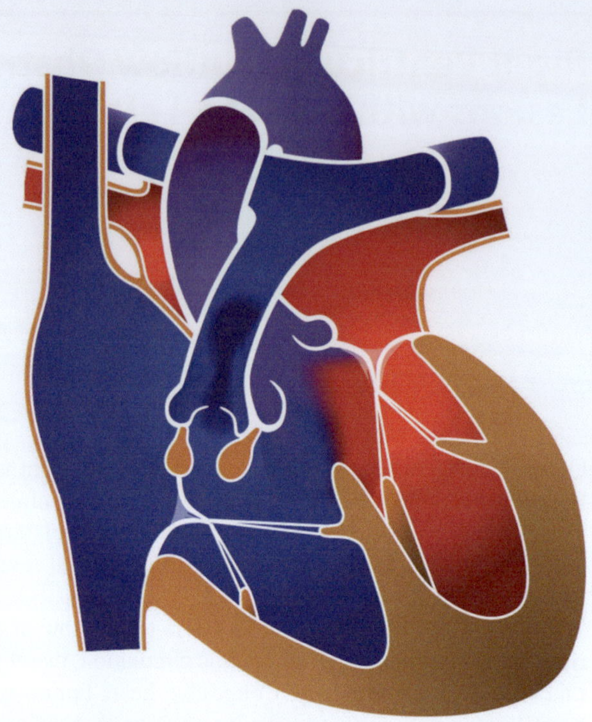

Fig. 16.1 Tetralogy of Fallot. The four components of tetralogy of Fallot are shown: obstruction of the right ventricular outflow, right ventricular hypertrophy, a large ventricular septal defect, and an aorta that overrides the ventricular septum

stenosis and narrowing of the branch pulmonary arteries. The ventricular septal defect is large and can be perimembranous, outlet, or subarterial in location. In tetralogy of Fallot with a subarterial defect, the outlet septum is fibrous rather than muscular in nature.

Associated cardiac anomalies in tetralogy Fallot include right-sided aortic arch (in 20%) and coronary arterial anomalies. The most common coronary arterial anomaly is anomalous origin of the left anterior descending artery arising from the right coronary artery, which has surgical implications as the artery crosses the right ventricular outflow tract anteriorly.

16.1.2 Pathophysiology

The haemodynamic consequences of tetralogy of Fallot are determined mainly by the severity of the right ventricular outflow obstruction. As the right ventricular outflow obstruction is usually significant, equalization of the right and left ventricular systolic pressures occurs. When the resistance of emptying into the pulmonary circulation exceeds that of the systemic circulation, blood in the right ventricle empties into the aorta (right-to-left shunt) and results in cyanosis clinically. When the outflow obstruction is less severe, a balanced situation may occur with no net shunting in either direction (the so-called 'pink Fallot'). When the obstruction is mild, left-to-right shunt predominates and the haemodynamic consequences in this group of 'pink Fallot' patients are those of a large ventricular septal defect. Uncommonly, partial coverage of the ventricular septal defect by tricuspid valve aneurysm limits the right-to-left shunt, improves cyanosis, and leads to a supra-systemic level of right ventricular systolic pressure.

16.1.3 Clinical Manifestations

The timing of presentation and severity of cyanosis are related to the degree of pulmonary stenosis. In newborn babies with severe infundibular stenosis, the pulmonary circulation is duct-dependent, and cyanosis occurs within hours after birth. Most of the children with tetralogy of Fallot are acyanotic at birth and present with cyanosis in infancy due to progressive infundibular stenosis. In older children, squatting on exercise is characteristic. Squatting reduces right-to-left shunting of blood by increasing the systemic vascular resistance and promotes pulmonary arterial flow by increasing the systemic venous return.

Signs of tetralogy of Fallot are those of right ventricular outflow obstruction (Table 16.1). Heart failure is usually not a feature of tetralogy of Fallot but may be present in the so-called 'pink Fallot' with minimal degree of pulmonary stenosis (mimicking the presentation of a large ventricular septal defect).

Hypercyanotic or tet spell is a potentially left-threatening complication (Table 16.2). It is characterized by unprovoked intense episodes of cyanosis,

Table 16.1 Signs of tetralogy of Fallot

Signs	Origins
Cyanosis	Cyanosis worsens with increasing severity of the right ventricular outflow obstruction
Right ventricular impulse	Right ventricular pressure overloading
Single S2	Soft and inaudible P2
An ejection systolic murmur at the left upper sternal border	Related to pulmonary stenosis and not ventricular septal defect

Table 16.2 Clinical features and management of hypercyanotic spell

Clinical features	Management
Irritability	Hold and calm the baby
Prolonged crying	Maintain knee-chest position
Hyperpnoea	Subcutaneous / intravenous morphine
Intense cyanosis	Intravenous sodium bicarbonate
Loss of consciousness	Intravenous esmolol / propranolol
Decreased murmur intensity	Intravenous vasoconstrictor (phenylephrine)
	Intravenous fluid bolus
	For severe spell
	Intubate and paralyze
	Emergency shunt operation

hyperpnoea and irritability, and may result in the loss of consciousness, convulsion, and brain damage. Hypothesized mechanisms include spasm of the right ventricular outflow tract, fall in systemic vascular resistance, and increased sympathetic activity with tachycardia-induced decrease in right ventricular preload.

In patients with chronic severe cyanosis, the risk of stroke and brain abscess formation is increased.

16.1.4 Investigations

CXR: The cardiac silhouette has a characteristic boot shape (coeur-en-sabot), with elevation of the cardiac apex due to right ventricular hypertrophy and concavity of the left upper cardiac border (pulmonary bay) due to a small pulmonary trunk. The presence a right-sided aortic arch exaggerates the concavity. The pulmonary vascular markings may be reduced, normal or increased, depending on the severity of right ventricular outflow obstruction.

ECG: Electrocardiogram shows right axis deviation and right ventricular hypertrophy.

Echocardiography: Echocardiography demonstrates the four components of tetralogy of Fallot, enables the assessment the size of the pulmonary valve annulus, size and stenosis of branch pulmonary arteries, patency of the arterial duct, origins of the coronary arteries, and sidedness of the aortic arch, and provides an estimation of peak systolic pressure gradient across the right ventricular outflow tract (Fig. 16.2).

CT: Computed tomography is usually not required. It may be useful in some patients to define the origins and course of coronary arteries (when echocardiographic assessment fails), large aortopulmonary collaterals (uncommon in tetralogy of Fallot with pulmonary stenosis), patency of the systemic-to-pulmonary arterial shunt, and shunt-associated pulmonary arterial distortion.

Genetic evaluation: Genetic testing for 22q11.2 microdeletion and assessment for associated features of DiGeorge syndrome is required (Chap. 62).

16.1.5 Management Strategy

The management strategy of neonates and infants with severe cyanosis and recurrent cyanotic spells differs among centres. In some, primary surgical repair is contemplated regardless of the age or size of patients. In others, the strategy of oral propranolol to manage hypercyanotic spell and palliative surgical or transcatheter interventional procedures to augment pulmonary flow is adopted in young infants with severe cyanosis or uncontrolled cyanotic spells, in patients with hypoplastic pulmonary arteries, and in premature or low body weight babies until corrective surgery after 3–4 months of age. These palliative procedures include insertion of a modified Blalock-Taussig shunt, balloon dilation and stenting of the right ventricular outflow, and stenting of the arterial duct.

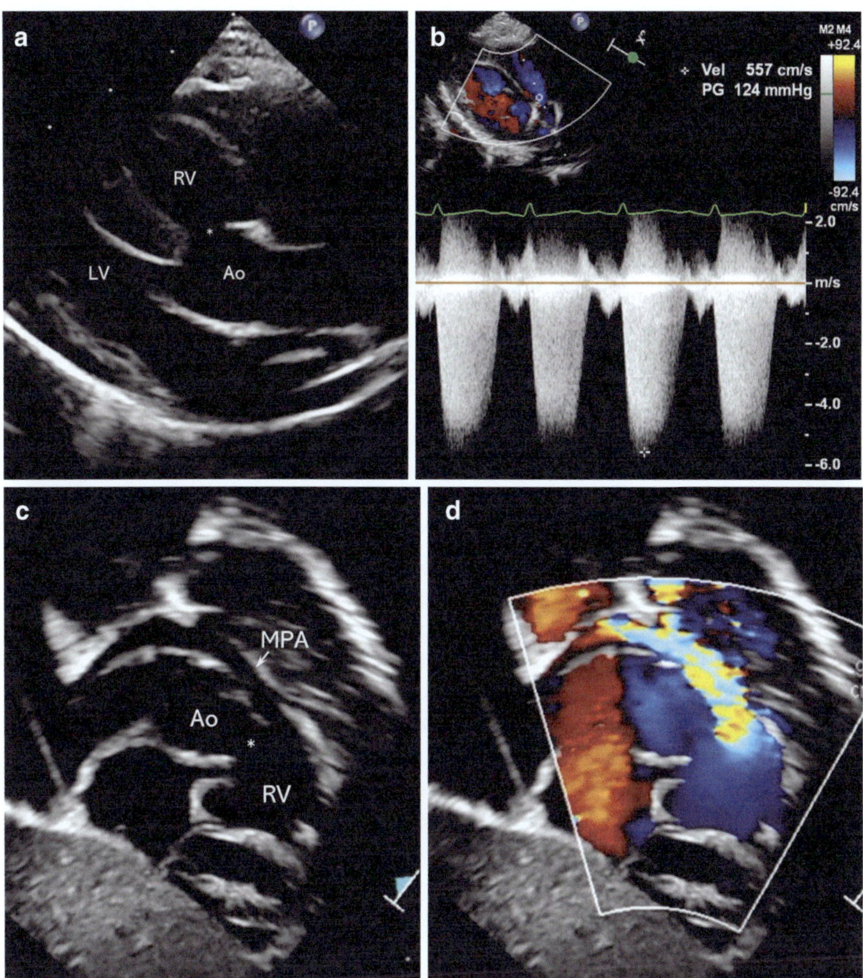

Fig. 16.2 Echocardiographic assessment of tetralogy of Fallot. (**a**) Parasternal long axis view showing the ventricular septal defect (asterisk) and overriding aorta (**b**) Continuous wave Doppler echocardiography reveals a significant pressure gradient across the right ventricular outflow (**c**) Subcostal anterior oblique view demonstrating the ventricular septal defect (asterisk) and hypoplasia of the pulmonary valve annulus and main pulmonary artery (**d**) Colour flow mapping reveals high velocity flow across the right ventricular outflow (Abbreviations: *Ao* aorta, *LV* left ventricle, *MPA* main pulmonary artery, *RV* right ventricle)

Corrective surgery involves repair of the ventricular septal defect and enlargement of the right ventricular outflow by resection of infundibular muscle with insertion of a patch across the pulmonary annulus (transannular patch) where indicated. The placement of a transannular patch results in free pulmonary regurgitation. There are increasing attempts in the current era to preserve the pulmonary valve at the expense of modest degree of residual right ventricular outflow obstruction. The maintenance or creation of an interatrial communication is common in anticipation of development of low cardiac output syndrome secondary to restrictive right ventricular physiology (Chap. 27).

16.1.6 Postoperative Considerations

Important postoperative complications include low cardiac output syndrome and cardiac arrhythmias.

The low cardiac output syndrome after repair of tetralogy of Fallot is characterized by tachycardia (sinus or junctional ectopic tachycardia), low blood pressure, high central venous pressure, normal left atrial pressure, oliguria, and metabolic acidosis. Residual significant right ventricular outflow obstruction and left-to-right shunt must be excluded. Most commonly, this complication is due to postoperative restrictive right ventricular physiology (Chap. 27). Postoperative arrhythmias include complete heart block and junctional ectopic tachycardia.

Initial intensive care management includes standard fluid restriction, boluses of fluid to maintain right ventricular preload in the presence of restrictive right ventricular physiology, maintenance of a sinus rhythm, judicious use of inotropes and inodilators to avoid excessive tachycardia and severe vasodilation (although low dose milrinone infusion may have lusitropic effect on the right ventricle), and diuretics. Systemic vasoconstrictor is used to maintain the systemic perfusion pressure. In some centres, esmolol infusion is used postoperatively in the hope of slowing the heart rate to increase diastolic filling time and hence the right ventricular stroke volume. Patients should be ventilated with a low mean airway pressure and extubated early if possible. The low cardiac output syndrome and right-to-left shunt through the interatrial communication usually begin to improve after 48 hours as the right ventricular compliance improves over 48 to 72 hours postoperatively.

16.1.7 Long-Term Monitoring

Despite reparative surgery, follow up is required for the monitoring of long-term morbidities, which include chronic pulmonary regurgitation and its functional consequences (Chap. 15), ventricular and atrial arrhythmias, residual structural lesions (obstruction or aneurysmal dilation of the right ventricular outflow, branch pulmonary arterial stenosis, leak across the patched ventricular septal defect), tricuspid regurgitation, and progressive dilation of the aortic root (Chap. 33).

16.2 Tetralogy of Fallot with Absent Pulmonary Valve Syndrome

Congenital absence of the pulmonary valve is a rare cardiac malformation. It occurs commonly in association with tetralogy of Fallot. This combination of lesions is termed tetralogy of Fallot with absent pulmonary valve syndrome.

Rarely, absence of pulmonary valve is associated other types of congenital heart disease, which include atrial septal defect, atrioventricular septal defect, double-outlet right ventricle, coarctation and interruption of the aortic arch, transposition of the great arteries, and persistent arterial duct. The section focuses on tetralogy of Fallot with absent pulmonary valve syndrome.

16.2.1 Anatomy

Absent pulmonary valve syndrome has been reported to occur in about 3–5% of patients with tetralogy of Fallot. Tetralogy of Fallot with absent pulmonary valve syndrome has the typical anatomy of ventricular septal defect, overriding of aorta, variable degrees of pulmonary stenosis, and right ventricular hypertrophy (Fig. 16.3). The cardinal feature is rudimentary development or absence of pulmonary valvar tissue. The hypoplastic pulmonary annulus and narrow infundibulum cause varying degree of pulmonary stenosis.

An arterial duct is almost always absent in tetralogy of Fallot with absent pulmonary valve syndrome. The absence of an arterial duct has been proposed to play a pathogenetic role in the abnormal development of the pulmonary valve by altering the flow haemodynamics in the developing pulmonary artery.

Marked dilation of the main pulmonary trunk and branch pulmonary arteries can occur in utero, which is probably related to increased pulmonary arterial pulsatility due to significant pulmonary regurgitation or increased pulmonary blood due to the relatively mild pulmonary stenosis. Marked dilation of the pulmonary arteries causes extrinsic compression of the trachea and bronchi and tracheobronchomalacia.

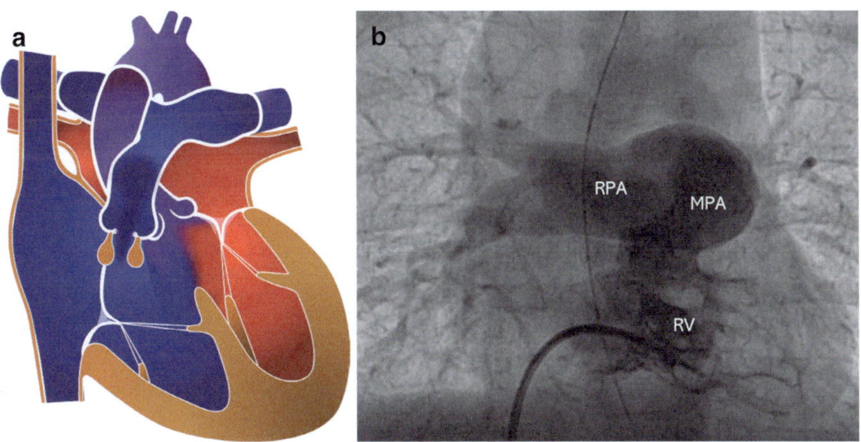

Fig. 16.3 Tetralogy of Fallot with absent pulmonary valve syndrome. (**a**) Illustration of tetralogy of Fallot with absent pulmonary valve syndrome (**b**) Angiographic demonstration of gross dilation of main pulmonary artery and right pulmonary artery (*MPA* main pulmonary artery, *RPA* right pulmonary artery, *RV* right ventricle)

16.2.2 Pathophysiology

Heart failure may occur in utero and cause hydrops fetalis and fetal demise. Postnatally, the pathophysiology is similar to that of tetralogy of Fallot. Additionally, depending on severity of pulmonary arterial dilation, varying degrees of extrinsic compression of the trachea and bronchi and tracheobronchomalacia are usually present.

16.2.3 Clinical Manifestations

The initial presentation depends on severity of extrinsic compression of the airway and tracheobronchomalacia. About half of the patients present at birth or soon afterwards with respiratory symptoms, which range from mild stridor to severe shortness of breath. Babies without significant airway obstruction have presentations similar to patients with tetralogy of Fallot.

The signs are those of tetralogy of Fallot. Two additional signs are unique to tetralogy of Fallot with absent pulmonary valve syndrome: (a) obvious respiratory distress and occasional stridor in babies with significant airway obstruction, and (b) a to-and-fro murmur (Table 16.3).

16.2.4 Investigations

CXR: The cardiac silhouette is boot-shaped as in tetralogy of Fallot with elevation of the cardiac apex due to right ventricular hypertrophy. Cardiomegaly is caused by right ventricular dilation and, in the presence of significant left-to-right shunt when pulmonary stenosis is mild, left ventricular dilation. The silhouette of the aneurysmally dilated main pulmonary trunk and branch pulmonary arteries can sometimes be appreciated. Air-trapping due to airway obstruction may be present.

Table 16.3 Signs of tetralogy of Fallot with absent pulmonary valve syndrome

Signs	Origins
Cyanosis	Degree of cyanosis varies with the severity of the right ventricular outflow obstruction
Right ventricular impulse	Right ventricular pressure and volume overloading
Single S2	Absent P2
To-and-fro murmur at the left upper sternal border	An ejection systolic murmur followed by an early diastolic murmur related to concomitant pulmonary stenosis and regurgitation
Respiratory distress and stridor	Extrinsic compression of the trachea and bronchi and tracheobronchomalacia and left-to-shunt if the pulmonary stenosis is mild

ECG: Electrocardiogram shows right axis deviation and right ventricular dilation and hypertrophy.
Echocardiography: Echocardiographic assessment demonstrates the anatomy of tetralogy of Fallot and rudimentary or absent pulmonary valvar tissue and provides an assessment of severity of pulmonary stenosis and regurgitation, right ventricular dilation, and aneurysmal dilation of the main pulmonary trunk and branch pulmonary arteries. Hyperinflation of the lungs may, however, limit the acoustic window.
CT: Computed tomography is useful for the delineation of dilation of the pulmonary arteries, including the distal branches, their relationship with the tracheobronchial tree, and severity of extrinsic compression of the airway.
Flexible bronchoscopy: This demonstrates extrinsic tracheobronchial compression and the malacic component of the airway narrowing.
Genetic evaluation: Genetic testing for 22q11.2 microdeletion and assessment for associated features of DiGeorge syndrome is required (Chap. 62).

16.2.5 Management Strategy

For patients with no respiratory distress, which suggests the absence of significant airway compression or malacia, the standard management of tetralogy of Fallot applies. In these patients, surgical reduction of the enlarged pulmonary arteries may not be necessary.

For patients with significant airway compromise, early operation during the neonatal period is required. Different surgical approaches have been adopted. These include (a) surgical reduction (plication and partial excision) of pulmonary arteries to decrease their diameters with or without performance of the Lecompte manoeuvre (translocation of the pulmonary arteries anterior to the aorta) and (b) removal of the main pulmonary trunk and proximal branch pulmonary arteries with replacement using a homograft. Additional procedures including pulmonary arteriopexy with or without aortopexy and stenting of the malacic airway may be required.

16.2.6 Postoperative Considerations

The postoperative cardiac issues are those after repair of tetralogy of Fallot. Respiratory management of the malacic airways and other complications including air trapping and lung atelectasis requires fine manipulation of the positive end expiratory pressure and mean airway pressure and frequent airway suction. Long-term ventilation with tracheostomy is required in patients with severe tracheobronchomalacia.

16.2.7 Long-Term Monitoring

While survival after surgery has improved in the current era, patients with significant airways abnormalities continue to have significant morbidity and mortality despite cardiac surgery. The need for long-term ventilation is required in about one-third of the patients.

16.3 Pulmonary Atresia with Ventricular Septal Defect

Pulmonary atresia with ventricular septal defect has the intracardiac anatomy of that of tetralogy of Fallot, but with pulmonary atresia rather than pulmonary stenosis. This malformation is commonly regarded as the extremely end of the spectrum of tetralogy of Fallot and is hence also termed 'tetralogy of Fallot with pulmonary atresia'.

16.3.1 Anatomy

Pulmonary atresia with ventricular septal defect shares most of the components of tetralogy of Fallot with pulmonary stenosis. Right ventricular hypertrophy, ventricular septal defect (usually perimembranous, but can also be muscular or subarterial), and an overriding aorta are typically present. It differs, however, from tetralogy of Fallot with pulmonary stenosis in two main aspects: (a) complete atresia of the right ventricular outflow, and (b) the wide spectrum of pulmonary arterial abnormalities and variable pulmonary arterial supply (Fig. 16.4).

Atresia of the right ventricular outflow is usually caused by complete muscular obliteration of the infundibulum with absence of the main pulmonary trunk. Less commonly, there is pulmonary valve atresia, and the main pulmonary trunk is present. The latter type of atresia is amenable to initial palliative transcatheter perforation.

For the pulmonary arterial anatomy, the intrapericardial native right and left pulmonary arteries may be present and can be confluent or non-confluent. In the most severe cases of pulmonary atresia with pulmonary atresia, native pulmonary arteries are absent. Blood supply to the lungs is derived from the systemic arterial circulation through the persistent arterial duct and/or multiple aortopulmonary pulmonary collateral arteries (MAPCAs). 'Unifocal' blood supply to the lungs refer to all lung segments being supplied by the confluent branch pulmonary arteries, whereas 'multifocal' supply refers to the situation when different parts of the lung are supplied by more than one source.

Three major patterns of pulmonary arterial supply to the lungs in pulmonary atresia with ventricular septal defect are recognized. These form the basis of classification of the cardiac malformation by the Congenital Heart Surgery Nomenclature and Database Project (Table 16.4) Given the variation in the pulmonary arterial

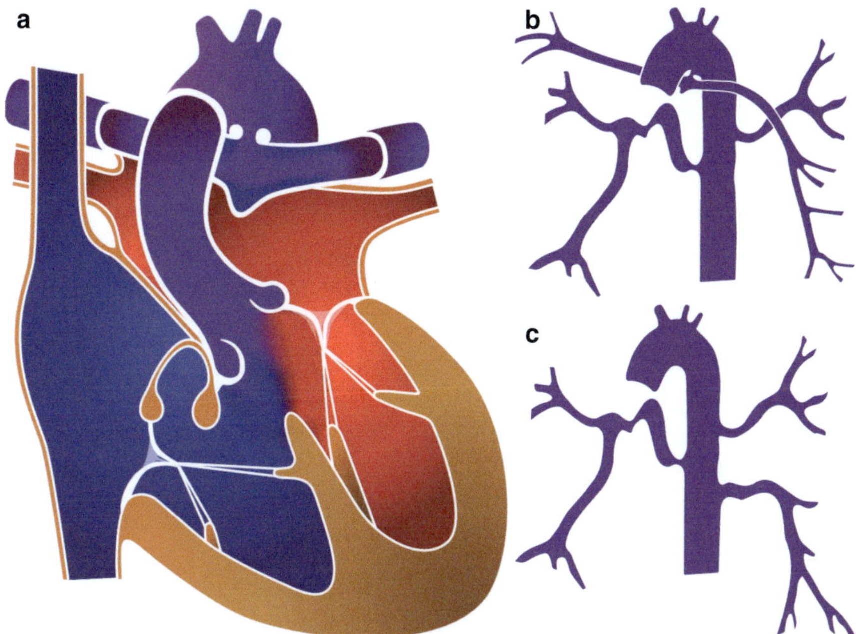

Fig. 16.4 Pulmonary atresia with ventricular septal defect. Atretic pulmonary outflow with (**a**) type A (**b**) type B and (**c**) type C pattern of pulmonary arterial supply

Table 16.4 Classification of pulmonary atresia with ventricular septal defect based on the pattern of pulmonary arterial supply to the lungs

Type	Description
A	Presence of native pulmonary arteries (usually confluent and supplied by a unilateral arterial duct, but rarely non-confluent and supplied by bilateral arterial ducts) and no MAPCAs
B	Confluent native pulmonary arteries coexisting with MAPCAs (the confluent native pulmonary arteries usually do not supply all pulmonary segments and MAPCAs supply those not perfused by the native pulmonary arteries)
C	Absence of native pulmonary arteries with all the lung segments being supplied by MAPCAs

anatomy and pulmonary arterial supply, pulmonary atresia with ventricular septal defect is regarded as one of the most complex congenital heart conditions to manage.

16.3.2 Pathophysiology

As the right ventricular outflow is atretic, there is right-to-left shunting of the entire systemic venous return through the ventricular septal defect into the aorta. Mixing of pulmonary and systemic venous blood occurs at the aorta. Distribution of aortic blood between the systemic and pulmonary circulation depends on the relative resistance of the two circulations. High pulmonary blood flow, due to a large arterial duct supplying the confluent pulmonary arteries or large MAPCAs, leads to high systemic oxygen saturation and heart failure. The high flow through large MAPCAs can further lead to development of pulmonary vascular disease. On the other hand, constriction of the arterial duct or progressive localized stenoses of the MAPCAs limits pulmonary arterial flow and causes poor systemic oxygenation.

16.3.3 Clinical Manifestations

Most neonates with pulmonary atresia and ventricular septal defect present with cyanosis within a few hours after birth due to ductal closure (duct-dependent pulmonary circulation). In babies with large MAPCAs, cyanosis may not be obvious and heart failure may develop at 4–6 weeks of age when the pulmonary vascular resistance drops. With time, however, many of these babies develop progressive cyanosis as they begin to outgrow the source of pulmonary blood supply with concomitant progressive stenoses of the MAPCAs.

The physical findings are similar to those of tetralogy of Fallot, except for the absence of the murmur of pulmonary stenosis. In patients with abundant aortopulmonary collaterals, continuous collateral murmurs are audible (Table 16.5).

16.3.4 Investigations

CXR: The cardiac silhouette has a characteristic boot shape (coeur-en-sabot). Right ventricular hypertrophy elevates the cardiac apex, while severe hypoplasia or absence of the pulmonary trunk and a right-sided aortic arch, occurring in 50% of patients, cause pronounced concavity of the left upper cardiac border. When the pulmonary blood flow is limited as a result of ductal constriction or stenosed MAPCAs, the vascular markings are diminished (oligaemic lung fields). In the presence of MAPCAs, the pulmonary vascular markings appear uneven as the perfused regions depend on the course, position, and size of the collaterals.
ECG: Electrocardiogram shows right axis deviation and right ventricular hypertrophy.

Table 16.5 Signs of pulmonary atresia with ventricular septal defect

Signs	Origins
Cyanosis	Degree of cyanosis depends on the amount of pulmonary flow via the arterial duct and/or aortopulmonary collaterals
Right ventricular impulse	Right ventricular pressure overloading
Single S2	Absent P2 as the pulmonary outflow is atretic
Absence of cardiac murmur or soft systolic/continuous murmur	Soft murmurs are related to flow through an arterial duct and/or aortopulmonary collaterals

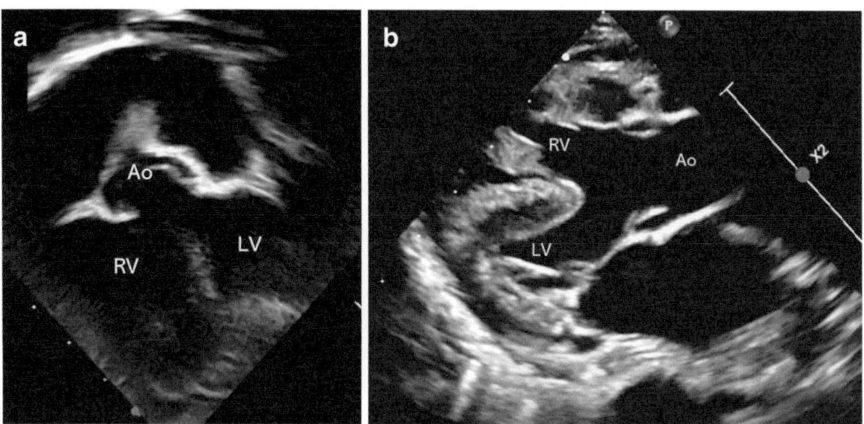

Fig. 16.5 Echocardiographic assessment of pulmonary atresia with ventricular septal defect. (**a**) Five-chamber and (**b**) parasternal long-axis views showing overriding of the aorta and a large ventricular septal defect (*Ao* aorta, *RV* right ventricle, *LV* left ventricle)

Echocardiography: Echocardiography demonstrates the ventricular septal defect and overriding aorta (Fig. 16.5), the type of atresia (membranous versus muscular) of the right ventricular outflow, the anatomy and size of the native pulmonary arteries, patency of the arterial duct, sidedness of the aortic arch, and presence or absence of aortopulmonary collateral flow. However, detailed delineation of aortopulmonary collaterals can only be achieved using cardiac catheterization, computed tomography, or magnetic resonance imaging.

Cardiac catheterization: Cardiac catheterization with angiography aims to define (a) the source of pulmonary supply, (b) the anatomy of the native pulmonary arteries and lung segments being supplied, and (c) the origin, course, and stenoses of MAPCAs, their connections with the native pulmonary arteries, and lung segments being supplied (Fig. 16.6a, b).

CT: Computed tomography angiography is increasingly used to define the anatomy of native pulmonary arteries and origins and distribution of the MAPCAs (Fig. 16.6c, d). The dataset can further be used for 3D printing for better planning of interventions.

Genetic evaluation: Genetic testing for 22q11.2 microdeletion and assessment for associated features of DiGeorge syndrome is required (Chap. 62).

16.3.5 Management

In most of the babies, intravenous prostaglandin E infusion is required to maintain ductal patency before the next stage of management. The subsequent management strategy is individualized and based on (a) whether native pulmonary arteries are present, (b) the size of native pulmonary arteries if present, and (c) the pattern of pulmonary arterial supply.

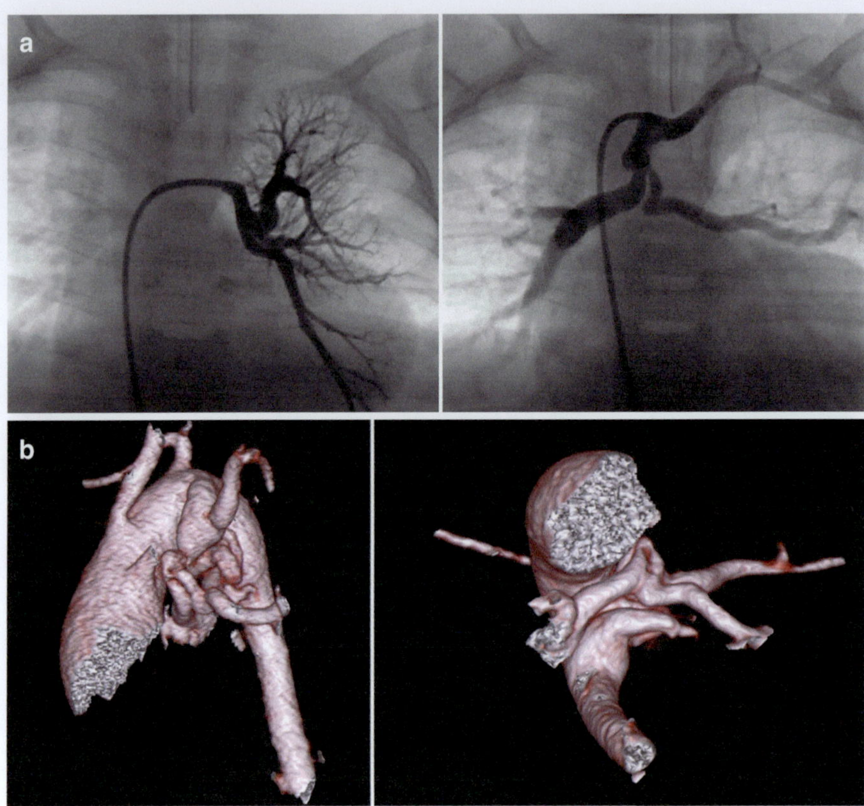

Fig. 16.6 Angiographic and CT imaging of MAPCAs. (**a**) Angiographic and (**b**) computed tomographic illustrations of MPACAs in an infant with pulmonary atresia with ventricular septal defect

Good-sized native pulmonary arteries with unifocal supply from the arterial duct: Options include (a) insertion of a systemic-to-pulmonary arterial shunt in the neonatal period with definitive surgery in the first few years of life, and (b) neonatal repair with closure of ventricular septal defect and placement of a right ventricle-to-pulmonary artery valved conduit.

Hypoplastic native pulmonary arteries with unifocal supply from the arterial duct: The initial palliative procedure aims to augment pulmonary arterial growth. Options include insertion of a systemic-to-pulmonary arterial shunt, implantation of a ductal stent, or perforation of the atretic pulmonary valve when present with stenting of the right ventricular outflow.

MAPCAs with native pulmonary arteries: It is important to define whether the MAPCAs constitute a dual blood supply or the sole supply to certain pulmonary segments, based on which different management approaches are adopted (Fig. 16.7). While debates on the unifocalization (to anastomose the MAPCAs to the native pulmonary arteries) versus 'rehabilitation' (with a central shunt) approach to

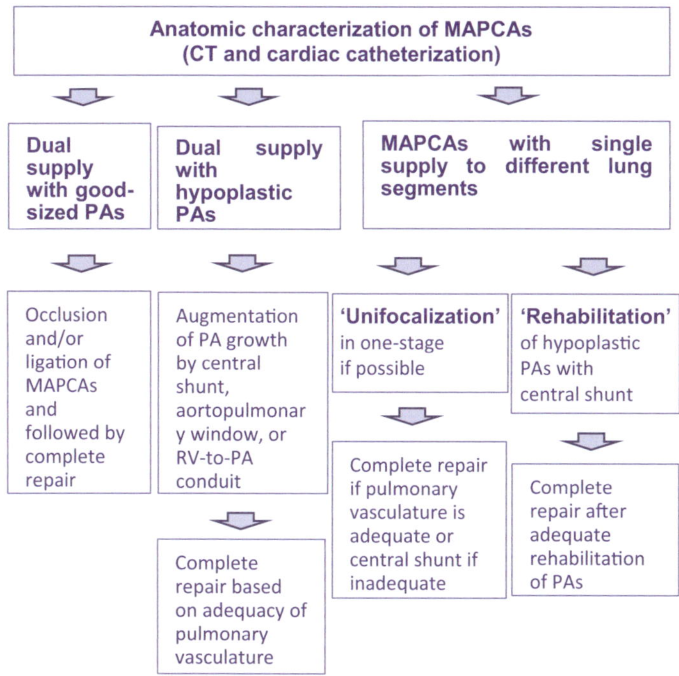

Fig. 16.7 Management based on characterization of MAPCAs. *MAPCAs* multiple aortopulmonary collaterals, *PAs* pulmonary arteries, *RV* right ventricle

manage MPACAs with single supply to different lung segments are ongoing, many centres regard these approaches as complementary in the management of this complex congenital heart lesion.

MAPCAs only with no native pulmonary arteries: This is the most difficult type to manage. Conservative management with palliative measures to improve systemic oxygen saturation (shunt insertion, balloon dilation and stenting of stenosed MAPCAs) when necessary has been adopted in some centres, with the ultimate aim of heart-lung transplantation. Unifocalization of MAPCAs to a central pulmonary confluence, created using a prosthetic or pericardial tube and supplied by a shunt, has also been attempted.

Decision to close the ventricular septal defect: Complete surgical repair involves closure of the ventricular septal defect and placement of an appropriately sized conduit between the right ventricle and the pulmonary artery confluence. This is feasible, however, only if the pulmonary arteries are of satisfactory sizes and supplying adequate lung segments. When closure of the defect is not deemed possible, a central shunt or a restricted right ventricular-to-pulmonary arterial conduit is placed as the source of pulmonary blood flow. Further surgical and/or transcatheter rehabilitation of the pulmonary arteries is required before closure of the defect can be contemplated.

16.3.6 Postoperative Considerations

The postoperative considerations depend on the type of initial intervention. Issues on the balance between pulmonary and systemic flow and the optimal SaO2 after shunting are discussed in Chap. 54. For patients who have undergone unifocalization, measures to optimize pulmonary flow (similar to those described after shunting) may be required. For patients after total repair, the important postoperative complications and initial intensive care management are similar to those after repair of tetralogy of Fallot.

16.3.7 Long-Term Monitoring

Most patients require multiple surgical and transcatheter interventions for rehabilitation of the pulmonary arteries. The chance of successful complete repair has been reported to vary between 40–80%. There are patients who never become candidates for definitive repair because of poor development of the native pulmonary arteries or the unifocalized MAPCAs despite aggressive rehabilitation. For patients who have undergone complete repair, follow up is required for the monitoring of long-term morbidities including conduit dysfunction and other issues as described for repaired tetralogy of Fallot.

16.4 Pulmonary Atresia with Intact Ventricular Septum

Pulmonary atresia with intact ventricular septum is characterized by complete obstruction of the right ventricular outflow tract. This is a heterogeneous congenital cardiac malformation with variations in tricuspid valvar abnormalities, right ventricular hypoplasia, and coronary arterial anomalies. The heterogeneities in anatomy and physiology pose significant challenges in the management of this congenital heart disease.

16.4.1 Anatomy

In pulmonary atresia with intact ventricular septum, complete obstruction of the right ventricular outflow tract is due to imperforation of pulmonary valve or complete muscular obliteration of the infundibulum (Fig. 16.8).

The right ventricle is usually hypoplastic and hypertrophied, although rarely the right ventricle can be grossly dilated and thin walled when the tricuspid valve is severely dysplastic or having severe Ebstein malformation with significant tricuspid regurgitation. In describing the hypoplastic right ventricles, the terms tripartite, bipartite, and unipartite have been used. The normal right ventricle is tripartite and consists of inlet, apical trabecular, and outlet components. In pulmonary atresia

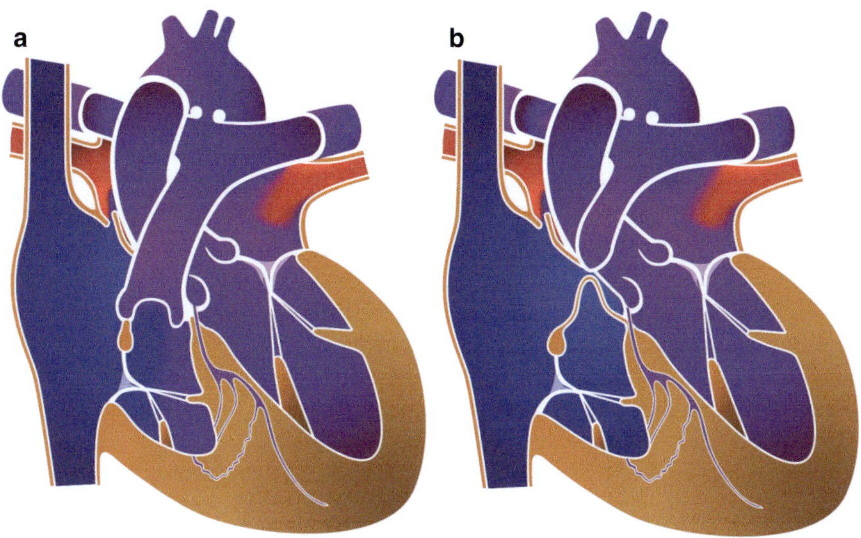

Fig. 16.8 Pulmonary atresia with intact ventricular septum. (**a**) Complete obstruction of the right ventricular outflow tract due to imperforation of pulmonary valve (**b**) Complete muscular obliteration of the infundibulum

Table 16.6 Partite classification of the right ventricle

Partite	Frequency	Description
Tripartite	About 60%	Consists of inlet, apical trabecular, and outlet components
Bipartite	About 30%	With only inlet and outlet components due to hypertrophic overgrowth of the apical trabecular component
Unipartite	About 5% to 10%	Severely hypoplastic right ventricle with only an inlet component due to muscular obliteration of both the apical and outlet components

with intact ventricular septum, one or two of the components may be obliterated by the severely hypertrophic myocardium (Table 16.6).

The tricuspid valve is usually small, incompetent (but stenotic in some), and abnormal. Its size parallels the degree of right ventricular hypoplasia. Abnormalities include dysplasia of the leaflets, malformation of the valvar apparatus, and Ebstein malformation.

Fistulous communications between the coronary arteries and right ventricular sinusoids may develop, most commonly in association with severe right ventricular hypoplasia, for decompression of the hypertensive right ventricle. Coronary arterial abnormalities include coronary arterial stenoses or interruptions, and atresia of the aortocoronary connection. Recognition of these coronary arterial abnormalities is important given the physiologic and management implications of a right ventricular-dependent coronary circulation as discussed below.

16.4.2 Pathophysiology

Complete obstruction of the right ventricular outflow causes severe pressure overloading of the right ventricle. The systolic pressure generated by the right ventricle may exceed that of the left ventricle, as no ventricular septal defect is present to equalize the pressures between the two ventricles (in contrast to pulmonary atresia with ventricular septal defect). Blood within the hypertensive right ventricle is usually emptied into the right atrium via tricuspid regurgitation. In patients with right ventriculo-coronary fistulous communications, blood in the right ventricle may empty through these communications into the ascending aorta during systole.

Right ventricular-dependent coronary circulation describes the reliance of the coronary blood flow on retrograde blood flow from the right ventricular cavity. It occurs in the presence of coronary arterial stenoses, coronary arterial interruptions, or atresia of the aortocoronary connection, all of which limit or prevent normal antegrade perfusion of the myocardium from the aorta. Recognition of this phenomenon has two implications: (a) surgical or transcatheter decompression of the right ventricle is contraindicated because decompression of the hypertensive right ventricle may lead to coronary artery steal, myocardial ischaemia and infarction, and sudden cardiac death, and (b) supply of deoxygenated blood from the right ventricle to the coronary arterial circulation may contribute to ventricular dysfunction in the long term.

There is obligatory right-to-left shunting of the systemic venous return from the right to the left atrium through the oval foramen. As the arterial duct represents the sole source of pulmonary blood supply, its patency is essential for survival (duct-dependent pulmonary circulation).

16.4.3 Clinical Manifestations and Findings

Neonates with pulmonary atresia and intact ventricular septum usually present within few hours after birth as the arterial duct closes (duct-dependent pulmonary circulation). Less commonly, shortness of breath may be present in babies with severe tricuspid regurgitation. Although this defect is associated with right ventricular outflow obstruction, the associated right ventricular hypoplasia leads to the absence of a right ventricular impulse. Murmurs may not be audible. If present, they are related to ductal flow and tricuspid regurgitation (Table 16.7).

Table 16.7 Signs of pulmonary atresia with intact ventricular septum

Signs	Origins
Cyanosis	Degree of cyanosis depends on the size of the arterial duct
Left ventricular impulse	Enlargement of the left ventricle as it receives both the systemic and pulmonary venous return; by contrast, right ventricular impulse is absent as the right ventricle is usually hypoplastic
Single S2	Absent P2 as the pulmonary outflow is atretic
A pansystolic murmur at the left lower sternal border or a soft systolic or continuous murmur at the left upper sternal border	Tricuspid regurgitation causes the pansystolic murmur, while ductal flow causes the soft systolic or continuous murmur

16.4.4 Investigations

CXR: The heart size may be normal or enlarged on the chest radiograph. In the presence of severe tricuspid regurgitation, the right atrium is grossly enlarged. The pulmonary vascular markings are usually diminished.

ECG: Electrocardiogram shows right atrial dilation, paucity of right ventricular forces, and left ventricular dominance.

Echocardiography: Echocardiography confirms the diagnosis and the type of pulmonary atresia (valvar versus infundibular) and enables the assessment of the adequacy of the obligatory right-to-left shunt through the patent oval foramen or atrial septal defect and ductal flow to supply the pulmonary circulation (Fig. 16.9). Further echocardiographic evaluation should focus on the definition of the heterogenous anatomic features that would guide management: (a) right ventricular morphology (partite classification), (b) right ventricular size (area of right ventricle, tricuspid valve z score, tricuspid-to-mitral valve annulus ratio), (c) severity of tricuspid valvar regurgitation and malformation, and (d) fistulous communications between the coronary arteries and right ventricular sinusoids (abnormal Doppler colour flow signals within the right ventricular myocardium) and (e) origins of the coronary arteries from the sinuses of Valsalva.

Cardiac catheterization: Cardiac catheterization is performed (a) in neonates suitable to undergo transcatheter intervention, and (b) in patients suspected to have right ventricular-dependent coronary circulation to define the coronary arterial anatomy.

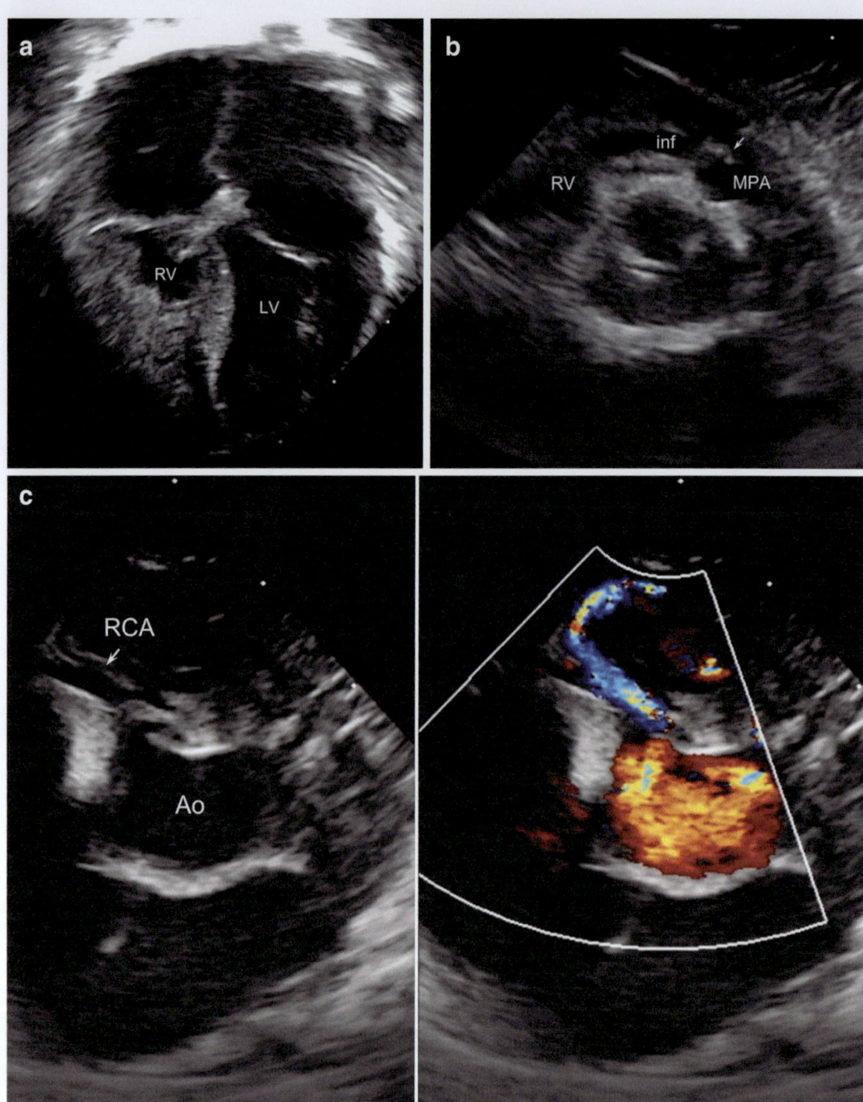

Fig. 16.9 Echocardiographic assessment of pulmonary atresia with intact ventricular septum. (**a**) A hypoplastic bipartite right ventricle with hypertrophic overgrowth of the apical trabecular component (**b**) Echocardiographic demonstration of an atretic pulmonary valve (arrow) (**c**) 2D echocardiography demonstrating dilation of the right coronary artery and colour flow mapping showing right ventriculo-coronary communications (Abbreviations: *Ao* aorta, *inf* infundibulum, *LV* left ventricle, *MPA* main pulmonary artery, *RV* right ventricle)

16.4.5 Management Strategy

Initial stabilization: Intravenous prostaglandin E is given to maintain ductal patency. In neonates with a restrictive atrial communication that limits the cardiac output, which is uncommon due to an obligatory right-to-left shunt in utero, balloon atrioseptostomy is performed. The haemodynamic status of the patients is otherwise usually stable.

Subsequent management algorithm: The next step in the management algorithm depends on several factors: (a) size of the right ventricle, (b) type of pulmonary atresia (membranous versus muscular), and (c) presence or absence of right ventricular-dependent coronary circulation (Fig. 16.10).

Heterogeneities of the anatomy of pulmonary atresia with intact ventricular septum lead to variations in management among centres. There are no universally agreed definitions of mild hypoplasia of the right ventricle that can support a biventricular or a one-and-a-half ventricular circulation or severe hypoplasia that would predict the need for univentricular repair. This is further discussed in the chapter on borderline right ventricle (Chap. 32). Nonetheless, the general management principles as shown in Fig. 16.10 apply.

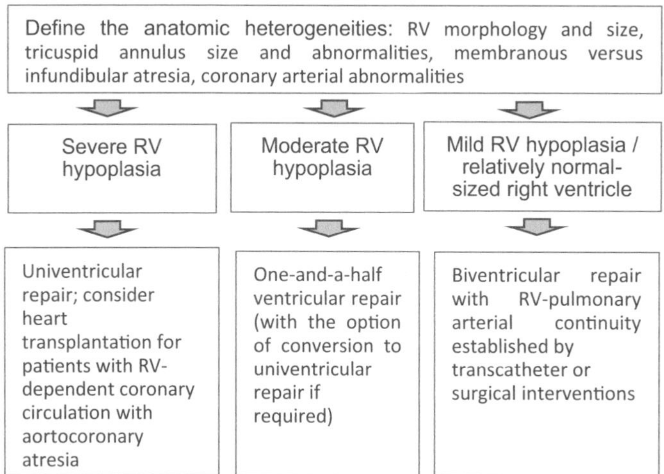

Fig. 16.10 Management algorithm of pulmonary atresia with intact ventricular septum. *RV* right ventricular

16.4.5.1 Univentricular Palliation

With a severely hypoplastic right ventricle, a modified Blalock-Taussig shunt or stenting of the arterial duct is initially performed and followed by univentricular repair later in childhood. Anatomic factors that indicate the need for univentricular repair are listed in Box 16.1.

Box 16.1 Anatomic Factors that Indicate the Need for Univentricular Repair

- Unipartite right ventricle
- Tricuspid valve z score < −5
- Tricuspid annulus/mitral annulus <0.5
- Minimal or mild tricuspid regurgitation
- Severe right ventricular dysfunction with right ventricular dilation
- Right ventricular-dependent coronary circulation

In neonates with a right ventricular-dependent coronary circulation due to aorto-coronary atresia, the high mortality despite univentricular palliation has prompted some centres to offer heart transplantation as a treatment option.

16.4.5.2 Biventricular Repair

With a mild hypoplastic or relatively normal-sized right ventricle, biventricular repair with establishment of right ventricular-pulmonary arterial continuity is the treatment of choice. Anatomic factors that favour biventricular repair are listed in Box 16.2.

When incorporation of a mildly hypoplastic right ventricle into a biventricular circulation is considered feasible, continuity between the right ventricle and the pulmonary trunk is established. For pulmonary valve atresia, the options include transcatheter radiofrequency or CTO (chronic total occlusion) wire-assisted pulmonary valvotomy followed by balloon valvoplasty (Fig. 16.11) and surgical pulmonary valvotomy. For infundibular atresia, surgical reconstruction of the right ventricular outflow is required.

Box 16.2 Anatomic Factors that Favour Biventricular Repair

- Tripartite right ventricle
- Tricuspid valve z score > −2
- Tricuspid annulus/mitral annulus >0.8
- Absence of right ventricular-dependent coronary circulation
- Moderate to severe tricuspid regurgitation

Despite establishment of a patent right ventricular outflow, the poorly compliant, hypertrophic, and relatively hypoplastic right ventricle may still limit diastolic

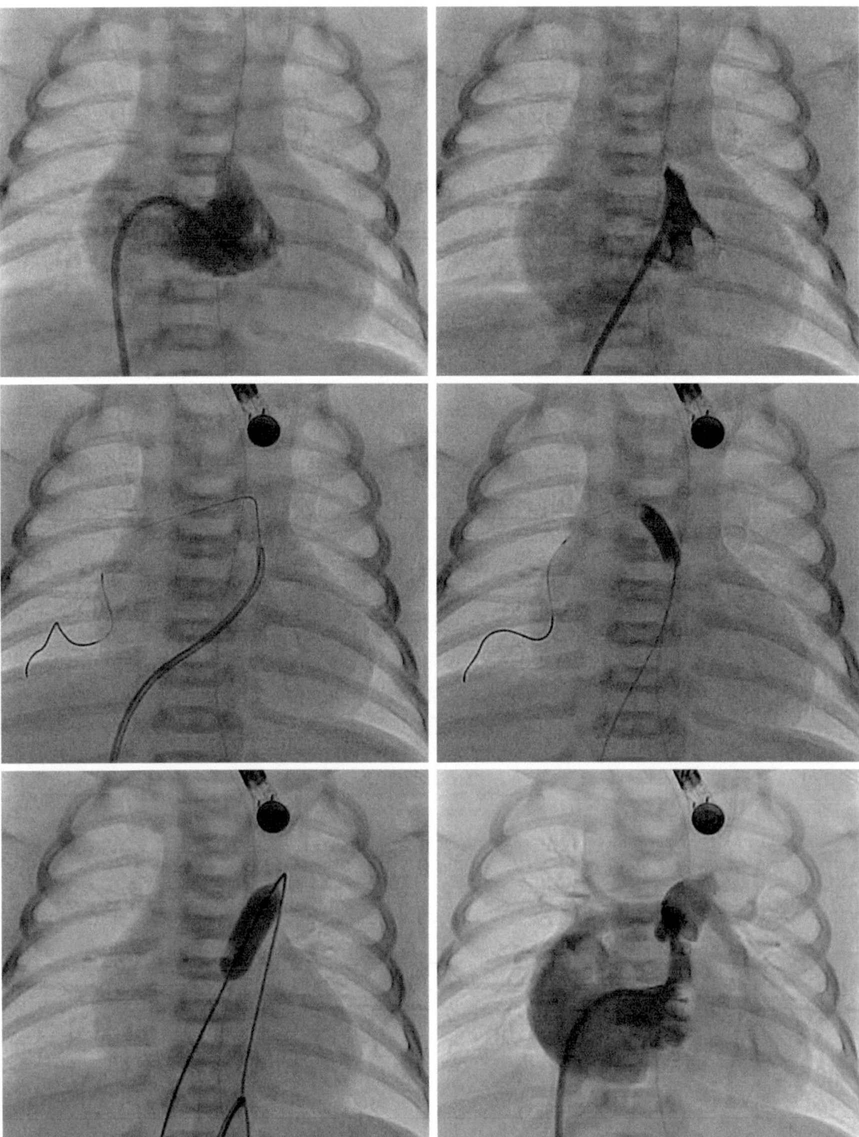

Fig. 16.11 Transcatheter management of pulmonary valve atresia. Right ventricle-to-pulmonary artery continuity is established by perforation of the atretic pulmonary valve by radiofrequency wire followed by serial balloon angioplasty

filling, thereby promoting right-to-left shunting through the interatrial communication to cause cyanosis. Maintenance of prostaglandin E may be required for 1–2 weeks after intervention to maintain systemic oxygenation and to assess the ability of the right ventricle to support the biventricular circulation.

In most of the patients with relatively normal-sized right ventricle, prostaglandin E can be weaned off successfully. If the atrial communication remains patent, completion of biventricular circulation is achieved later by transcatheter device occlusion of the communication.

There are patients with borderline right ventricles who are dependent on prostaglandin E. Insertion of systemic-to-pulmonary arterial shunt or stenting of the arterial duct to maintain adequate pulmonary blood flow may be required. In some centres, stenting of the arterial duct is performed at the same time as transcatheter perforation of the pulmonary valve to shorten hospital stay. In patients with adequate growth of the right ventricle, completion of a biventricular circulation can be achieved later by occlusion of the shunt or stented duct and the atrial communication. On the other hand, patients with poor growth of the borderline hypoplastic right ventricle require one-and-a-half ventricular repair.

16.4.5.3 One-and-a-Half Ventricular Repair

One-and-a-half ventricular repair involves the establishment of a patent right ventricular outflow, partial closure of the interatrial communication and a superior cavopulmonary anastomosis (bidirectional Glenn shunt). The bidirectional Glenn shunt provides a source of pulmonary blood flow from the superior caval vein (which constitutes about 50% of the total venous return in infants and 35% from about 6 years onward), while the borderline right ventricle blood pumps blood returning from the inferior caval vein into the pulmonary arteries.

In some centres, right ventricular overhaul (resection of right ventricular myocardium to enlarge the cavity size) is performed to promote ventricular growth and increase the success of biventricular repair. Nonetheless, the initial enthusiasm has been tempered by the lack of growth of the tricuspid valve annulus and data showing that exercise capacity is similar between patients with borderline right ventricle after one-and-a-half and those after univentricular repair. In many centres, these patients, usually with tricuspid valve z score < -2 and approaching z score of -5, are candidates for direct univentricular repair.

Further echocardiographic and haemodynamic assessments after one-and-a-half ventricular repair include the growth of the right ventricle, right atrial pressure and dilation, magnitude of right-to-left atrial shunt, systemic oxygen saturation, and pulmonary arterial pressure. Based on the results, the next step of management can either be (a) closure of the interatrial communication (if right ventricular growth is satisfactory and trial of balloon occlusion of the communication does not reduce cardiac output or cause significant right atrial hypertension), (b) maintaining the one-and-a-half ventricular circulation (some growth of the right ventricle, reasonable systemic oxygen saturation, but rise of right atrial pressure upon trial of balloon occlusion of the interatrial communication), or (c) conversion to univentricular repair (right ventricle remains hypoplastic with progressive worsening of systemic oxygen saturation due to significant right-to-left atrial shunt and inadequacy of the bidirectional Glenn shunt).

16.4.6 Postoperative and Post-catheter Considerations

For patients requiring insertion of a systemic-to-pulmonary arterial shunt or stenting of the arterial duct, potential complications include shunt or stent thrombosis, shunt migration, and pulmonary over- or under-circulation (Chap. 54).

In patients with right ventriculo-coronary fistulous communications, but without a right ventricular-dependent coronary circulation, opening of the right ventricular outflow with decompression of the hypertensive right ventricle may cause transient myocardial ischaemia (when the predominant systolic coronary flow transits to diastolic coronary flow).

Postoperative issues and management after bidirectional Glenn shunt and Fontan procedure are discussed in Chaps. 19 and 30.

16.4.7 Long-Term Monitoring

Adoption of different approaches to cater for this board spectrum of cardiac malformation has resulted in a survival of 60–90% at 10 years after interventions. Long-term issues in patients undergoing univentricular repair are those of the Fontan procedure. In patients who have undergone one-and-a-half or biventricular repair, long-term morbidity is related to right atrial hypertension and distention (atrial arrhythmias and chronic liver congestion), cyanosis (after one-and-half ventricular circulation or after biventricular circulation with an interatrial communication), and the need for pulmonary valve replacement with or without tricuspid valve repair (in patients with severe pulmonary regurgitation).

Transposition of the Great Arteries 17

In a structurally normal heart, the aorta arises from the morphologic left ventricle while the pulmonary artery arises from the morphologic right ventricle (concordant ventriculoarterial connection). Transposition of the great arteries, on the other hand, is characterized by discordant ventriculoarterial connection.

17.1 Anatomy

In TGA, the aorta arises from the right ventricle, while the pulmonary trunk arises from the left ventricle (Fig. 17.1a). The aorta is usually lying anterior and to the right of the pulmonary trunk. The most common associated cardiac lesion is a ventricular septal defect. Other associations include left ventricular outflow obstruction at the valvar and subvalvar levels (subpulmonary obstruction), subaortic obstruction, and coarctation of the aorta (which is usually occurring in association with a ventricular septal defect, anterior deviation of the outlet muscular septum, and a bicuspid aortic valve).

The coronary arteries arise from the aortic sinus(es) that face the pulmonary trunk. The Leiden Convention is a commonly used system to describe the coronary arterial patterns regardless of the position of the great arteries. Based on this system, the surgeon is standing in the aortic nonfacing sinus, with sinus 1 being the right-hand facing sinus and sinus 2 as the left-hand facing sinus. The usual pattern refers to the left coronary artery arising from sinus 1 and bifurcates into the left circumflex and anterior descending arteries (1LCx), while the right coronary artery arises from sinus 2 (2R). A variant pattern (e.g. single coronary artery, intramural arterial course) has been associated in the past with higher postoperative risk. Possible coronary arterial patterns as imaged by echocardiography are shown in Fig. 17.2.

Y.-f. Cheung, *Congenital and Paediatric Acquired Heart Disease in Practice*, https://doi.org/10.1007/978-981-99-2862-0_17

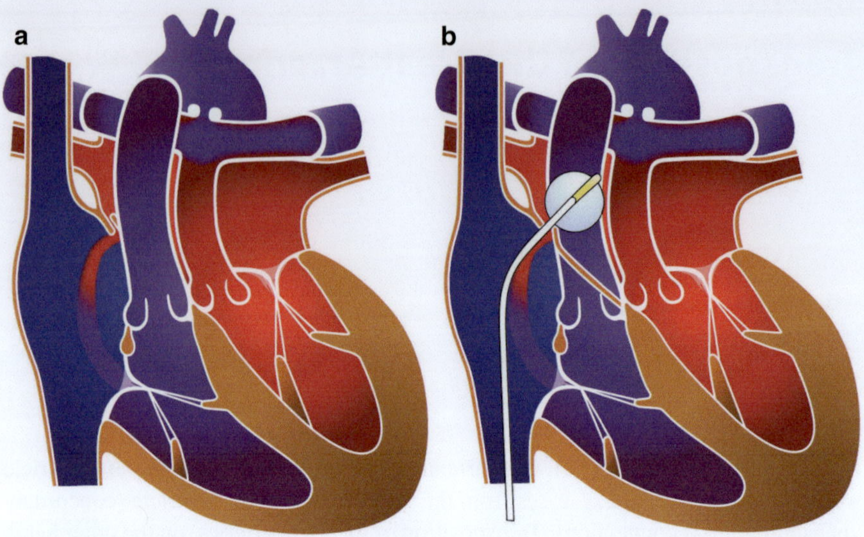

Fig. 17.1 Transposition of the great arteries. (**a**) Transposition of the great arteries with a parallel circulation and two sites of mixing (oval foramen and arterial duct). (**b**) Inflation of the balloon in the left atrium for performing balloon atrioseptostomy

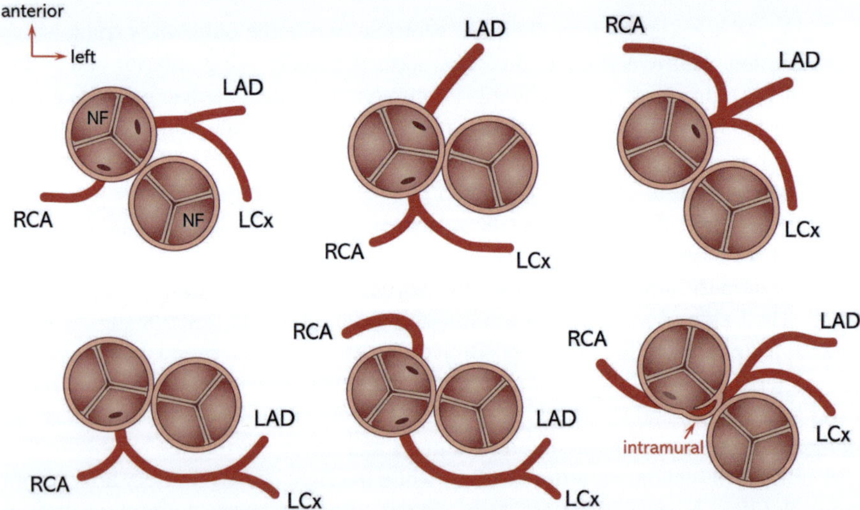

Fig. 17.2 Possible coronary arterial patterns based on echocardiography. Note that echocardiographic view differs from the surgeon's view and hence a way to designate the sinus based on echocardiography is having the echocardiographer to sit in the pulmonary nonfacing sinus with the right-hand facing aortic sinus being sinus 1 and left-hand facing aortic sinus being sinus 2 (*NF* nonfacing, *LCA* left coronary artery, *LCx* left circumflex artery, *RCA* right coronary artery)

17.2 Pathophysiology

The primary pathophysiologic abnormality in transposition of the great arteries is separation of the systemic and pulmonary circulations, leading to inadequate oxygen supply to the tissues. The systemic and pulmonary circulations are functioning in parallel, as contrast to the normal circulations that function in series. In the absence of mixing between the two circulations, the oxygenated pulmonary venous return is unable to enter the systemic circulation, while the deoxygenated systemic venous return fails to reach the lungs for oxygenation.

To be compatible with postnatal life, anatomic sites for the mixing of the two circulations are essential. These sites include a patent oval foramen or an atrial septal defect, an associated ventricular septal defect, and a persistent arterial duct. The extent of intercirculatory mixing depends on the number of anatomical sites, their size, and pulmonary blood flow. Hence, severe systemic hypoxaemia occurs with a small interatrial communication and worsens with postnatal closure of the arterial duct. A small and restrictive atrial communication further predisposes to pulmonary arterial hypertension before and after arterial switch operation. The presence of a large ventricular septal defect may improve intercirculatory mixing, although the increased flow to the lungs may cause early onset of heart failure.

With postnatal decrease in pulmonary vascular resistance, the left ventricular pressure and mass may decrease to the extent that the left ventricle may not be able to support the systemic circulation after arterial switch operation if performed too late after birth.

17.3 Clinical Manifestations

Newborns with transposition of the great arteries present with cyanosis soon after birth. Without adequate intercirculatory mixing, the babies will die of severe hypoxaemia. In the presence of adequate mixing, the cyanosis may be relatively mild. With progressive drop in pulmonary vascular resistance after birth, symptoms of heart failure with shortness of breath and poor feeding occur usually after the first week of life due to pulmonary over circulation. The auscultatory findings are non-specific (Table 17.1).

Table 17.1 Signs of transposition of great arteries

Signs	Origins
Cyanosis	Degree of cyanosis depends on the adequacy of the sites for mixing of systemic and pulmonary circulations
Signs of heart failure develop within the first week	Progressive increase in pulmonary flow with decrease in pulmonary vascular resistance after birth
Right ventricular impulse	Pressure overloading of the right ventricle as it is supporting the systemic circulation
Loud and single S2	Closure sound of the anteriorly positioned aortic valve
No murmur or a non-specific ejection systolic murmur	

17.4 Investigations

CXR: The characteristic radiographic features are an oval cardiac silhouette ('egg-on-side' appearance), a narrow mediastinal shadow, and increased pulmonary vascular markings. The abnormal antero-posterior relationship of the aorta and the pulmonary trunk and stress-related thymic involution account for narrowing of the superior mediastinum.

ECG: The electrocardiographic findings are typically normal for age.

Echocardiography: Echocardiography confirms the diagnosis by demonstrating parallel arrangement of the great arteries with the pulmonary trunk arising posteriorly from the left ventricle and the aorta arising anteriorly from the right ventricle, enables the assessment of associated cardiac abnormalities (in particular ventricular septal defect), adequacy of mixing at the arterial ductal and interatrial communication, and coronary arterial pattern and allows the monitoring of balloon atrioseptostomy (Fig. 17.3).

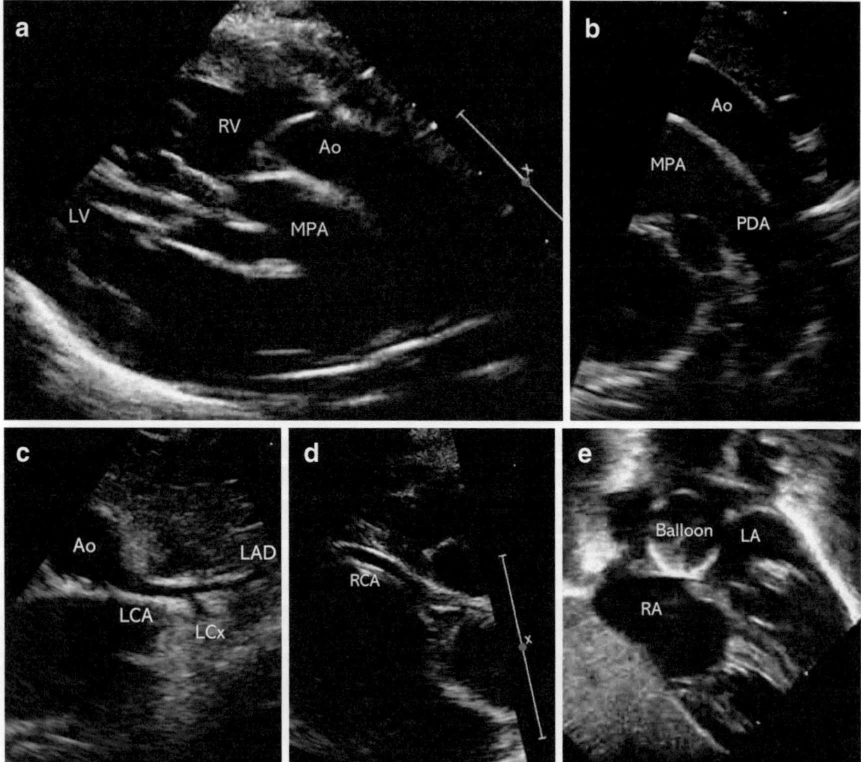

Fig. 17.3 Echocardiographic assessment of TGA. (**a**) Parasternal long-axis view and (**b**) suprasternal view showing parallel arrangement of the two great arteries (**c**) Left and (**d**) right coronary arteries are shown using the parasternal short axis (**e**) Echocardiographic monitoring of balloon atrioseptostomy (*Ao* aorta, *MPA* main pulmonary artery, *LA* left atrium, *LAD* left anterior descending artery, *LCA* left main coronary artery, *LCx* left circumflex artery, *LV* left ventricle, *MPA* main pulmonary artery, *PDA* persistent arterial duct, *RA* right atrium, *RCA* right coronary artery, *RV* right ventricle)

17.5 Management Strategy

Initial management aims at promoting intercirculatory mixing at two levels: (1) the ductal level by intravenous prostaglandin E infusion, and (2) the atrial level by performing balloon atrial septostomy (Figs. 17.1b and 17.3e).

17.5.1 TGA with an Intact Ventricular Septum

Arterial switch operation (also called Jatene operation named after Dr Adib Jatene, the Brazilian surgeon who successfully performed the surgery in 1975), is the treatment of choice (Fig. 17.4). This is usually performed within the first week of life, but best after day two to allow for the postnatal drop in pulmonary vascular resistance. The surgery involves transection and reanastomosis of the great arteries, so that the left ventricle supports the neoaorta and the right ventricle supports the neopulmonary trunk. The LeCompte manoeuvre, described in 1981, involves mobilization of the bifurcation of the pulmonary arteries anterior to the neoaorta. The coronary arteries with buttons of aortic tissue are reimplanted in the neoaortic root.

In some parts of the world, babies with transposition of the great arteries may present late beyond the second to third month of life, at a time when afterload to the left ventricle has decreased. Decreased left ventricular thickness, mass, and volume may result in acute left ventricular failure after arterial switch operation. Options for these infants include (1) retraining of the left ventricle by pulmonary arterial banding followed by arterial switch operation, (2) arterial switch operation with post operative mechanical circulatory support, and (3) atrial switch operation (Chap. 25).

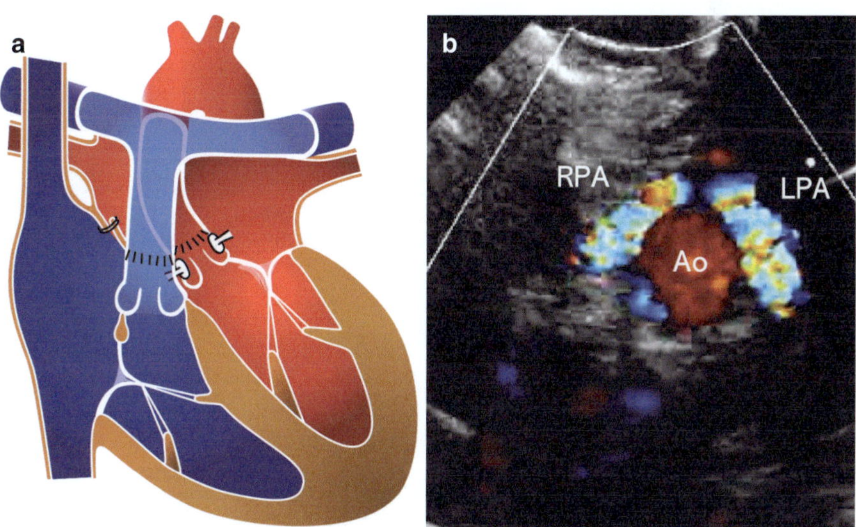

Fig. 17.4 Arterial switch operation and echocardiographic assessment. (**a**) Arterial switch operation. (**b**) Colour flow mapping demonstrating the bifurcation of the pulmonary arteries anterior to the neoaorta after LeCompte manoeuvre (*Ao* aorta, *LPA* left pulmonary artery, *RPA* right pulmonary artery)

17.5.2 TGA with Ventricular Septal Defect and/or Aortic Arch Obstruction

Arterial switch operation is performed as described. The ventricular septal defect, if moderate to large in size, is repaired at the time of arterial switch operation. Mild obstruction of the left ventricular outflow can be managed by muscle resection. Associated coarctation or interruption of the aortic arch is also repaired as a one-stage operation.

17.5.3 TGA with Severe Left Ventricular Outflow Obstruction

Patients with severe left ventricular outflow obstruction, which usually occurs in association with a large ventricular septal defect, require alternative surgical approaches (Box 17.1).

Box 17.1 Surgical Management of TGA with Severe Left Ventricular Outflow Obstruction

Rastelli Procedure

- Patching the ventricular septal defect to the aorta to direct blood flow from the left ventricle to the aorta
- Closure of pulmonary valve with division of the pulmonary trunk
- Establishment of right ventricle-pulmonary artery continuity with a valved conduit

Reparations à l'ètage Ventriculaire (REV) Procedure

- Excision of outlet septum
- Patching the ventricular septal defect to the aorta to direct blood flow from the left ventricle to the aorta
- LeCompte manoeuvre to mobilize the pulmonary trunk anteriorly with suturing of posterior rim of the pulmonary trunk to the right ventriculotomy and pericardial patch reconstruction of the anterior pulmonary trunk

Nikaidoh Procedure

- Harvesting of the aorta with the coronary arteries by right ventriculotomy and leaving a rim of muscle beneath the aortic valve
- Excision of the stenotic pulmonary valve and incision of outlet septum to widen the left ventricular outflow tract
- Posterior translocation of aortic root with suturing it to the left ventricular outflow
- Closure of the ventricular septal defect
- Right ventricular outflow reconstruction with a valved conduit or with LeCompte manoeuvre and an anterior pericardial patch

17.6 Postoperative Considerations

The postoperative course is usually relatively stable after timely arterial switch operation with the left ventricle coping with the systemic circulation. Important postoperative complications include low cardiac output syndrome, coronary artery complications, and bleeding issues. Transient low cardiac output syndrome may occur at about 6–18 h, with a nadir at 9–12 h, postoperatively. For severe left ventricular dysfunction, coronary insufficiency should be excluded. Reopening of the closed sternum with inspection of the coronary arterial anastomosis may be required. If extracorporeal membrane oxygenation support is required, residual lesions must be excluded by cardiac catheterization.

Initial intensive care management includes standard fluid restriction, inotropic support with low dose milrinone and adrenaline infusion. The threshold for peritoneal dialysis should be low to ensure negative fluid balance. Chylothorax may develop with reintroduction of enteral feeding and should be managed accordingly (Chap. 59).

17.7 Long-Term Monitoring

Long-term follow up for neoaortic root dilation and regurgitation, pulmonary stenosis due to supravalvar and branch pulmonary arterial stenosis and hypoplasia of the pulmonary trunk (due to inadequate mobilization of the pulmonary arteries), and coronary arterial complications including stenosis or even occlusion is required.

Truncus Arteriosus 18

Truncus arteriosus is an uncommon congenital heart condition characterized by a common arterial trunk arising from the ventricles. As with other conotruncal defects, DiGeorge syndrome (Chap. 62) is a common association.

18.1 Anatomy

In truncus arteriosus, a single trunk arises from the ventricle and gives rise to coronary arteries, pulmonary arteries, and aorta (Fig. 18.1). Based on the Collet and Edwards classifications, four types are described (Table 18.1).

A ventricular septal defect is almost always present, although the defect may be restrictive. Rarely, the ventricular septum is intact, and the trunk arises then usually from the right ventricle. The truncal valve usually overrides the ventricular septum and connects to both ventricles. The truncal valve, consisting of two to five cusps, may be dysplastic, stenotic and/or regurgitant. Other associated cardiac anomalies include coarctation and interruption of the aorta.

Y.-f. Cheung, *Congenital and Paediatric Acquired Heart Disease in Practice*, https://doi.org/10.1007/978-981-99-2862-0_18

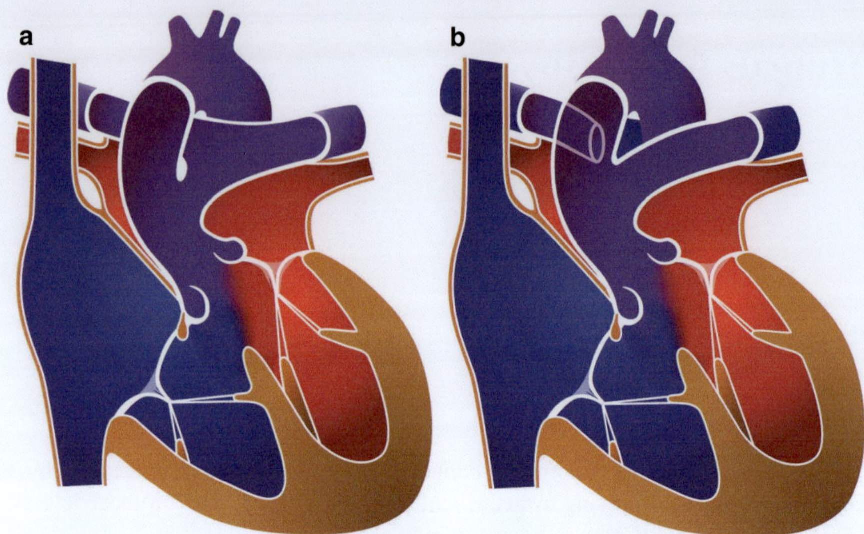

Fig. 18.1 Types of truncus arteriosus. (**a**) Type I truncus arteriosus (**b**) Type II truncus arteriosus

Table 18.1 Classification of truncus arteriosus

Type	Description
I	A single pulmonary trunk arises from the trunk and bifurcates into the right and left pulmonary arteries
II	The right and left pulmonary arteries arise in close proximity from the dorsal wall of the trunk
III	The pulmonary arteries arise separately from the lateral wall of the trunk
IV	Absence of intrapericardial pulmonary arteries and the pulmonary branches arise from the descending aorta (no longer regarded as truncus arteriosus, but rather categorized under pulmonary atresia with ventricular septal defect)

18.2 Pathophysiology

As the trunk mostly arises from both ventricles and the ventricular septal defect is large, the right and left ventricular systolic pressures are equal. Truncus arteriosus constitutes a common-mixing situation in which systemic deoxygenated blood from the right ventricle mixes with oxygenated blood from the left ventricle at the level of the trunk. The oxygen contents of the blood in the aorta and pulmonary arteries are hence identical.

The haemodynamics in truncus arteriosus, albeit a cyanotic heart lesion, are similar to those of large left-to-right shunts. As the origin of the pulmonary arteries from the trunk is usually non-stenotic, the pulmonary flow significantly increases with reduction of pulmonary vascular resistance after birth.

The haemodynamic consequences are (1) minimal or mild degree of cyanosis (large portion of oxygenated blood available for mixing due to increased pulmonary venous return), (2) prominent features of heart failure (pulmonary arterial congestion, increased pulmonary venous return causing volume overloading of the left heart), (3) large pulse pressure (diastolic runoff to the pulmonary arteries), and (4) development of pulmonary hypertension (high pulmonary flow and increased pulmonary vascular resistance due to medial hypertrophy of the pulmonary arterioles) and Eisenmenger syndrome (if left unrepaired).

18.3 Clinical Manifestations

Mild cyanosis, which may escape notice, occurs shortly after birth. With progressive decrease in pulmonary vascular resistance, symptoms of heart failure become obvious at 1–2 months of age. Cyanosis becomes milder or even absent and the clinical picture mimics that of a large left-to-right shunt. The dilated single arterial trunk accounts for the physical signs of a loud and single second heart sound and an ejection systolic click (Table 18.2).

Table 18.2 Signs of truncus arteriosus

Signs	Origins
Signs of heart failure	Appears as pulmonary vascular resistance decreases
Mild cyanosis	Degree of cyanosis is inversely related to pulmonary flow
Bounding pulses	Runoff to the pulmonary arteries from the aorta during diastole
Hyperactive praecordium with biventricular impulses	LV volume overloading with RV pressure overloading
Loud and single S2	Closure of the single truncal valve
Ejection click	Opening of the truncal valve
An ejection systolic murmur at the left sternal border	High flow across the truncal valve

18.4 Investigations

CXR: The typical radiographic findings of cardiomegaly and pulmonary plethora are similar to those of large left-to-right shunts. The enlarged cardiac chambers are the left atrium and the left ventricle. The thymic shadow may be absent in patients with DiGeorge syndrome.

ECG: Electrocardiogram shows evidence of biventricular overloading (right ventricular pressure overloading with left ventricular volume overloading).

Echocardiography: Echocardiography confirms the diagnosis, defines the type by demonstrating the truncal origins of the pulmonary arteries, and enables the assessment of the morphology and stenosis and/or regurgitation of the truncal valve (Fig. 18.2).

Genetic evaluation: Genetic testing for 22q11.2 microdeletion and assessment for associated features of DiGeorge syndrome is required.

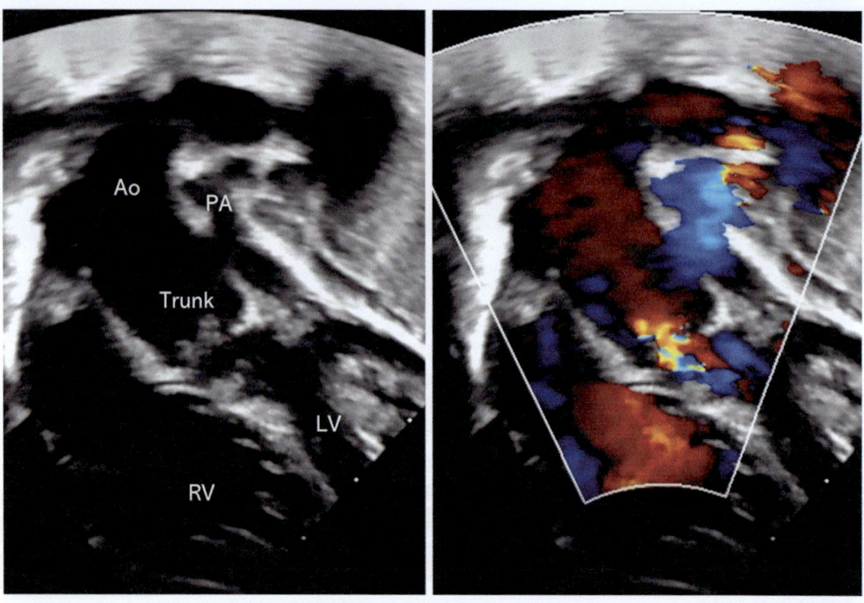

Fig. 18.2 Echocardiographic assessment of truncus arteriosus. Subcostal view showing type I truncus arteriosus and truncal valve regurgitation (*Ao* aorta, *LV* left ventricle, *PA* pulmonary artery, *RV* right ventricle)

18.5 Management Strategy

Medical treatment of the congestive heart failure is required. Reparative surgery with closure of the ventricular septal defect and placement of a valved conduit, either a homograft or Contegra (heterologous bovine jugular venous graft) between the right ventricle and the pulmonary arteries should be performed in early infancy. Coarctation or interruption of the aorta, when present, is also repaired.

Management of truncal valvar regurgitation remains challenging. Mild or even moderate degree of truncal valvar regurgitation is usually managed conservatively. However, repair or rarely replacement of severely regurgitant truncal valve may be required.

18.6 Postoperative Considerations

The perioperative morbidity and mortality are high given the proneness to develop severe pulmonary hypertension and truncal valvar abnormalities. Historically, the mortality was reported as high as 40%. Even recent data suggest a mortality of about 10%. The need to repair coarctation or interruption of the aorta increases the surgical mortality.

The postoperative course is commonly complicated by low cardiac output syndrome and reactive pulmonary hypertension. Initial intensive care management includes fluid restriction, milrinone and adrenaline infusion, inhaled nitric oxide, and diuretics. In patients with DiGeorge syndrome, the serum calcium level requires close monitoring and hypocalcaemia should be timely corrected.

18.7 Long-Term Monitoring

Monitoring of conduit and truncal valve function is required. Replacement of the conduit when significant conduit dysfunction occurs has been the definitive treatment in the past. Increasingly, transcatheter intervention (balloon angioplasty, stenting, or percutaneous pulmonary valve replacement) is used in selected patients. Truncal valve replacement may be required on follow up, especially in patients who require initial valve repair.

Functionally Univentricular Heart 19

The term 'univentricular heart' has created much controversy, given that (1) majority of the so-called univentricular hearts have an additional non-functional rudimentary chamber, and (2) a staged management approach towards univentricular repair (Fontan procedure) is adopted also for hearts with two ventricles with one ventricle being severely hypoplastic, for example pulmonary atresia with intact ventricular septum and severe hypoplasia of the right ventricle (Chap. 16), hypoplastic left heart syndrome (Chap. 21), and unbalanced atrioventricular septal defect (Chap. 11). Given these considerations, these cardiac entities are better described as 'functionally' univentricular hearts.

19.1 Anatomy

In general, functionally univentricular heart has one dominant ventricular chamber (Fig. 19.1) and, in most patients, an additional non-functional rudimentary chamber is present.

The combination of atrial arrangement, atrioventricular connection, ventricular morphology, and ventriculoarterial connection can vary among patients (Table 19.1).

Y.-f. Cheung, *Congenital and Paediatric Acquired Heart Disease in Practice*, https://doi.org/10.1007/978-981-99-2862-0_19

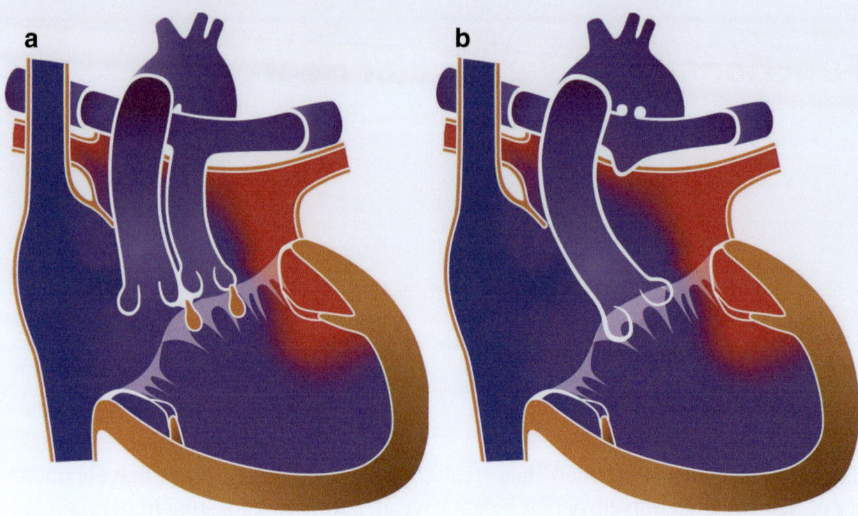

Fig. 19.1 Functionally univentricular heart. (**a**) Double-outlet functional single ventricle (**b**) Functionally univentricular heart with pulmonary atresia

Table 19.1 Anatomic segments in functionally univentricular hearts

Segment	Description
Atrial arrangement	Usual Mirror-imaged Isomeric in heterotaxy syndrome (Chap. 20)
Atrioventricular connection	Absent right-sided connection (tricuspid atresia) Absent left-sided connection (mitral atresia) Double-inlet (when the dominant ventricle supports both atrioventricular junction)
Main ventricular chamber morphology	A dominant morphologic right ventricle with a rudimentary morphologic left ventricle A dominant morphologic left ventricle with a rudimentary right ventricle A solitary indeterminate ventricle
Ventriculoarterial connection	Concordant (the great arteries arising from their respective morphologic ventricles) Discordant (aorta arising from the morphologic right ventricle and pulmonary artery arising from the morphologic left ventricle) Double-outlet from the dominant ventricular chamber (with or without pulmonary stenosis at the valvar and/or subvalvar level) Single outlet with pulmonary atresia

19.2 Pathophysiology

The major haemodynamic consequence is mixing of systemic and pulmonary venous blood in the dominant ventricle. The oxygen content of blood in the aorta is identical to that in the pulmonary arteries. The degree of pulmonary outflow obstruction determines the magnitude of pulmonary flow. The amount of pulmonary flow is related inversely to the severity of cyanosis and directly to the severity of congestive heart failure.

Severe cyanosis hence occurs in patients with significant pulmonary outflow obstruction and who are duct-dependent. On the other hand, the clinical picture of heart failure predominates in patients without pulmonary outflow obstruction. In between these extremes, patients may have a balanced haemodynamic status with the pulmonary flow being neither too excessive nor too limited. This occurs when the pulmonary stenosis is moderate in degree.

19.3 Clinical Manifestations

The clinical presentation depends on the severity of pulmonary outflow obstruction. Neonates with pulmonary atresia or severe pulmonary stenosis present soon after birth with cyanosis as the arterial duct closes. On the other hand, in patients with no pulmonary outflow obstruction, the cyanosis is mild and features of heart failure predominate. The symptoms and signs of congestive heart failure become apparent usually by 1–2 months of age when the pulmonary vascular resistance drops. Patients with a balanced haemodynamic status, on the other hand, have mild cyanosis and absence of heart failure. The physical signs are likewise determined mainly by the severity of pulmonary outflow obstruction (Table 19.2).

Table 19.2 Signs of univentricular hearts

Signs	Origin
Cyanosis	Related inversely to pulmonary blood flow
Signs of heart failure	Related to high pulmonary blood flow
Single S2	Suggestive of associated pulmonary stenosis or atresia
An ejection systolic murmur at the left upper sternal border	Suggestive of associated pulmonary stenosis

19.4 Investigations

CXR: The radiographic findings are variable. The heart may be located in the right or the left hemithorax, and the heart size may be normal or enlarged. The pulmonary vascular markings depend on the degree of pulmonary stenosis. In the presence of moderate to severe stenosis, the lung fields appear oligaemic. The abdominal visceral arrangement may also be abnormal, as in patients with heterotaxy syndrome (Chap. 20).

ECG: The electrocardiographic findings are likewise variable, depending on the position of heart, the atrial arrangements, and the relative dominance of the right and left ventricular masses.

Echocardiography: Echocardiographic assessment should adopt a sequential segmental approach to define the atrial arrangement (inferred from location of inferior caval vein and aorta relative to the spine), atrioventricular connection, ventricular morphology, and ventriculoarterial connection (Fig. 19.2a, b). Further assessment aims to determine severity of atrioventricular regurgitation, severity of pulmonary outflow obstruction and patency of the arterial duct in duct-dependent circulation.

Cardiac catheterization: Diagnostic cardiac catheterization is not usually required for initial diagnosis. This is commonly performed as part of the preoperative assessment of haemodyanamics, cardiac anatomy, and adequacy of the pulmonary vasculature prior to bidirectional Glenn shunt and Fontan procedure (Fig. 19.2c, d).

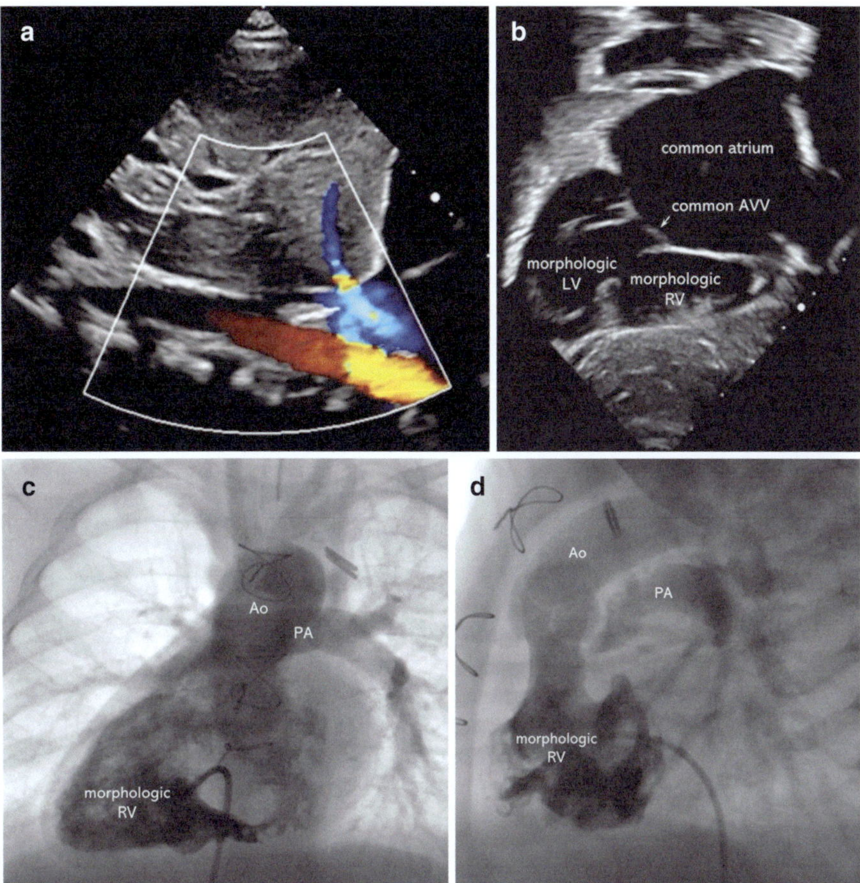

Fig. 19.2 Imaging of functionally univentricular heart. (**a**) An anterior inferior caval vein (blue) and a posterior aorta (red) arrangement suggests right atrial isomerism. (**b**) The common atrium and a large complete atrioventricular septal defect with deficient ventricular septum is characteristic in right atrial isomerism. (**c**) Anteroposterior and (**d**) lateral projections of ventricular angiogram demonstrating the morphologic right ventricle supporting two great arteries with severe subpulmonary stenosis (*Ao* aorta, *AVV* atrioventricular valve, *LV* left ventricle, *PA* pulmonary artery, *RV* right ventricle)

19.5 Management Strategy

The primary aim of management of functionally univentricular heart is to achieve an optimal outcome after Fontan procedure, which in turn depends on (1) a low central venous pressure (satisfactory pulmonary arterial arborization, good pulmonary arterial growth with absence of significant stenosis, low pulmonary vascular resistance, absence of pulmonary venous obstruction) and (2) satisfactory output from the functional single ventricle (absence of significant systolic and diastolic dysfunction, ventricular outflow obstruction, and atrioventricular valvar regurgitation).

Patients undergoes staged management (Fig 19.3) towards eventual conversion to a Fontan circulation (Chap. 30): (1) a first stage palliation in the neonatal period to achieve balanced and satisfactory pulmonary and systemic blood flow, (2) a second stage palliation at 4–6 months of age with superior cavopulmonary (bidirectional Glenn) shunt, and (3) the third stage with completion of Fontan circuit at 3–5 years of age.

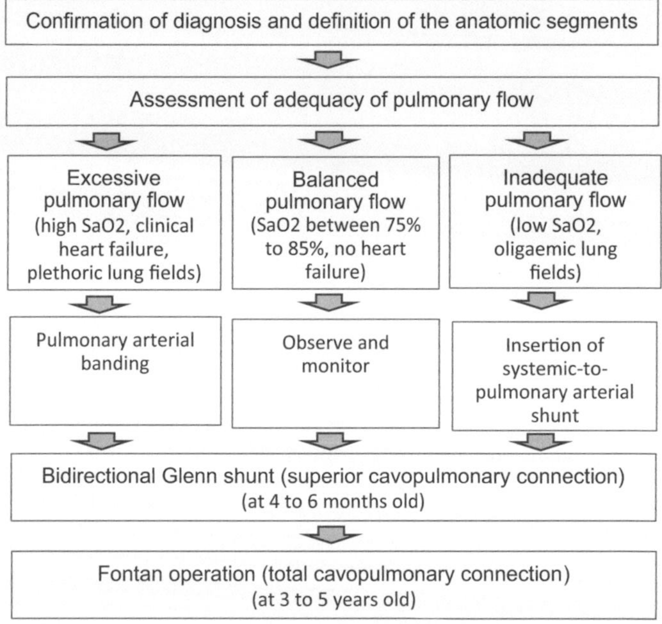

Fig. 19.3 Management algorithm of functionally univentricular hearts. SaO2 arterial oxygen saturation

19.5.1 First Stage Palliation

The aim of a first stage palliation in the neonatal period is to achieve balanced and satisfactory pulmonary and systemic blood flow (Chap. 29). This initiation step may be insertion of a systemic-to-pulmonary arterial shunt (usually a modified Blalock-Taussig shunt) (Fig. 19.4a), pulmonary arterial banding (Fig. 19.4b), or observation and monitoring alone.

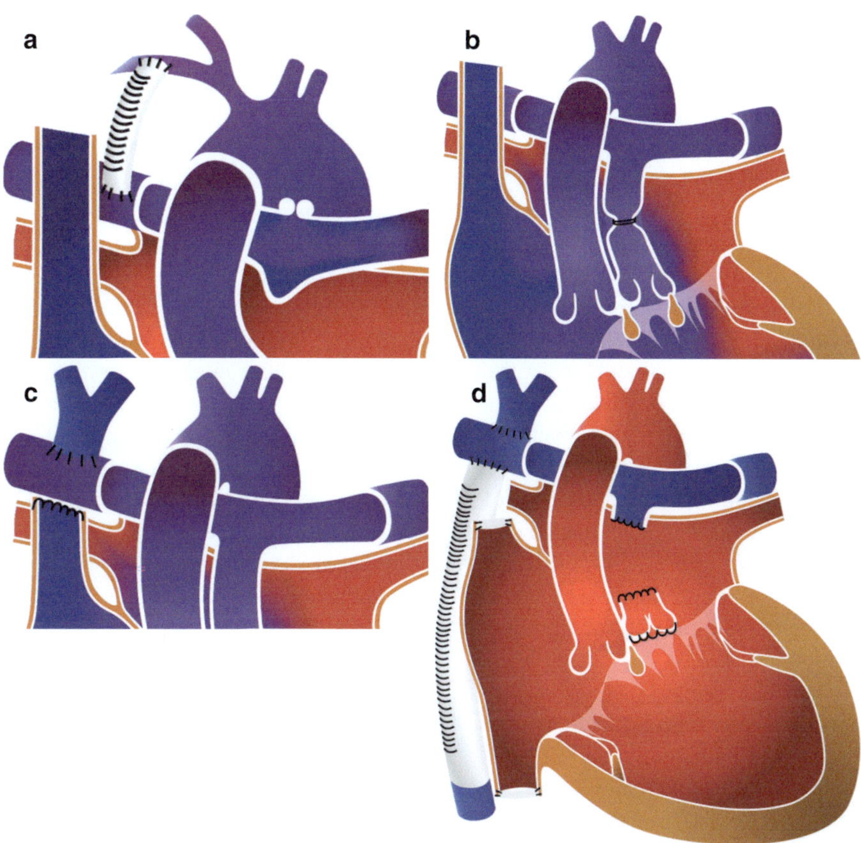

Fig. 19.4 Staged surgical management of functionally univentricular hearts. (**a**) Modified Blalock-Taussig shunt. (**b**) Pulmonary arterial banding. (**c**) Bidirectional Glenn shunt. (**d**) Fontan procedure

19.5.2 Bidirectional Glenn Shunt (Superior Cavopulmonary Connection)

The second stage involves a bidirectional Glenn shunt (superior cavopulmonary connection), which is usually performed at the age of 4–6 months (Fig. 19.4c). This involves the anastomosis of the superior caval vein to the right pulmonary artery, thereby permitting blood to flow from the superior caval vein into both the right and left pulmonary arteries. In the presence of bilateral superior caval veins as in heterotaxy syndrome, bilateral bidirectional Glenn shunts are performed. Satisfactory functioning of the bidirectional Glenn shunt requires the presence of low pulmonary vascular resistance.

Benefits of this second-stage palliation include: (1) volume unloading of the functional single ventricle (as the superior caval venous blood flows directly into the pulmonary circulation), (2) decrease in ventricular work and ventricular stroke volume, and (3) obligatory systemic venous flow from the superior caval vein (about 50% of the total venous return in infants) to maintain systemic oxygenation (with SaO_2 maintained at about 85%). The physiology after a bidirectional Glenn shunt is further discussed in Chap. 29.

In patients with antegrade pulmonary flow from the ventricle prior to bidirectional Glenn shunt, it remains controversial whether this antegrade flow should be interrupted at the time of surgery. Proponents of maintaining antegrade flow suggest several advantages in doing so: (1) improvement of systemic arterial oxygen saturation, (2) promotion of pulmonary arterial growth after bidirectional Glenn shunt, (3) pulsatile flow reduces pulmonary vascular resistance, and (4) provision of 'hepatic factor' to minimize development of pulmonary arteriovenous malformations. On the other hand, the maintenance of antegrade flow constitutes a volume load while early volume unloading is considered to confer haemodynamic benefits to the functional single ventricle. Data remain conflicting on whether the maintenance or interruption of antegrade pulmonary flow may improve long-term clinical outcomes.

19.5.3 Completion of Fontan Circuit

The principle of the final stage of univentricular repair by the Fontan procedure is to channel the remaining systemic venous blood from the inferior caval vein (in additional to the superior caval venous blood) directly into the pulmonary circulation with separation of the systemic from the pulmonary venous return (Fig. 19.4d). This channelling is achieved either by baffling of the right atrium with an intraatrial patch or the use of an extracardiac conduit. The surgical evolution and refinement of the Fontan procedure and its physiology are further discussed in Chap. 30.

The Fontan procedure is performed usually at 3–5 years age. With Fontan completion, the systemic venous return into the pulmonary circulation is driven by the central venous pressure, change in intrathoracic pressure during inspiration, suction force generated by relaxation of the systemic ventricle, and the peripheral skeletal muscle pump.

Detailed preoperative evaluation to assess the suitability of completion of the Fontan circuit is required (Box 19.1).

Box 19.1 Preoperative Evaluation and Interventions Before Fontan Procedure

ECG
- Rhythm

Echocardiography
- Ventricular function
- Atrioventricular valvar regurgitation
- Ventricular outflow obstruction
- Other significant structural lesions (e.g. systemic and pulmonary venous stenosis, pulmonary arterial stenosis)

Cardiac Catheterization
- Haemodynamic parameters: mean superior caval venous pressure, mean pulmonary arterial pressure, transpulmonary gradient, pulmonary vascular resistance, systemic ventricular end-diastolic pressure, systemic ventricular outflow gradient, Qp:Qs ratio
- Angiography: pulmonary arterial size and arborization, pulmonary venous return, systemic ventricular outflow obstruction, hepatic and inferior caval venous drainage, aortopulmonary and venovenous collaterals
- Interventions: pulmonary arterial balloon angioplasty and stenting, embolization of arteriovenous and venovenous collaterals

An effective Fontan circulation depends on several important factors that have to be optimized before surgery: (1) sinus rhythm, (2) mean pulmonary arterial pressure <15 mmHg, (3) low pulmonary vascular resistance <4 Wood · units m^2, (4) normal pulmonary arterial size and arborization and with no distortion, (5) unobstructed pulmonary venous return, (6) satisfactory ventricular function, (7) absence or minimal atrioventricular valvar regurgitation, and (8) absence of systemic ventricular outflow obstruction.

Less favourable factors, while regarded as contraindication in the past, can be modified in the current era with medications (pulmonary vasodilators), transcatheter interventions (balloon angioplasty and stent implantation for pulmonary arterial stenosis, embolization of arteriovenous and venovenous collaterals), and surgery (repair or replacement of atrioventricular valve and relief of residual systemic ventricular outflow obstruction).

Some centres create a fenestration routinely at the level of the intraatrial baffle or the extracardiac conduit during Fontan completion, while others adopted this only in high-risk patients. The creation of a fenestration, which allows right-to-left shunting of blood, can increase ventricular preload and cardiac output and reduce systemic venous pressure after the Fontan procedure. Duration of postoperative pleural effusion due to systemic venous hypertension may also be shortened by creation of a fenestration.

19.6 Postoperative Considerations

19.6.1 First Stage Palliation

The issues on balancing between pulmonary and systemic flow and optimizing SaO_2 after systemic-to-pulmonary arterial shunting are discussed in Chaps. 29 and 54. Initiation of heparin infusion early after surgery (when bleeding is not an issue) followed by oral aspirin therapy until takedown of the shunt is practised in many centres.

19.6.2 Bidirectional Glenn Shunt

Potential issues after bidirectional Glenn shunt are related to an increase in venous pressure in the upper part of the body. These include headache, systemic hypertension (may be related to an increase in intracranial pressure secondary to systemic venous hypertension), facial and upper limb swelling, and pleural effusion.

Initial intensive care management includes standard fluid restriction, early establishment of spontaneous breathing and extubation, medical treatment of systemic hypertension, diuretics and, if necessary, pulmonary vasodilator for increased superior caval venous pressure and congestion of the upper part of the body. Initiation of heparin infusion early after surgery (when bleeding is not an issue) followed by oral aspirin therapy until Fontan completion is usually adopted for thromboprophylaxis.

19.6.3 Post Fontan Procedure

Potential complications after Fontan procedure include low cardiac output syndrome, cardiac arrhythmias including sinus node dysfunction, atrial arrhythmias, and junctional ectopic tachycardia (less common after extracardiac conduit Fontan procedure), off target SaO_2 with significant hypoxaemia (Chap. 54), and transient liver dysfunction.

In Fontan patients, the most important factors that determines cardiac output are transpulmonary flow and systemic ventricular filling. Hence, measures that reduce pulmonary vascular resistance and ensure adequate intravascular volume load and ventricular filling are important early after operation.

Initial intensive care management include standard fluid restriction, boluses of volume to ensure adequate volume load (a central venous pressure of 12–15 mmHg is commonly required) in the first 24 h of surgery, early establishment of spontaneous breathing and extubation, maintenance of atrioventricular synchrony, and low dose milrinone and adrenaline in the presence of ventricular dysfunction with or without atrioventricular regurgitation (to augment contractility and reduce afterload, but need to avoid tachycardia that may impair ventricular filling). Continuation of fluid restriction and diuresis are necessary to manage systemic venous congestion and shorten the duration of pleural effusion. Oral pulmonary vasodilators may be considered in patients with high Fontan circuit pressure in association with significant right-to-left shunt through the fenestration and/or prolonged pleural effusion.

With stabilization of the haemodynamics and recovery of liver dysfunction, thromboprophylaxis with warfarin or aspirin, depending on institutional practice and patient risk factors, should be started. Preliminary data suggest the possibility of using an oral direct factor Xa inhibitor (NOAC, non-vitamin K antagonist oral anticoagulants or DOAC, direct oral anticoagulants) for thromboprophylaxis in paediatric and adult post Fontan patients.

19.7 Long-Term Monitoring

Long-term issues pertaining to the unique physiology after Fontan procedure require life-long monitoring and management and are discussed in Chap. 30.

Heterotaxy Syndrome 20

'Heterotaxy' is a term with its origin from the Greek words 'heteros' (meaning 'other than') and 'taxis' (meaning 'arrangement'). Heterotaxy syndrome is a rare condition characterized by abnormal arrangement of the thoracic and abdominal organs that departs from the usual arrangement of the right-left axis (often referred to as 'situs solitus') in normal individuals.

Disorders of the left-right axis determination during embryogenesis, with ciliary dysfunction probably playing a contributory role, result in heterotaxy syndrome. An association between primary ciliary dyskinesia (with some patients harbouring mutations in *DNAI1* and *DNAH5* that encode the outer arm dynein proteins) and heterotaxy syndrome has been shown.

20.1 Anatomy

In the usual arrangement of the thoracic and abdominal organs normal body, right-left asymmetry is the norm. On the other hand, in heterotaxy syndrome, isomerism of these organs is present. The term 'isomerism' is derived from the Greek words 'iso' (meaning 'equal') and *meros (*meaning 'part').

In congenital cardiac malformation, isomerism pertains to the description of atrial appendages (Table 20.1). In right atrial isomerism, morphologic right atrial appendages are present on both sides of the heart. In left atrial isomerism, morphologic left atrial appendages are present on both sides.

Y.-f. Cheung, *Congenital and Paediatric Acquired Heart Disease in Practice*, https://doi.org/10.1007/978-981-99-2862-0_20

Table 20.1 Features of the atrial appendages

	Right atrial appendage	Left atrial appendage
Pectinate muscle	The pectinate muscle extends around the atrioventricular junction to meet at the crux	The pectinate muscle is contained within the tubular appendages
Morphology of appendage	Triangular shape with a broad junction with the smooth-walled component of the atrium	Tubular shape with a narrow or constricted junction with the smooth-walled component of the atrium
Terminal crest	Present	Absent

Table 20.2 Symmetric features of body structures in atrial isomerism

	Right atrial isomerism	Left atrial isomerism
Bronchus	Short right main stem bronchus Tracheobronchial angle >135°	Long left main stem bronchus Tracheobronchial angle <135°
Pulmonary lobulation	Three lobes	Two lobes
Spleen	Absence of spleen	Polysplenia
Liver	Central liver	Central liver Biliary atresia may occur

For other organs and structures of the body, paired structures on opposite sides may be symmetrical and mirror images of each other (Table 20.2 and Fig. 20.1). However, there can be discordance between the arrangement of atrial appendages and bronchial and splenic arrangements.

In clinical practice, the recognition and diagnosis of atrial isomerism is based on the findings of abnormal relationships between the inferior caval vein and aorta (as described below), symmetric features of body structures (Table 20.2), associated cardiac malformations (Table 20.3), and extracardiac anomalies (Table 20.4).

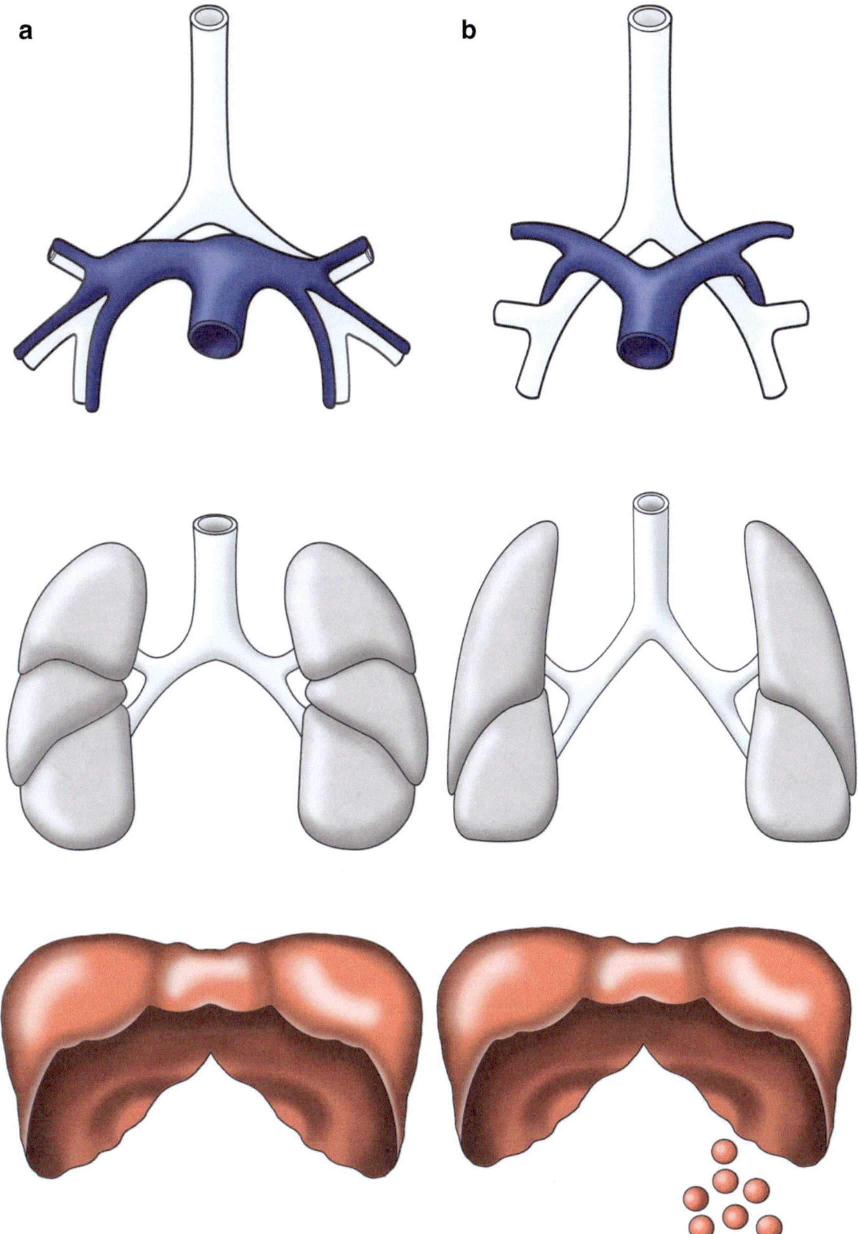

Fig. 20.1 Symmetry of body structures and organs in heterotaxy syndrome. (**a**) Right atrial isomerism. (**b**) Left atrial isomerism

Table 20.3 Associated cardiac malformations and electrophysiologic abnormalities in atrial isomerism

	Right atrial isomerism	Left atrial isomerism
Atrial septum	Severely deficient atrium septum with almost a common atrium	Maybe intact or severely deficient
Atrioventricular junction	Usually with complete atrioventricular septal defect	Can have intact ventricular septum or complete atrioventricular septal defect
Ventricles	Predominantly a functional single ventricle (single or double-outlet)	Can have two ventricles or a functional single ventricle
Ventricular outflow obstruction	Pulmonary stenosis or atresia is common	Coarctation of the aorta can occur
Pulmonary venous abnormalities	Total anomalous pulmonary venous drainage (unobstructive or obstructive) is common	Partial anomalous pulmonary venous connection can occur
Systemic venous abnormalities	Absent coronary sinus Bilateral superior caval veins	Interruption of inferior caval vein with azygous continuation to the superior caval vein
Electrophysiologic abnormalities	Twin sinus and atrioventricular nodes with supraventricular tachyarrhythmias	Hypoplastic or absent sinus node with sinus node dysfunction, atrial arrhythmias, and atrioventricular block

Table 20.4 Extracardiac anomalies in atrial isomerism

	Right atrial isomerism	Left atrial isomerism
Central nervous system	Neural tube defects (rare)	–
Liver and gastrointestinal system	Gut malrotation	Gut malrotation Biliary atresia
Immune abnormalities	Absence of splenic function	Splenic function can be abnormal despite polysplenia
Renal anomalies	Horseshoe kidney, solitary kidney, ectopic or duplication of ureters	Similar renal anomalies as in right atrial isomerism

20.2 Pathophysiology and Clinical Features

The pathophysiology and clinical features vary and depend on the cardiac malformations associated with the type of isomerism.

In patients with right atrial isomerism, the pathophysiology and features are usually those of a functional single ventricle (Chap. 19), anomalous pulmonary venous connection (Chap. 37), and duct-dependent pulmonary circulation due to pulmonary atresia.

In patients with left atrial isomerism, on the other hand, the pathophysiology and features vary as these patients can have a functionally single ventricle or a biventricular circulation with haemodynamically insignificant lesions (e.g. isolated interruption of inferior caval vein with azygous continuation to the superior caval vein).

Other clinical manifestations are associated with extracardiac abnormalities. These include recurrent sinus and respiratory tract infections (due to associated ciliary dysfunction in right and left isomerism), sepsis with bacteraemia due to encapsulated organisms (related to asplenia in right isomerism or abnormal splenic function even with the presence of polysplenia in left isomerism), jaundice (as a presenting symptom of biliary atresia in left atrial isomerism), and bowel obstruction (due to gut malrotation in right and left atrial isomerism).

20.3 Investigations

CXR: Chest radiographic findings reflect the underlying pathophysiology of the associated cardiac malformations. Additional information includes the bronchial arrangement and central liver.

ECG: The electrocardiogram shows findings that reflect the underlying electrophysiologic abnormalities.

Echocardiography: Echocardiographic assessment is used to diagnose atrial isomerism. In right atrial isomerism, the inferior caval vein and aorta are located on the same side of the spine and run adjacent to each other or having an anteroposterior relationship. In left atrial isomerism, azygous continuation of the inferior caval vein, running posterior to the aorta, with drainage into the superior caval vein can be demonstrated.

Cardiac catheterization: Invasive cardiac catheterization is rarely necessary for initial diagnostic purpose. Haemodynamic assessment later is required for the staged univentricular repair in patients with a functional single ventricle.

Evaluation of splenic function: Radionuclide scan is useful for assessment of functional splenic tissues. The presence of Howell-Jolly bodies in peripheral blood smear suggests asplenia.

Assessment of gut malrotation: Contrast study for gut malrotation is not routinely performed unless bowel obstruction is suspected.

20.4 Management Strategy

20.4.1 Cardiac Malformations

The management depends on the associated cardiac malformations. Most of the patients (almost all patients with right atrial isomerism and about 50–75% of those with left atrial isomerism) require staged univentricular repair for functional single ventricles. Patients who can be managed using biventricular repair are likely those with left atrial isomerism.

There are several unique surgical issues in patients with isomerism undergoing univentricular repair:

1. Pulmonary arteriovenous malformations may develop after Kawashima procedure (Box 20.1) in patients with left atrial isomerism and worsen systemic oxygen saturation. This is due to the lack of supply of 'hepatic factors' (nature being unknown) to the pulmonary circulation. Completion of Fontan circuit requires inclusion of hepatic veins to the pulmonary arteries.
2. Bilateral bidirectional Glenn shunt is required for patients with bilateral superior caval veins. The growth of the pulmonary arterial segment between the anastomotic sites may be hypoplastic and requires arterioplasty upon completion of the total cavopulmonary connection.
3. Obstructed pulmonary venous return and significant atrioventricular valvar regurgitation constitute high-risk surgical repair in patients with right atrial isomerism.
4. Bilateral hepatic venous drainage with separate drainage from the inferior caval vein of the left hepatic veins into the atrium can occur in right atrium isomerism. This right-to-left hepatic shunt may cause systemic oxygen desaturation after Fontan completion and necessitate surgical ligation or transcatheter device occlusion of the right-to-left hepatic shunts or reinclusion of residual hepatic venous drainage into the Fontan circuit.

Box 20.1 Kawashima Procedure

- Performed in patients with left isomerism having azygous continuation of interrupted inferior caval vein to the superior caval vein
- Procedure involves a bidirectional Glenn shunt with additional ligation or transection of the pulmonary trunk
- The superior caval vein drains a greater proportion (about 80–85%) of the systemic venous return as blood from the lower part of body is also channelled to the superior caval vein
- The deoxygenated hepatic venous and coronary sinus blood drains to the systemic ventricle and cause mild degree of oxygen desaturation
- Worsening of oxygen saturation suggests development of pulmonary arteriovenous malformations

20.4.2 Extracardiac Anomalies

Extracardiac anomalies contribute to morbidity and mortality in patients with atrial isomerism and need to be carefully managed:

1. Antibiotic prophylaxis is required for patients with absent or severely decreased splenic function (Box 20.2).

2. Pneumococcal, meningococcal, and *Haemophilus influenzae* type B vaccinations are required for patients with absence or severely decreased splenic function. Annual influenza vaccination reduces the risk of secondary bacterial, in particular pneumococcal, infection.
3. Gut malrotation predisposes to acute intestinal obstruction, which requires surgical intervention. Prophylactic surgery is, however, usually not indicated.
4. Kasai procedure is required in patients with left atrial isomerism and associated biliary atresia.

Box 20.2 Antibiotic Prophylaxis for Patients with Absent or Severely Decreased Splenic Function

- Phenoxymethylpenicillin (pen VK) 125 mg BD (<3 years) or 250 mg BD (≥3 years) or amoxycillin 10 mg/kg BD (maximum 250 mg/dose)
- If sensitive to beta-lactam antibiotics, azithromycin 5 mg/dose once daily (maximum 250 mg once daily)
- Until 5 years of age although some would recommend lifelong antibiotic prophylaxis

20.5 Postoperative Considerations

The postoperative management and complications are mostly those described after different stages of univentricular repair. In patients with right atrial isomerism, important postoperative issues include pulmonary hypertension (for those with obstructed anomalous pulmonary venous connection), severe common atrioventricular valvar regurgitation, and supraventricular tachyarrhythmias.

20.6 Long-Term Monitoring

The long-term outcomes depend on the complexity of the cardiac and extracardiac anomalies in patients with heterotaxy syndrome and the type of surgery repair. The highest risk patients are those having right atrial isomerism with obstructed pulmonary venous return, severe common atrioventricular valvar regurgitation, and ventricular dysfunction. Heart transplantation may be an option for these patients. Development of cardiac arrhythmias should be monitored and managed accordingly. Vaccinations, antibiotic prophylaxis, and family education are important to reduce the morbidity and mortality related to sepsis.

21 Hypoplastic Left Heart Syndrome

Hypoplastic left heart syndrome comprises lesions with varying degree of hypoplasia of the left-sided cardiac structures that cannot support the systemic circulation.

21.1 Anatomy

Hypoplastic left heart syndrome is characterized by underdevelopment of the mitral valve apparatus, the left ventricle, and the aorta. The hypoplastic mitral valve is stenotic or atretic, the left ventricle is slit-like, and the aortic valve is atretic or severely hypoplastic and stenotic (Fig. 21.1a). The ascending aorta is diminutive and associated coarctation of the aorta is common. The coronary arteries arise normally from the hypoplastic aortic root.

The oval foramen is patent and non-restrictive in most of the patients. In the rare situation of a restrictive atrial communication or an intact atrial septum, blood is forced to empty the left atrium through the levoatrial cardinal vein (an embryologic remnant of the fetal venous system that connects the pulmonary venous drainage with the caval venous system, e.g. innominate vein or superior cavel vein) or the fenestrated roof of the coronary sinus.

Y.-f. Cheung, *Congenital and Paediatric Acquired Heart Disease in Practice*, https://doi.org/10.1007/978-981-99-2862-0_21

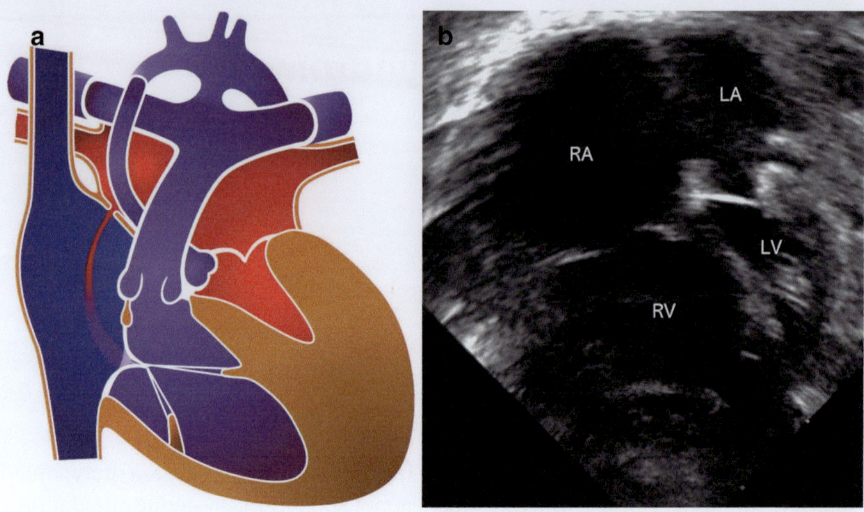

Fig. 21.1 Hypoplastic left heart syndrome. (**a**) Illustration of hypoplastic left heart syndrome. (**b**) Echocardiographic demonstration of the hypoplastic left ventricle, hypoplastic mitral valve and atrial septal defect (*LA* left atrium, *LV* left ventricle, *RA* right atrium, *RV* right ventricle)

21.2 Pathophysiology

Blood in the left atrium flows to the right atrium through a patent oval foramen or an atrial septal defect as the left ventricular inflow is obstructed. Rarely, when the atrial communication is restrictive or the atrial septum is intact, left atrial hypertension develops despite decompression of the left atrium by way of the levoatrial cardinal vein or the fenestrated roof of the coronary sinus. This causes arterialization of the pulmonary veins and lymphangiectasia.

There is no cardiac output from the left ventricle and the sole source of systemic blood supply is from the right ventricle through the dilated main pulmonary trunk and the arterial duct (duct-dependent systemic circulation). The ascending aorta and its branches (coronary and cranial arteries) are therefore perfused in a retrograde manner.

21.3 Clinical Presentation and Findings

Although cyanosis occurs as a result of the right-to-left shunt through the arterial duct, the predominant clinical manifestation is that of severe left ventricular outflow obstruction (Chap. 13). Hence, neonates with hypoplastic left heart syndrome

Table 21.1 Signs of hypoplastic left heart syndrome

Signs	Origins
Signs of heart failure and poor perfusion	Usually within the first week of life
Weak peripheral pulses	The pulse volume may be variable, depending on the size of the arterial duct
RV impulse	Right ventricle supports both the systemic and pulmonary circulations
Single S2	Atresia of the aortic valve
Ejection click	Dilation of the pulmonary trunk
Heart murmur	Either absent or non-specific

typically presents with early-onset heart failure, usually within the first week of life, due to closure of the arterial duct (duct-dependent systemic circulation). The signs are those of low cardiac output syndrome (Table 21.1). Heart murmur is either absent or non-specific. Hypoplastic left heart syndrome should be included in the list of differential diagnoses in neonates presenting with shock (Chap. 1).

21.4 Investigations

CXR: The typical radiographic features are cardiomegaly and increased pulmonary vascular markings. The right atrium and right ventricle are enlarged. The increased pulmonary vascular markings are related to pulmonary plethora and, when the atrial communication is small and restrictive, pulmonary venous congestion.
ECG: Electrocardiogram shows right axis deviation and right ventricular hypertrophy. Coronary insufficiency due to inadequate retrograde aortic flow may cause ST-segment depression and T wave inversion.
Echocardiography: Echocardiography defines the hypoplastic left-sided cardiac structures, patency and size of the arterial duct, size of the interatrial communication, patency of the levoatrial cardinal vein if the interatrial communication is restrictive, systemic right ventricular function, and competency of the tricuspid valve (Fig. 21.1b)

21.5 Management Strategy

Initial stabilization: Initial stabilization aims at optimizing the systemic perfusion by intravenous infusion of prostaglandin E, inotropic support, and correction of metabolic acidosis. The size of the interatrial communication has implications on the next steps in management; (1) severely restrictive atrial communication: balloon atrioseptostomy to relieve pulmonary venous congestion and to increase cardiac output is required, (2) mildly restrictive atrial communication: no active interventions are required until the first stage of palliative intervention, and (3) large atrial communication: this requires early intervention as it predisposes to early heart failure due to high pulmonary flow when the pulmonary vascular resistance decreases. systemic hypoperfusion with coronary insufficiency, and multiorgan failure.

Management of neonatal heart failure: The management aims to limit pulmonary flow, increase systemic flow, and reduce congestion by: (1) positive pressure ventilation with room air and avoidance of respiratory of alkalosis, (2) giving low dose inodilator, inotropes, and/or systemic vasodilators, and (3) prescription of diuretics.

Neonatal surgical interventions: Surgery aims at staged univentricular repair with eventual utilization of the functional right ventricle to support the systemic circulation.

The first stage surgical intervention performed in the neonatal period is the Norwood procedure (Fig. 21.2a). The proximal end of the transected pulmonary trunk and the hypoplastic native aorta are used to reconstruct a new ascending aorta and aortic arch (neoaorta). The pulmonary blood flow is supplied either by a

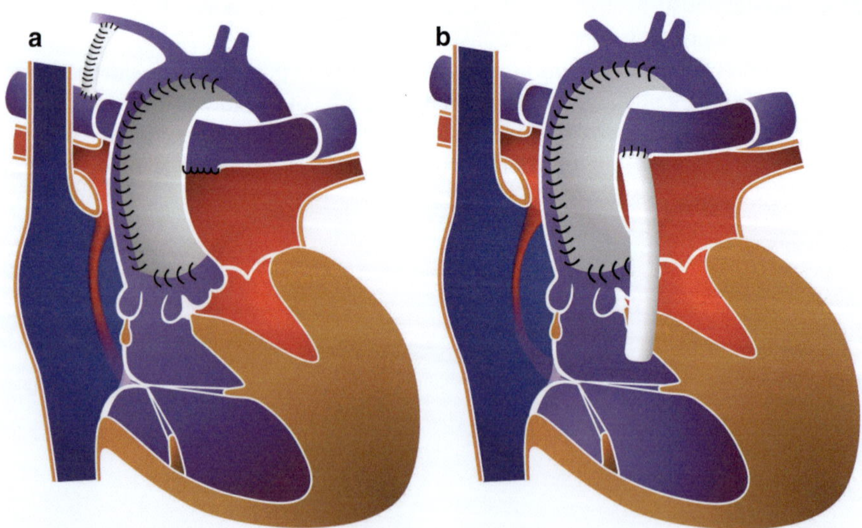

Fig. 21.2 Norwood procedure and Sano shunt. (**a**) Illustration of the Norwood procedure. (**b**) Sano modification of the Norwood procedure

modified Blalock-Taussig shunt or a Sano shunt (a conduit interposed between the right ventricle and the distal end of the pulmonary trunk (Fig. 21.2b). Issues related to imbalance of pulmonary and systemic flow after a modified Blalock-Taussig shunt are highlighted in Chaps. 29 and 54. Sano shunt, on the other hand, is associated with more stable postoperative haemodynamics, higher diastolic blood pressure, and lower risk of coronary steal and myocardial ischaemia. Placement of a Sano shunt, however, requires right ventriculotomy with potential impact of systemic right ventricular function.

Some centres adopt a hybrid procedure as the first stage of palliation that does not require cardiopulmonary bypass. The hybrid procedure consists of (1) bilateral banding of the pulmonary arteries, (2) stenting of the arterial duct, and (3) enlargement of the interatrial communication by balloon atrioseptostomy or stenting (Fig. 21.3). A more extensive stage two repair as described below is, however, required after an initial hybrid procedure. Recently, a first stage palliative procedure, which is completely percutaneous, with endoluminal banding of the branch pulmonary arteries using manually modified microvascular plugs as pulmonary flow restrictors and stenting of the arterial duct has been described.

Minimization of interstage mortality: Patients after the first stage palliation remain at risk of interstage mortality, which occurs at a rate of about 10%. Causes of death include shunt complications (stenosis or thrombosis), imbalance of pulmonary and systemic blood flow (with pulmonary overcirculation and systemic

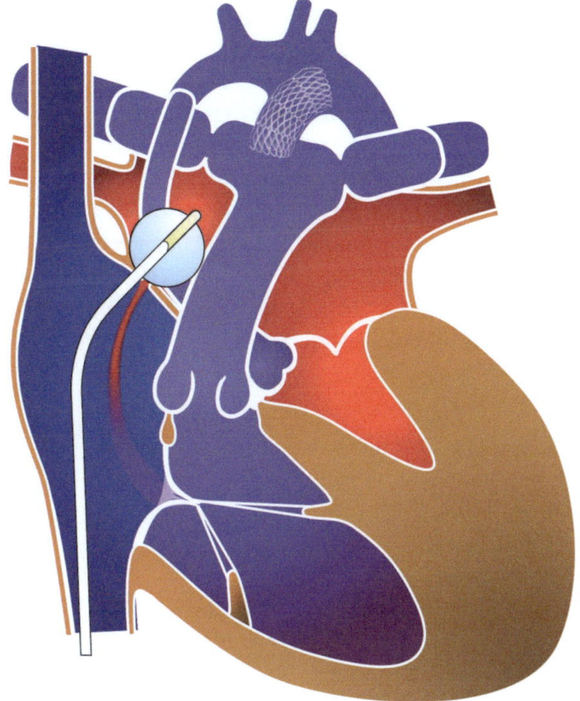

Fig. 21.3 Hybrid approach for hypoplastic left heart syndrome. Illustration showing bilateral banding of pulmonary arteries, stenting of arterial duct, and enlargement of the interatrial communication in stage 1 hybrid palliation of hypoplastic left heart syndrome

hypoperfusion, which causes coronary insufficiency), cardiac arrhythmias, residual lesions (e.g. recoarctation of the aorta), and ventricular dysfunction with significant tricuspid regurgitation. Institution of home monitoring programme with close attention to daily body weight and oxygen saturation and early alert of the medical personnel has significantly reduced the interstage mortality.

Second and third stages of palliative surgery: The second stage with bidirectional Glenn shunt and the third stage with completion of the Fontan procedure are similar to those described for staged repair of functionally univentricular hearts (Chap. 19).

For patients who had the hybrid procedure at the first stage of palliation, a more extensive stage two repair with removal of ductal stent and pulmonary arterial bands, reconstruction of the neoaorta, and repair of the branch pulmonary arteries in addition to the bidirectional Glenn shunt is required.

Other management options: Heart transplantation may be required in some patients between Norwood procedure and bidirectional Glenn shunt and in some before completion of the Fontan procedure. Given the high surgical risks and mortality and the uncertainties of the long-term outcomes, the parental decision of opting not for surgery after a thorough discussion should be respected.

21.6 Postoperative Considerations

Postoperative issues and intensive care after the three different stages of palliations are those described for functionally univentricular hearts (Chap. 19).

21.7 Long-Term Monitoring

Survival after the Norwood procedure is about 60–70%. Survivors are at risk for neurodevelopmental impairment. Available data, albeit limited, suggest similar neurodevelopmental outcomes at 4 years of age between patients after Norwood procedure and those after hybrid intervention as the first stage of palliation. Long-term issues pertaining to the unique physiology after Fontan procedure require life-long monitoring and management and are discussed in Chap. 30.

22 Ebstein Anomaly

Ebstein anomaly is a very rare congenital heart disease but is the most common congenital malformation of the tricuspid valve. Dr. Wilhelm Ebstein, a German physician, described this malformation in 1866 in a 19-year-old man with cyanosis, dyspnoea, palpitations, jugular venous distension, and cardiomegaly.

22.1 Anatomy

The normal tricuspid valve consists of three leaflets, namely the anterior, inferior (posterior), and septal leaflets. Failed delamination of tricuspid valve leaflets during embryogenesis results in adherence of the valve leaflets to the myocardium. The consequence is displacement of the leaflets away from the usual position at the atrioventricular junction (Fig. 22.1a). The most commonly involved leaflet is the septal leaflet, followed by the inferior leaflet, while the anterior leaflet usually retains its normal hinge at the atrioventricular junction. In severe cases, both the septal and inferior leaflets appear rudimentary, dysplastic, thickened, while the anterior leaflet is redundant, deformed, and may be fenestrated. The anterior leaflet may also combine with the inferior leaflet to form a valve curtain. The chordae tendineae are short and poorly formed.

While downward displacement of the tricuspid valve leaflets has been used to describe this anomaly, the septal and inferior leaflets assume in essence a spiral rotation inferiorly into the right ventricle, hence rotating the tricuspid orifice away

Y.-f. Cheung, *Congenital and Paediatric Acquired Heart Disease in Practice*, https://doi.org/10.1007/978-981-99-2862-0_22

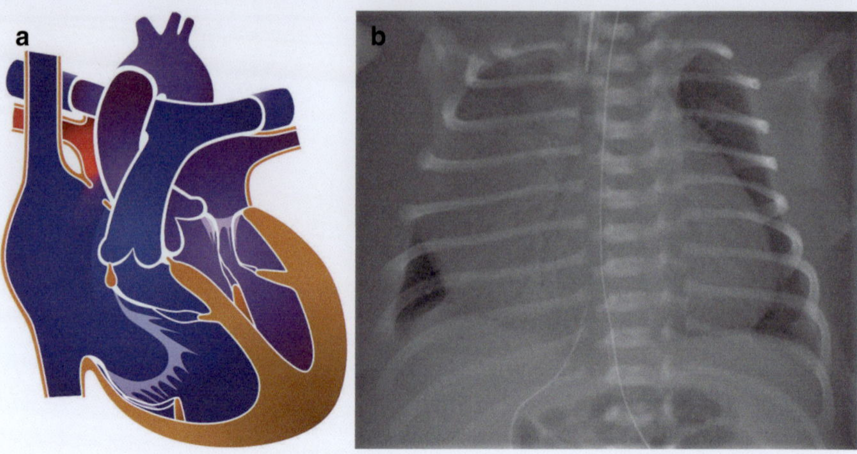

Fig. 22.1 Ebstein anomaly. (**a**) Illustration of Ebstein anomaly. (**b**) Chest radiograph showing the characteristic wall-to-wall heart in severe Ebstein anomaly

Table 22.1 Carpentier classification of Ebstein anomaly

Type	Description
A	Anterior leaflet is large and moving freely, septal and posterior leaflets are moderately displaced, functional right ventricular volume is adequate, atrialized right ventricle is small
B	Anterior leaflet is large and moving freely, septal and posterior leaflets are markedly displaced, functional right ventricle is small, atrialized right ventricle is large
C	Restricted anterior leaflet motion, septal and posterior leaflets are markedly displaced and may be severely hypoplastic, functional right ventricle is very small and may have poor contractility, atrialized right ventricle is large
D	Adherence of the anterior leaflet to the infundibulum and the trabecular portion of the right ventricle, almost complete atrialization of the poorly contractile right ventricle, restrictive opening between the atrialized right ventricle and infundibulum

from the usual atrioventricular junction. The orifice divides the right ventricle into a proximal atrialized portion, which is thin-walled and dilated, and a distal functional portion. Tricuspid valvar regurgitation is common. In some patients, severe tethering of the leaflets to the ventricular wall results in a stenotic keyhole opening. Fusion of the free edges of the leaflets may even result in tricuspid atresia in the setting of Ebstein malformation. Carpentier proposed a classification of the severity of Ebstein anomaly based on the anatomy of the valve leaflets and the right ventricle (Tables 22.1).

Almost all patients have an interatrial communication, usually in the form of a patent oval foramen. Association with pulmonary stenosis or atresia is common. Hypoplasia of the lungs may occur in the presence of severe Ebstein malformation due to gross dilation of the right atrium and the atrialized right ventricle.

22.2 Pathophysiology

The pathophysiological effects of Ebstein anomaly depends on severity of the valvar malformation, the size and contractile function of the functional right ventricle, and patency of the right ventricular outflow. Tricuspid regurgitation and stenosis cause right atrial dilation and hypertrophy. Left ventricular function may be impaired due to adverse ventricular-ventricular interaction (Chap. 28).

In the presence of pulmonary stenosis or structural pulmonary atresia, significant cyanosis occurs as a result of a large right-to-left atrial shunt. Contraction of the atrialized portion of the right ventricle may further increase the severity of right-to-left atrial shunt. Functional pulmonary atresia due to ineffective right ventricular forward flow may occur in newborn babies with high pulmonary vascular resistance and severe tricuspid regurgitation.

On the other hand, if the tricuspid valvar malformation and regurgitation is less severe and obstruction to pulmonary flow is mild or absent, the shunt through the interatrial communication may be bidirectional and the degree of cyanosis is minimal.

22.3 Clinical Manifestations

Neonates with severe Ebstein anomaly present with significant cyanosis and heart failure, although the cyanosis may improve after a few days with reduction in pulmonary vascular resistance.

Patients with milder degree of tricuspid valvar malformation may have mild cyanosis, which may become undetectable as the pulmonary vascular resistance drops. They may present later in life with worsening cyanosis (increased right-to-left atrial shunting due to worsening of tricuspid regurgitation and/or right ventricular function), palpitation (supraventricular tachyarrhythmias due to right atrial dilation and associated Wolff-Parkinson-White syndrome that is present in about 25% of patients), and impaired exercise capacity.

Physical signs of cyanosis, heart failure, and a quadruple gallop rhythm are common in patients with severe Ebstein malformation (Table 22.2).

Table 22.2 Signs of severe Ebstein malformation

	Origins
Cyanosis	Right-to-left atrial shunt and right ventricular outflow obstruction
Signs of systemic venous congestion	Proportional to the severity of tricuspid regurgitation and tricuspid stenosis
Quadruple rhythm	
Split S1	The second component is related to tricuspid valve closure
Split S2	Right ventricular conduction delay
S3 and S4	Impaired right ventricular filling or vibration of tricuspid valve
A pansystolic murmur at left lower sternal border	Tricuspid regurgitation

22.4 Investigations

CXR: Massive cardiomegaly due to significant dilation of the right atrium and the atrialized portion of the right ventricle is characteristic of severe Ebstein malformation (wall-to-wall appearance) (Fig. 22.1b). The pulmonary vascular markings are diminished. In older children with less severe forms of Ebstein malformation, the cardiac size may be mildly enlarged or even normal.
ECG: Electrocardiogram shows right atrial dilation, small QRS voltages over the right praecordial leads reflecting diminished right ventricular forces and widening of QRS complex due to intraventricular conduction delay. Features of Wolff-Parkinson-White syndrome are present in about 25% of patients.
Echocardiography: Echocardiography demonstrates downward displacement of the tricuspid valve leaflets and permits the assessment of the severity of tricuspid regurgitation, tricuspid stenosis, and functional or structural right ventricular outflow obstruction (Fig. 22.2a, b). Detailed assessment of all the leaflets (size, mobility, and adherence to the right ventricular myocardium) with two- and three-dimensional echocardiography is important before valve repair. Other evaluation includes functional assessment of the right and left ventricles and the size of the atrial communication. Rarely, the presence of significant pulmonary regurgitation can lead to a circular shunt in neonates (Chap. 29).

An echocardiographic grading score for assessing severity of Ebstein malformation in neonates based on the apical four-chamber view at end-diastole has been proposed by Celermajer and colleagues (also referred to as the Great Ormond Street score, Table 22.3): (right atrial area + atrialized right ventricular area)/(functional right ventricular area + left atrial area + left ventricular area). This score carries prognostic information (a ratio >1.5 has been reported previously to be associated with 100% mortality), although the prognostic association may have changed with contemporary management strategy.
CMR: In older children and adolescents, cardiac magnetic resonance enables the assessment of right ventricular and left ventricular volumes and function and evaluation of the Ebstein valve rotation angle (a larger rotation angle has been reported to increase the risk of valve dehiscence after cone repair).

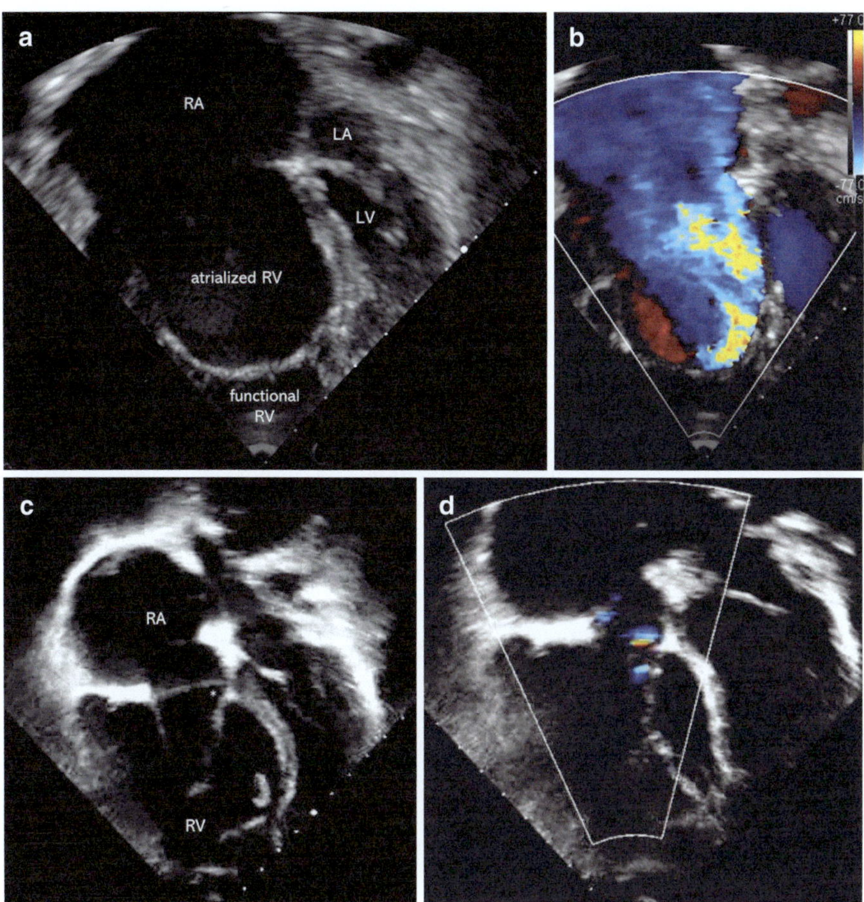

Fig. 22.2 Echocardiographic assessment of Ebstein anomaly before and after cone repair. (**a**) Echocardiographic demonstration of severe Ebstein anomaly with gross enlargement of the right atrium and atrialized right ventricle. (**b**) Colour flow mapping showing severe tricuspid regurgitation. (**c**) Echocardiographic appearance of the tricuspid valve after cone repair. (**d**) Colour flow mapping showing only mild tricuspid regurgitation after cone repair (*RA* right atrium, *RV* right ventricle, *LA* left atrium, *LV* left ventricle)

Table 22.3 Echocardiographic grading on severity of Ebstein malformation in neonates

Grade	Ratio
1	<0.5
2	0.5–0.99
3	1–1.49
4	>1.5

22.5 Management Strategy

22.5.1 Initial Stabilization

Newborn babies with severe Ebstein malformation may be critically ill with one of the following clinical scenarios:

1. Severe cyanosis due to associated structural pulmonary atresia or severe pulmonary stenosis: intravenous prostaglandin E infusion is required,
2. Severe cyanosis associated with functional pulmonary atresia: short duration of intravenous prostaglandin E infusion with gradual weaning as the pulmonary vascular resistance drops, and manoeuvres to reduce pulmonary vascular resistance (hyperventilation, high FiO_2, inhaled nitric oxide),
3. Severe heart failure with respiratory distress due to severe malformation of the tricuspid valve, severe tricuspid regurgitation, and cardiomegaly: ventilatory and inotropic support,
4. Systemic hypoperfusion due a circular shunt: ventilatory and inotropic support, and elimination of the circular shunt (Chap. 29).

22.5.2 Subsequent Management in Neonates and Infants

The next steps in the management algorithm are shown in Fig. 22.3. Many neonates with functional pulmonary atresia improve as the pulmonary vascular resistance drops and no further neonatal interventions are required. Further surgical

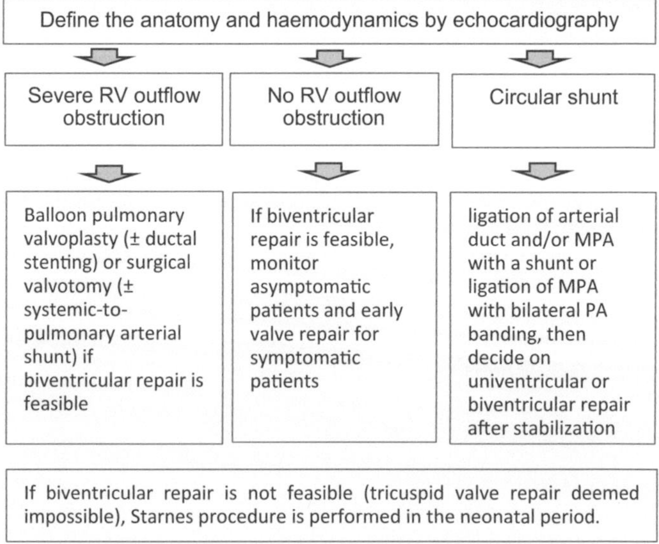

Fig. 22.3 Management algorithm of severe Ebstein anomaly in neonates. *MPA*, main pulmonary artery, *RV* right ventricular

interventions during the neonatal period are required in the presence of severe cyanosis, tricuspid regurgitation, cardiomegaly, and right heart failure. In the absence of these findings, the patient should be clinical stable and no neonatal interventions are required.

22.5.2.1 Univentricular Palliation in Neonates with Severe Ebstein Malformation

If tricuspid valve repair is not possible, these patients shall undergo a staged management towards eventual conversion to a Fontan circulation (Chap. 30): (1) the first stage palliation in the neonatal period is a Starnes procedure (right ventricular exclusion with fenestrated patch closure of the tricuspid valve, atrial septectomy, and insertion of a systemic-to-pulmonary arterial shunt), (2) a second stage palliation at 4–6 months of age with superior cavopulmonary (bidirectional Glenn) shunt, and (3) the third stage with completion of Fontan circuit at 3–5 years of age.

22.5.2.2 Repair of Tricuspid Valve

Tricuspid valve repair with reduction of the atrial communication, plication of the atrialized right ventricle, and right reduction atrioplasty can be performed as described below if deemed necessary. If possible, however, surgical repair of the tricuspid valve is generally avoided in the neonatal period.

22.5.3 Management in Older Children and Adolescents

Medical management of congestive heart failure and supraventricular tachycardia may be required. Surgical management consists of tricuspid valve repair, plication of the atrialized right ventricle, right reduction atrioplasty, and partial or total closure of the atrial communication. Indications for surgery in older children and adolescents are shown in Box 22.1.

Box 22.1 Indications for Surgical Repair of the Tricuspid Valve in Older Children and Adolescents with Ebstein Anomaly

- Worsening cyanosis
- Symptoms of heart failure
- Reduced exercise capacity
- Increasing cardiomegaly
- Progressive right ventricular dysfunction
- New onset or worsening of atrial tachyarrhythmias
- Paradoxical embolism

22.5.3.1 Repair of Replacement of Tricuspid Valve

Different techniques of tricuspid valve repair have been described. Cone reconstruction of the tricuspid valve has gained popularity in the current era. This involves the mobilization of all available leaflets from their abnormal attachments and rotating the leaflets in a clockwise direction to form a cone of valvar tissue, suturing together the valvar tissues, and finally reanchoring of the valve at the level of new tricuspid valve annulus. An additional annuloplasty is commonly performed. Tricuspid valve replacement remains to be an option if valve repair fails or is not possible.

22.5.3.2 Role of Bidirectional Glenn Shunt

A one-and-a-half ventricular repair (Chap. 32) with a bidirectional Glenn shunt is commonly considered in patients with significant right ventricular dilation and/or dysfunction and in those in whom the tricuspid valvar orifice becomes limited after surgical repair. A low pulmonary arterial pressure and resistance is, however, required, for the one-and-a-half ventricular repair.

Potential advantages of a bidirectional Glenn shunt in this setting include (1) unloading of the right ventricle, (2) provision of pulmonary flow and left ventricular preload independent of right ventricular function, and (3) reduction of flow across a relatively small tricuspid valvar orifice after tricuspid valve repair and annuloplasty. The need for further completion of the Fontan procedure in patients with Ebstein anomaly beyond infancy is uncommon.

22.5.3.3 Management of Arrhythmias

Electrophysiologic study is commonly performed in patients with Ebstein anomaly to identify accessory pathways. Patients with supraventricular tachycardia are managed by oral beta-blocker therapy (infants and younger children) and catheter ablation (in older children and adolescents). In older patients and adults with atrial fibrillation and flutter, right-sided or bi-atrial Maze procedure is performed at the time of surgical repair.

22.5.3.4 Heart Transplantation

Heart transplantation may be required for patients with severe biventricular dysfunction.

22.6 Postoperative Considerations

Postoperative issues and intensive care for neonates after Starnes procedure are those described for functionally univentricular heart (Chap. 19). For patients after repair of tricuspid valve, postoperative management includes inotropic support to optimize right ventricular function and maintenance of a low pulmonary vascular resistance to reduce right ventricular afterload.

22.7 Long-Term Monitoring

For patients managed by univentricular repair, long-term issues pertaining to the unique physiology after Fontan procedure require life-long monitoring and management (Chap. 30). For patients who have undergone repair or replacement of the tricuspid valve, long-term monitoring of the valvar function, right ventricular function and remodelling, left ventricular function, and atrial tachyarrhythmias is required.

Part IV

Other Diseases of the Right Heart

23 Double-Outlet Right Ventricle

Double-outlet right ventricle is a type of ventriculoarterial connection in which both great vessels (aorta and pulmonary artery) arise either predominantly or entirely from the right ventricle. This type of ventriculoarterial connection can occur in association with different types of atrial arrangements and atrioventricular connections and in biventricular or functionally univentricular hearts. This chapter focuses on the description of double-outlet right ventricle in the setting of a biventricular circulation with usual atrial arrangement and atrioventricular concordance.

23.1 Anatomy

With regard to the definition of a double-outlet right ventricle, there are three controversial aspects that have been debated over the years: (1) degree of overriding of the great vessels over the ventricular septum to arise from the right ventricle (50% versus 90% rule), (2) the need for the presence of mitral-aortic or mitral-pulmonary fibrous discontinuity, and (3) the need for the presence of bilateral coni (a subpulmonary conus and a subaortic conus). In the Congenital Heart Surgery Nomenclature and Database Project, the committees of the Society of Thoracic Surgeons and the European Society of Cardiothoracic Surgery adopted the more liberal requirement of the 50% rule with none of the other two features required for diagnosis of a double-outlet right ventricle.

A ventricular septal defect is almost always present in double-outlet right ventricle. The so-called 'ventricular septal defect' is in essence the channel that serves as an outlet for the left ventricle to empty blood to the right ventricle, the latter supporting the two great vessels. This is, however, not the defect to be closed in surgery. This defect is therefore better conceptualized as an 'interventricular communication' in the setting of a double-outlet right ventricle.

Based on the relationship of the ventricular septal defect to the great vessels (Fig. 23.1), different types of double-outlet right ventricle are recognized (Table 23.1).

Y.-f. Cheung, *Congenital and Paediatric Acquired Heart Disease in Practice*,
https://doi.org/10.1007/978-981-99-2862-0_23

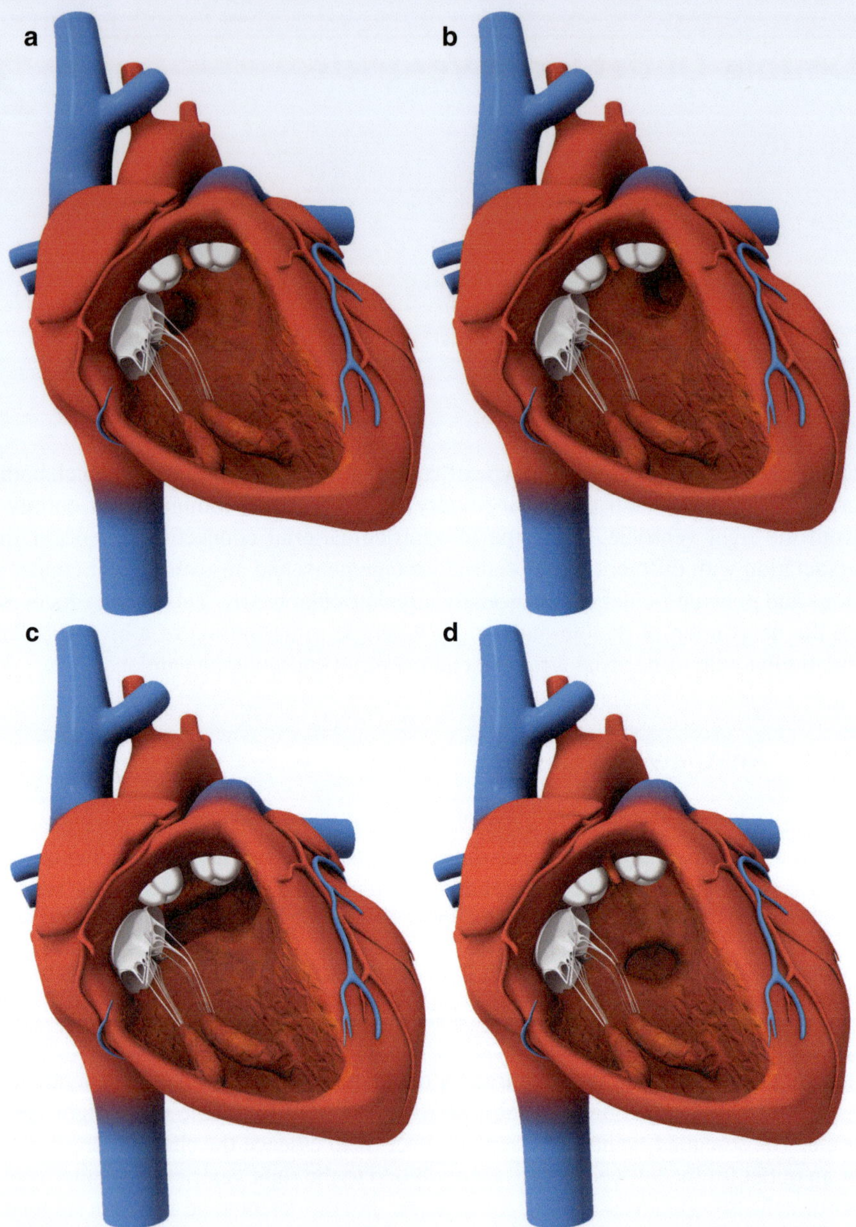

Fig. 23.1 Types of double-outlet right ventricle. Double-outlet right ventricle with (**a**) subaortic ventricular septal defect. (**b**) Subpulmonary ventricular septal defect (**c**) doubly committed subarterial ventricular septal defect and (**d**) remote (non-committed) ventricular septal defect

Table 23.1 Types of double-outlet right ventricle (DORV)

Type	Comments
DORV with subaortic ventricular septal defect (VSD)	aorta overrides the ventricular septum and spirals from the right to left relative to the pulmonary trunk
DORV with subaortic VSD and pulmonary stenosis	aorta overrides the ventricular septum and spirals from the right to left relative to the pulmonary trunk in conjunction with pulmonary stenosis, the most common type of DORV
DORV with subarterial VSD	absence of outlet septum, with both the aorta and pulmonary trunk overriding the ventricular septum
DORV with subpulmonary VSD	the pulmonary trunk overrides the ventricular septum, the aorta is to the right of and runs parallel to the pulmonary trunk (Taussig-Bing anomaly), the second most common type of DORV
DORV with remote VSD	The VSD is non-committed to either of the great vessels, the great vessels may run in a spiral or a parallel fashion with the aorta to the right of the pulmonary trunk

Associated cardiac lesions include pulmonary stenosis, atrial septal defect, persistent arterial duct, atrioventricular valvar abnormalities, and subaortic obstruction and coarctation of the aorta (especially in Taussig-Bing anomaly).

23.2 Pathophysiology and Clinical Features

The pathophysiology and clinical features depend on the location of the ventricular septal defect, the arrangement of the great arteries, the presence or absence of pulmonary or aortic stenosis, and associated cardiac lesions.

In double-outlet right ventricle, preferential streaming of blood through the ventricular septal defect (interventricular communication) is an important haemodynamic phenomenon, which has important implication on the mixing of oxygenated and deoxygenated blood: (1) in double-outlet right ventricle with subaortic ventricular septal defect, the oxygenated blood from the left ventricle preferentially streams to the aorta, thereby limiting the deoxygenated blood from the right ventricle to enter the systemic circulation, (2) in double-outlet right ventricle with subpulmonary ventricular septal defect, there is preferential streaming of the oxygenated blood from the left ventricle through the interventricular communication into the pulmonary artery, while deoxygenated blood from the right ventricle flows preferentially to the aorta.

Depending on mixing of the oxygenated blood with deoxygenated blood and the anatomy, the pathophysiology and clinical features mimic those of ventricular septal defect, tetralogy of Fallot, and transposition of the great arteries (Table 23.2).

Table 23.2 Pathophysiology and clinical features of double-outlet right ventricle (DORV) with different types of ventricular septal defect (VSD)

Type	Pathophysiology	Clinical features
DORV with subaortic or subarterial VSD	Mimics a large VSD	No significant cyanosis, symptoms and signs of heart failure
DORV with subaortic VSD and pulmonary stenosis	Mimics tetralogy of Fallot	Cyanosis with other signs of tetralogy of Fallot
DORV with subpulmonary VSD	Mimics transposition of the great arteries	Cyanosis with other signs of transposition of the great arteries
DORV with remote VSD	Mimics functional single ventricle with mixing of blood in the right ventricle	Cyanosis or symptoms and signs of heart failure depending on the presence or absence of pulmonary stenosis

23.3 Investigations

CXR: Chest radiographic findings reflect the underlying pathophysiology, mimicking those of a large ventricular septal defect, tetralogy of Fallot, of transposition of the great arteries.
ECG: The electrocardiographic findings reflect similarly the underlying pathophysiology, although the most consistent finding is right ventricular hypertrophy.
Echocardiography: Echocardiography demonstrates that both great arteries arise predominantly (>50% overriding) or entirely from the right ventricle and defines the location and size of the ventricular septal defect (interventricular communication), relationship of the defect to the outlet of the two great arteries, pulmonary stenosis, and other associated cardiac abnormalities. Echocardiography is also useful for the monitoring of balloon atrioseptostomy in Taussig-Bing anomaly.
CT and CMR: These imaging modalities help to define the location of remote ventricular septal defects relative to the arterial outlet and provide dataset for 3D printing that facilitates surgical decision and planning.

23.4 Management Strategy

The medical treatment and surgical interventions depend on the type of double-outlet right ventricle and pathophysiologic consequence (Fig. 23.2).

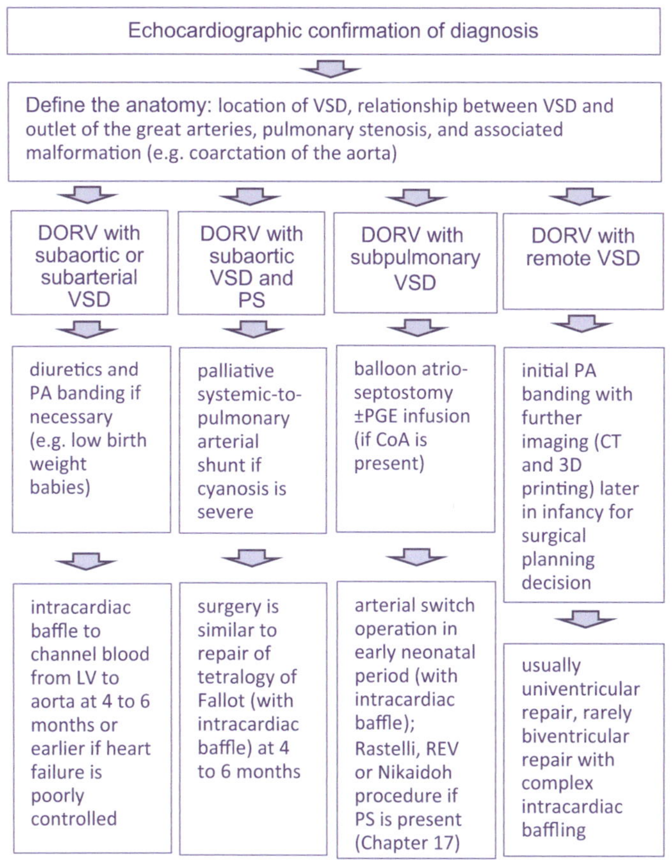

Fig. 23.2 Management strategy for double-outlet right ventricle. *LVOTO* left ventricular outflow tract obstruction, *PA* pulmonary arterial, *PS* pulmonary stenosis, *RV* right ventricular, *VSD* ventricular septal defect, *REV* réparation à l'ètage ventriculaire, *TV* tricuspid valve

23.5 Postoperative Considerations

The postoperative management and complications are similar to those encountered after repair of isolated ventricular septal defect (Chap. 11), repair of tetralogy of Fallot (Chap. 16), arterial switch operation for transposition of the great arteries (Chap. 17), and pulmonary arterial banding as the initial step in single ventricular palliation (Chap. 19), depending on the procedure used for the type of double-outlet right ventricle.

23.6 Long-Term Monitoring

Long-term complications related to the surgical strategies as described above require long-term monitoring. In patients requiring intracardiac baffling of blood from the left ventricle to the aorta (or neoaorta), subaortic obstruction occurs not uncommonly in the long term and requires reintervention.

Congenitally Corrected Transposition of the Great Arteries

24

Congenitally corrected transposition of the great arteries is characterized by discordant atrioventricular connection and discordant ventriculoarterial connection. This segmental combination can occur in the setting of usual or mirror-imaged atrial arrangement.

24.1 Anatomy

In congenitally corrected transposition of the great arteries, the morphologic right atrium is connected to the morphologic left ventricle through a mitral valve, while the morphologic left atrium is connected to the morphologic right ventricle through a tricuspid valve (Fig. 24.1a). The ventricles assume a side-by-side relationship and the cardiac mass and apex are often abnormally positioned, with mesocardia being found in about 25% of patients with congenitally corrected transposition of the great arteries.

The morphologic left ventricle gives rise to the pulmonary trunk, while the morphologic right ventricle gives rise to the aorta. The coronary arteries originate from the aortic sinus adjacent to the pulmonary trunk. In patients with usual atrial arrangement, the coronary arterial pattern is mirror image of that in a normal heart. Hence, the right-sided coronary artery, which supplies the subpulmonary morphologic left ventricle, assumes the pattern of a morphologic left coronary artery (with bifurcation into the anterior descending and circumflex branches). On the other hand, the left-sided coronary artery, which supplies the systemic morphologic right ventricle, assumes the pattern of a morphologic right coronary artery.

The conduction system in congenitally corrected transposition of the great arteries is abnormal. An anterior atrioventricular node replaces the usual posterior atrioventricular node to connect to the bundle of His, which continues as the

Y.-f. Cheung, *Congenital and Paediatric Acquired Heart Disease in Practice*, https://doi.org/10.1007/978-981-99-2862-0_24

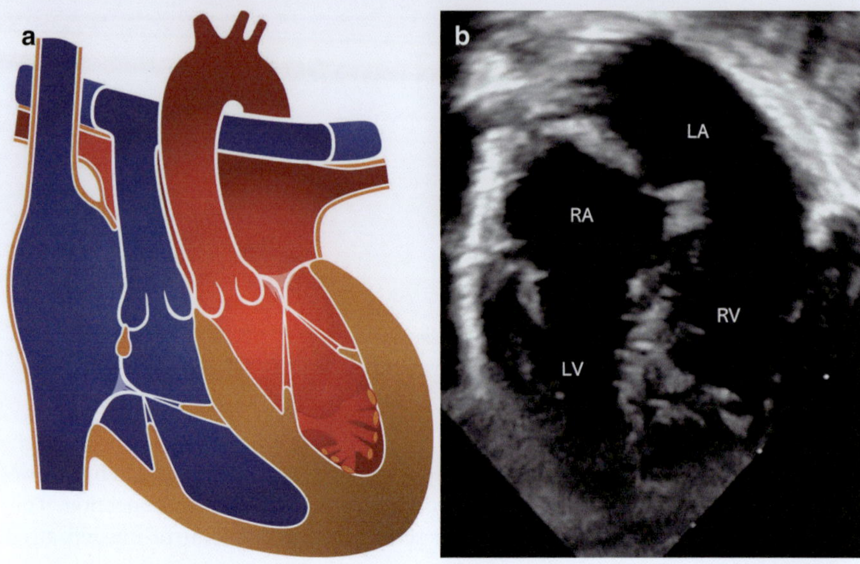

Fig. 24.1 Congenitally corrected transposition of the great arteries. (**a**) An illustration of congenitally corrected transposition of the great arteries. (**b**) Echocardiographic demonstration of the trabeculated systemic right ventricle on the left side and the morphologic left ventricle on the right side (*LA* left atrium, *LV* left ventricle, *RA* right atrium, *RV* right ventricle)

atrioventricular conduction bundle. Fibrosis of or damage to the abnormally long atrioventricular conduction bundle predisposes to development of spontaneous heart block or heart block after cardiac catheterization or surgery.

Associated cardiac malformations are present in the majority of patients. These include ventricular septal defect (50–70%) (usually perimembranous in location), left ventricular outflow obstruction (30–50%) (valvar pulmonary stenosis, subpulmonary stenosis related to muscles, membrane, or aneurysmal dilation of fibrous tissue derived from the membranous septum, and pulmonary atresia), and tricuspid valvar dysplasia with or without Ebstein malformation (about 30%).

24.2 Pathophysiology

In the absence of associated cardiac malformation, the circulatory physiology in congenitally corrected transposition of the great arteries is normal. Deoxygenated systemic venous blood drains from the morphologic right atrium into the morphologic left ventricle to enter the pulmonary circulation, while oxygenated pulmonary venous return to the systemic arterial circulation by way of the morphologic left atrium and morphologic right ventricle. In the presence of associated cardiac malformations, the pathophysiology reflects that of the different associated defects.

The morphologic right ventricle is the systemic ventricle and is vulnerable to progressive dysfunction. Possible mechanisms include alteration of ventricular geometry leading to progressive tricuspid regurgitation, alteration of pattern of myocardial deformation, myocardial fibrosis, and impairment of myocardium perfusion due to the single coronary arterial supply.

24.3 Clinical Manifestations and Findings

The clinical presentation of patients with congenitally corrected transposition of the great arteries depends on the associated cardiac abnormalities. Infants with a large ventricular septal defect and absence of significant left ventricular outflow obstruction present with heart failure. Newborn babies with a large ventricular septal defect and severe left ventricular outflow obstruction (pulmonary stenosis or atresia) present with cyanosis. Patients with a large ventricular septal defect and moderate degree of left ventricular (pulmonary) outflow obstruction have balanced haemodynamics and present with incidental finding of a cardiac murmur. Adolescents and adults may present for the first time with symptoms of heart failure due to severe tricuspid regurgitation and systemic right ventricular dysfunction. Complete heart block may occur at any age and cause heart failure and syncope.

Asymptomatic patients with normal examination findings may be diagnosed by antenatal echocardiographic assessment or postnatal echocardiographic examination for functional murmur or other reasons. The signs of congenitally corrected transposition of the great arteries are those of the associated cardiac abnormalities (Table 24.1).

Table 24.1 Signs of congenitally corrected transposition of the great arteries

Signs	Origins
Signs of heart failure	Depends on the size of ventricular septal defect and severity of left ventricular outflow obstruction
Cyanosis	Degree of cyanosis depends on the severity of left ventricular (pulmonary) outflow obstruction
Right ventricular impulse	Pressure overloading of the right ventricle as it is supporting the systemic circulation and volume overloading in the presence of significant tricuspid regurgitation
Loud and single S2	Closure sound of the anteriorly positioned aortic valve
Cardiac murmur	The nature depends on the presence of ventricular septal defect and tricuspid regurgitation (pansystolic murmur), left ventricular outflow obstruction (ejection systolic murmur), or absence of associated lesions (no murmur)

24.4 Investigations

CXR: Chest radiograph may reveal levocardia, mesocardia, or dextrocardia. Cardiomegaly may be due to a large left-to-right shunt through the ventricular septal defect, right ventricular dysfunction, or tricuspid regurgitation. Depending on the associated cardiac malformations, the lung fields may appear plethoric (a large ventricular septal defect with no significant pulmonary stenosis) or oligaemic (severe pulmonary stenosis or atresia).

ECG: Electrocardiogram shows the characteristic findings of reversal of the praecordial Q wave pattern with Q waves in the right praecordial leads due to right to left depolarization of the ventricular septum (opposite to that of normal). Varying degrees of atrioventricular block may be present.

Echocardiography: Echocardiographic diagnosis is made by demonstration of (1) systemic veins draining through the right atrium into a morphologic left ventricle (recognized by the fine trabeculations and a smooth wall), (2) pulmonary veins draining through the left atrium into a morphologic right ventricle (recognized by the coarse trabeculations) (Fig. 24.1b), (3) morphology of the mitral valve with the paired papillary muscles in the morphologic left ventricle, and (4) offsetting of the septal leaflet of the tricuspid valve in the morphologic right ventricle and its attachment to the ventricular septum. Echocardiography also shows parallel arrangement of the two great arteries. Further imaging should include the assessment of associated cardiac malformations including ventricular septal defect, left ventricular (pulmonary) outflow obstruction, and tricuspid valvar dysplasia or Ebstein malformation, function of the systemic right ventricle, and competency of the tricuspid (systemic atrioventricular) valve.

Cardiac catheterization: Cardiac catheterization is not usually required for initial diagnosis. Diagnostic catheterization is performed to assess haemodynamics prior to Fontan procedure (Fig. 24.2a, b) or after pulmonary arterial banding to determine the preparedness of the left ventricle.

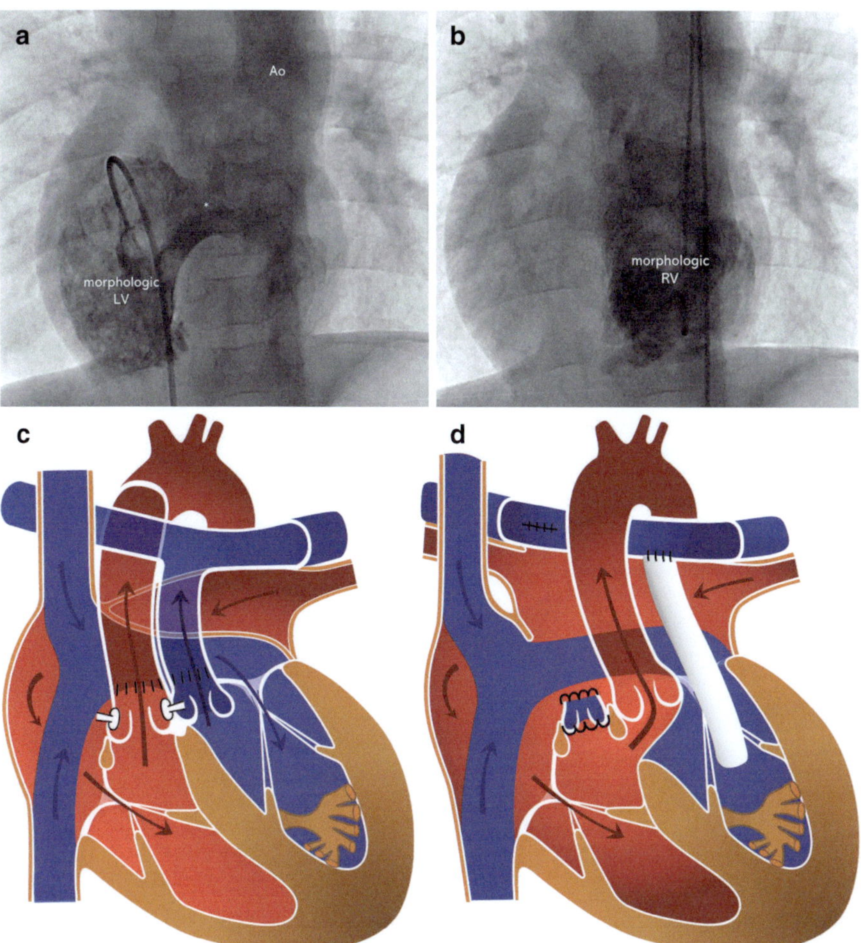

Fig. 24.2 Imaging and anatomic repair of congenitally corrected transposition of the great arteries. Angiographic illustrations of (**a**) a right-sided morphologic left ventricle that has fine trabeculations and a smooth wall and (**b**) a left-sided morphologic right ventricle with coarse trabeculations in a child with congenitally corrected transposition of the great arteries and associated ventricular septal defect (asterisk) and pulmonary atresia. (**c**) Double-switch operation. (**d**) Senning-Rastelli operation (*Ao* aorta, *LV* left ventricle, *RV* right ventricle)

24.5 Management Strategy

Management of congenital corrected transposition of the great arteries is challenging given the concerns of progressive systemic right ventricular dysfunction and the frequent associations with other significant cardiac malformations. The optimal surgical approach in terms of physiologic repair, anatomic repair, or Fontan palliation remains debatable. The management algorithm shown in Fig. 24.3 represents only a

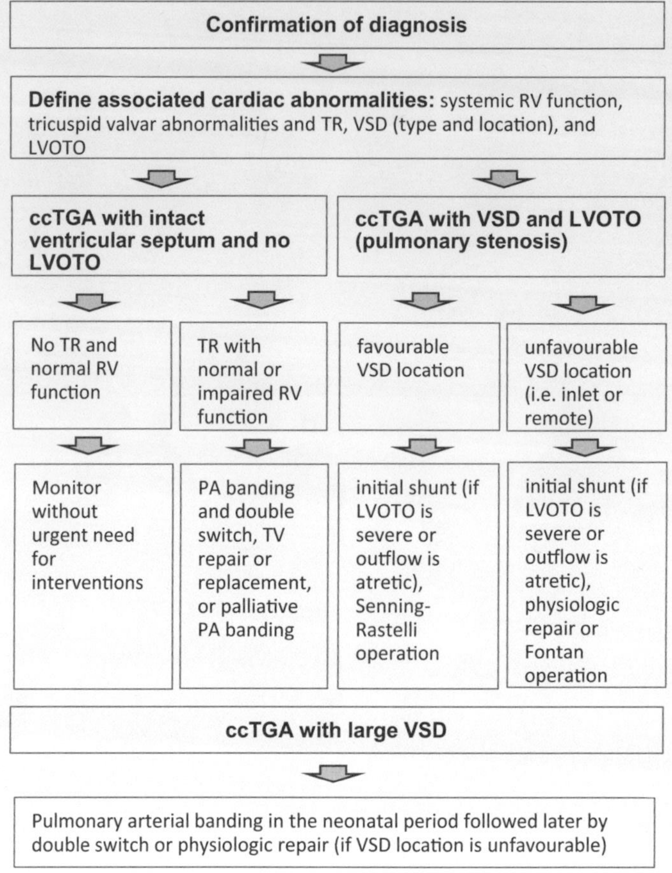

Fig. 24.3 Management algorithm of congenitally corrected transposition of the great arteries (ccTGA). *LVOTO* left ventricular outflow tract obstruction, *PA* pulmonary arterial, *RV* right ventricular, *TR* tricuspid regurgitation, *TV* tricuspid valve, *VSD* ventricular septal defect

framework and the final decision on management depends on the cardiac anatomy, ventricular function, age at presentation, clinical heart failure, patient and family decision, and centre expertise.

24.5.1 Palliative Interventions for Symptomatic Neonates

Neonates with severe left ventricular outflow (pulmonary) obstruction or pulmonary atresia require the insertion of a modified Blalock-Taussig shunt. In babies with a large unrestrictive ventricular septal defect refractory to medical therapy, pulmonary arterial banding to control heart failure is required before contemplating the next stage of definitive repair.

24.5.2 Definitive Repair

24.5.2.1 Physiologic Repair

Physiologic repair aims to correct the associated cardiac malformations but with maintenance of atrioventricular and ventriculoarterial discordance. This may involve (1) repair of the ventricular septal defect, (2) relief of left ventricular outflow obstruction by resection of subpulmonary muscular tissues, pulmonary valvotomy, or placement of a left ventricle-to-pulmonary artery conduit, and/or (3) tricuspid valve repair or replacement.

The morphologic right ventricle, however, continues to be the systemic right ventricle and remains vulnerable to the long-term complications of systemic ventricular dysfunction and tricuspid regurgitation. Maintenance of the morphologic left ventricular pressure at about half the systemic right ventricular by limited resection of the subpulmonary muscular tissues or using a smaller-sized left ventricle-to-pulmonary artery conduit may maintain the septal geometry and possibly lower the risk or postpone development of tricuspid regurgitation and right ventricular failure. In adolescents and adults with severe tricuspid regurgitation, tricuspid valve replacement should be performed before systemic right ventricular failure develops.

24.5.2.2 Anatomic Repair

The anatomic repair, although complicated and technically demanding, restores the morphologic left ventricle as the systemic ventricle. It is believed that the long-term outcome would improve with restoration of atrioventricular and ventriculoarterial concordance.

Types of anatomic repair: These include (1) a double switch (atrial switch with an arterial switch) for patients with an intact ventricular septum or a ventricular septal defect but with no left ventricular outflow obstruction (Fig. 24.2c), and (2) a Senning-Rastelli operation (with intraventricular rerouting of blood through the ventricular septal defect into the aorta and placement of a conduit from the morphologic right ventricle to the pulmonary arteries) for patients with ventricular septal defect and pulmonary stenosis or atresia (Fig. 24.2d). A variant of the anatomic repair is performance of a bidirectional Glenn shunt (Chap. 32) (or so-called 'hemi-Mustard' procedure) to channel the superior caval venous blood to the pulmonary artery, which can simplify the complex surgery and underload the morphologic right ventricle.

Preparedness of the left ventricle: The morphologic left ventricle usually involutes postnatally with decrease in pulmonary vascular resistance. However, the left ventricle remains pressure-loaded and is already primed to support the systemic circulation in three groups of patients: (1) patients with a large ventricular septal defect and pulmonary hypertension, (2) patients with initial pulmonary arterial banding to reduce the left-to-right shunt through a large ventricular septal defect, and (3) patients with severe left ventricular (pulmonary) outflow obstruction.

Pulmonary arterial banding: Pulmonary arterial banding aims to retrain of the involuted left ventricle beyond the neonatal period in preparation for anatomic repair. This procedure is challenging with unpredictable results and may cause left ventricular dysfunction. Endpoints used to gauge effective preparation of the left ventricle include a left ventricular systolic pressure of about 70–90% of systemic pressure and normalization of left ventricular mass. This procedure is more successful when performed during childhood.

24.5.2.3 Fontan Palliation

Fontan operation remains to be an option for patients with complex cardiac anatomy (e.g. straddling of atrioventricular valves over the ventricular septum, hypoplasia of either one of the ventricles, unfavourable location of the ventricular septal defect). Given the complexity of anatomic repair and the concern of systemic right ventricular dysfunction after physiologic repair, some centres opt for single ventricular palliation. As alluded to earlier, the optimal surgical approach in terms of physiologic repair, anatomic repair, or Fontan palliation remains debatable.

24.6 Long-Term Monitoring

Regardless of the type of definitive repair, complete heart block may develop in patients with congenitally corrected transposition of the great arteries.

After physiologic repair, close monitoring of systemic right ventricular function and tricuspid valvar regurgitation is required. Pulmonary arterial banding may reduce tricuspid regurgitation through ventricular-ventricular interaction (Chap. 28), palliate patients (especially adult patients who are more likely to fail to attain the goal of successful retraining of the left ventricle for anatomic repair), and provide a bridge to heart transplantation. The pooled results of studies to date fail to provide evidence of beneficial effects of medical therapy in patients with systemic right ventricular dysfunction.

After anatomic repair, systemic left ventricular dysfunction (which may be aggravated by right ventricular pacing in patients with complete heart block), complications of arterial switch operation (neo-aortic dilation and regurgitation), and complications after atrial switch operation (atrial arrhythmias and baffle obstruction and leakage) require long-term monitoring. Additionally, monitoring for progressive stenosis of the left ventricle-to-pulmonary artery conduit is necessary in patients who have undergone Senning-Rastelli operation. The need for long-term monitoring of patients after Fontan procedure is discussed in Chap. 30.

Transposition of the Great Arteries Post Atrial Switch Operation

25

The anatomy, pathophysiology, and contemporary management of transposition of the great arteries are discussed in Chap. 17. Although arterial switch operation has become the treatment of choice, there are adults who are being followed up in the grown-up congenital heart clinic who had undergone atrial switch operation for complete transposition of the great arteries in 1960s–1980s. Even in the present era, there are some children who may still be indicated for atrial switch operation as discussed below.

25.1 Atrial Switch Operations

The atrial switch operations represent physiologic repair of the transposition of the great arteries. These operations aim to direct the deoxygenated systemic venous blood to the mitral valve into the left ventricle, and the oxygenated pulmonary venous blood to the tricuspid valve into the right ventricle (Fig. 25.1). Hence, after atrial switch operations, systemic oxygenation is normalized, although the morphologic left ventricle remains to be the subpulmonary ventricle and the morphologic right ventricle continues to be the systemic ventricle.

25.1.1 Historical and Contemporary Perspectives

In 1957, Dr. Ake Senning performed the first atrial repair of complete transposition of the great arteries with baffling of the atria, using flaps of the atrial septum and right atrial free wall, to redirect systemic and pulmonary venous return to respectively the left and the right ventricles. In 1964, Dr. William Mustard described a simpler technique, which became more widely adopted, in which the atrial septum was completely excised, and an atrial patch baffle was placed to redirect venous

Y.-f. Cheung, *Congenital and Paediatric Acquired Heart Disease in Practice*, https://doi.org/10.1007/978-981-99-2862-0_25

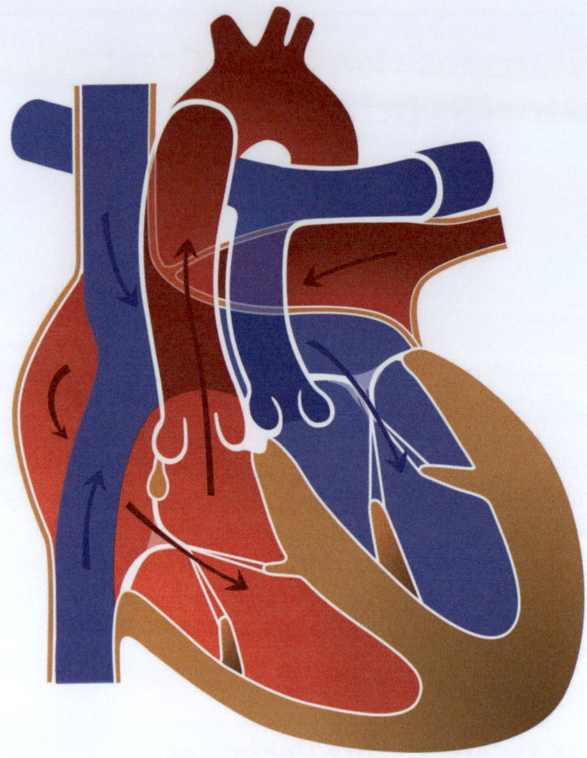

Fig. 25.1 Atrial switch operation. Illustration of the baffling of atria to direct the deoxygenated systemic venous blood to the left ventricle and oxygenated blood from the pulmonary veins to the right ventricle

return. Many of the patients who have undergone atrial switch operations are hence now in their fifth and sixth decades of life and monitored in the adult congenital heart clinic.

Although atrial switch operation has been almost completed replaced by arterial switch operation in the present era, there are situations where atrial repair may be considered: (1) infants with complete transposition of the great arteries who present late (Chap. 17), and (2) patients with congenitally corrected transposition who may be managed with double switch operation (Chap. 24).

25.1.2 Long-Term Complications

Patients after Senning and Mustard operations have similar survival. At 30 years of follow up, a heart transplantation-free survival rate of about 60% survival has been reported. Long-term complications are related to the right ventricle being the systemic ventricle, the use of atrial baffles, and atrial scarring (Box 25.1).

Box 25.1 Complications After Atrial Switch Operation

Systemic right ventricular dysfunction

Pre- and postcapillary pulmonary hypertension

Baffle complications
- baffle stenosis: right atrial-superior caval vein junction (more common after Mustard operation), pulmonary venous obstruction (more common after Senning operation), inferior baffle stenosis is uncommon
- baffle leak

Cardiac arrhythmias
- sinus node dysfunction
- atrial flutter and fibrillation
- ventricular tachycardia

25.2 Systemic Right Ventricular Dysfunction

Varying degrees of systemic right ventricular dysfunction are found in patients after atrial switch operations for transposition of the great arteries (Fig. 25.2). In older patients, right ventricular failure may develop and contribute to cardiac mortality.

Several factors contribute to dysfunction and failure of the systemic right ventricle after atrial switch operations: (1) coronary insufficiency that may be related to mismatch between right coronary arterial supply and systemic right ventricular hypertrophy and reduced vasodilator reserve of the coronary microcirculation, (2) myocardial fibrosis, (3) altered myocardial deformation pattern with predominant circumferential over longitudinal free wall shortening, but absence of torsion as found in the normal systemic left ventricle, (4) impaired atrioventricular transport due to non-contractile atrial baffles that limits systemic right ventricular preload, and (5) cardiomyopathy associated with tachycardias.

Systolic and diastolic dysfunction of the systemic right ventricle and impaired atrioventricular transport contribute further to late onset postcapillary pulmonary hypertension.

Tricuspid regurgitation occurs usually secondary to systemic right ventricular annular dilation and can lead to a vicious cycle that further worsens right ventricular dilation and tricuspid regurgitation.

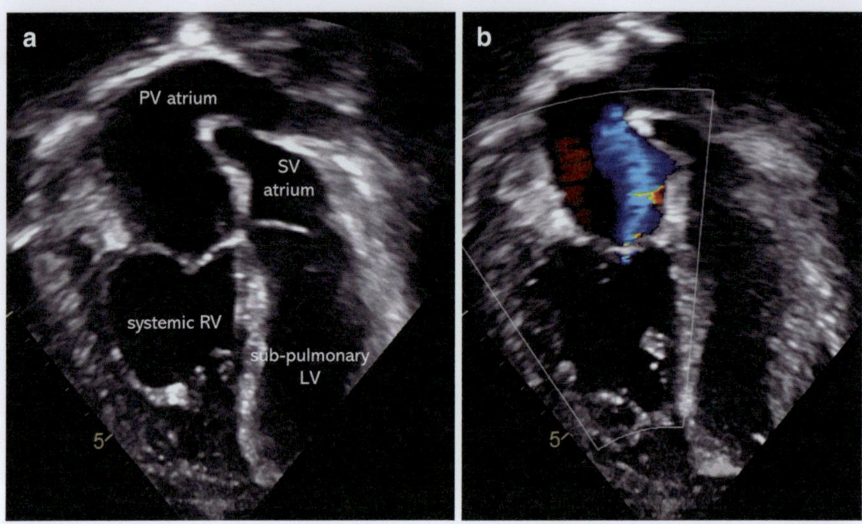

Fig. 25.2 Echocardiographic assessment after atrial switch operation. (**a**) Echocardiographic illustration of dilated systemic right ventricle and compressed subpulmonary left ventricle post atrial switch (**b**) Doppler colour flow mapping demonstrating moderate tricuspid valvar regurgitation (*LV* left ventricle, *PV* pulmonary venous, *RV* right ventricle, *SV* systemic venous)

25.3 Management Strategies for Long-Term Complications

Management of the following aspects is required on long-term follow up of patients after atrial switch operation: (1) systemic right ventricular dysfunction, (2) baffle complications, and (3) cardiac arrhythmias.

For patients with systemic right ventricular failure, retraining of the left ventricle to support the systemic circulation (by serial pulmonary arterial banding) followed by arterial switch operation and taking down of the atrial repair have been performed with success in some patients. Left ventricular failure may, however, occur after the banding procedure or after arterial switch operation. This practice has therefore not been widely adopted. On other hand, pulmonary arterial banding as a more definitive palliation has been advocated.

Other management options include medical treatment, transcatheter interventions, and device therapies (Box 25.2). Nonetheless, there is no definite evidence to date of beneficial effects of medical therapy for systemic right ventricular dysfunction.

Box 25.2 Management of Long-Term Complications After Atrial Switch Operation

Systemic right ventricular dysfunction and failure

- empirical use of heart failure medications
- cardiac resynchronization therapy
- pulmonary arterial banding ± arterial switch operation and takedown of atrial repair
- ventricular assist device
- heart transplantation

Baffle problems

- surgical or transcatheter closure of baffle leak
- surgical or transcatheter (balloon dilation and stenting) relief of baffle stenosis

Cardiac arrhythmias

- pacing for bradycardias
- medical control of tachycardias
- catheter ablation

Uhl Anomaly

26

Uhl anomaly is an extremely rare cardiac malformation, which is characterized by complete or partial absence of the right ventricular myocardium. This condition was first described in 1952 by Dr. Henry Uhl. The 'parchment heart' with thin and dilated ventricles, described by Dr. William Osler in 1905, may perhaps also be referring to a similar condition. Uhl anomaly can occur sporadically or in families.

26.1 Anatomy

In Uhl anomaly, the myocardium in the parietal wall of the right ventricle is absent and the epicardial and endocardial layers oppose against each other. The ventricular septum, septomarginal trabeculation, and the papillary muscles of the tricuspid valve are, on the other hand, normally muscularized. Although considered initially as developmental failure of the right ventricular myocardium during embryogenesis, recent data suggest apoptosis of right ventricular cardiomyocytes after completion of cardiac development as the culprit.

Uhl anomaly needs to be differentiated from Ebstein anomaly and arrhythmogenic right ventricular cardiomyopathy. In Uhl anomaly, the tricuspid valve is not dysplastic and has normal hinge points at the right atrioventricular junction, while tricuspid valve abnormalities are characteristic of Ebstein malformation (Chap. 22). In arrhythmogenic right ventricular cardiomyopathy (previously called arrhythmogenic right ventricular dysplasia), the characteristic anatomic features are localized or generalized dilation of the right ventricle, myocardial thinning in the regions of dilation, with variable extent of replacement of right ventricular myocardium by fibrofatty tissue.

Y.-f. Cheung, *Congenital and Paediatric Acquired Heart Disease in Practice*, https://doi.org/10.1007/978-981-99-2862-0_26

26.2 Pathophysiology

The pathophysiological consequence of Uhl anomaly is impairment of right ventricular contraction and diastolic filling (restrictive physiology). Right ventricular failure increases right atrial and systemic venous pressure and causes systemic venous congestion. Functional pulmonary atresia due to ineffective right ventricular forward flow may occur in newborn babies with high pulmonary vascular resistance. Right-to-left shunting of blood through the patent oval foramen leads to cyanosis.

26.3 Clinical Presentation and Findings

Neonates may present with significant cyanosis and right heart failure, although the cyanosis and heart failure may improve with reduction in pulmonary vascular resistance. In older patients, symptoms and signs of right heart failure are the main clinical features. By contrast to patients with arrhythmogenic right ventricular cardiomyopathy, patients with Uhl anomaly seldom present with cardiac arrhythmias.

Clinical features that help to distinguish Uhl anomaly from arrhythmogenic right ventricular cardiomyopathy are shown in Table 26.1.

Table 26.1 Clinical features that help to distinguish Uhl anomaly from arrhythmogenic right ventricular cardiomyopathy (ARVC)

Clinical features	Uhl anomaly	ARVC
Timing of presentation	Childhood	Adolescence and adulthood
Sex difference	None	More common in males
Family history	Absent	May be present
Clinical presentation	Right heart failure	Arrhythmias, syncope, or sudden death
Risk for sudden death	Low	High
Electrocardiographic findings	Non-specific, although epsilon wave may be present	Localized QRS prolongation (>110 ms) in right praecordial leads (V_1–V_3) and epsilon wave (characteristic of ARVC)

26.4 Investigations

CXR: Chest radiograph shows cardiomegaly due to right atrial and right ventricular dilation. In neonates with high pulmonary vascular resistance and functional pulmonary atresia, the lung fields appear oligaemic.
ECG: Electrocardiogram shows evidence of right atrial and right ventricular dilation. Epsilon (ε) wave (an electric signal of depolarization between the end of QRS complex and the beginning of the T wave due to slow intraventricular conduction through the abnormal right ventricle) may be seen in the right praecordial leads (epsilon wave is a characteristic finding in arrhythmogenic right ventricular cardiomyopathy).
Echocardiography: Echocardiographic assessment shows a thin right ventricular free wall with absence of myocardium, impaired contractility and restrictive filling of the right ventricle, right atrial dilation, and normal attachment of the tricuspid valve to the right atrioventricular junction. In neonates with cyanosis, echocardiographic evaluation for functional atresia of the pulmonary valve, patency and size of the arterial duct, and right-to-left atrial shunting is required.
CMR: Characteristic cardiac magnetic resonance findings include global dyskinesia of a thin-walled right ventricle, absence of myocardium at the right ventricular free wall, absence of fibrofatty infiltration (which is present in arrhythmogenic right ventricular cardiomyopathy), normal attachment of the tricuspid valve to the right atrioventricular junction (for exclusion of Ebstein anomaly), and normal left ventricular myocardium,

26.5 Management Strategy

A short duration of intravenous prostaglandin E infusion is indicated for neonates with severe cyanosis early after birth when the pulmonary vascular resistance is high. Diuretics for congestive right heart failure are usually required. Different surgical approaches including (1) right ventricular exclusion with atrial septectomy and a bidirectional Glenn shunt (superior cavopulmonary anastomosis), (2) one-and-a-half ventricular repair with partial right ventriculectomy and bidirectional Glenn shunt, and (3) cardiac transplantation have been adopted.

26.6 Long-Term Monitoring

The long-term outcome after surgery is unclear and prognosis of this rare cardiac malformation remains poor.

Part V

Unique Congenital Cardiac Physiology

Restrictive Right Ventricular Physiology 27

The concept of right ventricular restrictive physiology was introduced initially to describe the poorly compliant or stiff right ventricle in patients after repair of tetralogy of Fallot. This has also been described after interventions for other congenital heart disease with right ventricular outflow obstruction and varying degrees of right ventricular hypertrophy and hypoplasia (e.g. critical pulmonary stenosis, pulmonary atresia with intact ventricular septum).

27.1 Antegrade Diastolic Pulmonary Flow

Assessment of right ventricular compliance by conventional noninvasive Doppler echocardiography or even by invasive evaluation of the end-diastolic pressure-volume relationship is challenging and may be invalid (as the right ventricle is not a closed system in diastole).

The phenomenon of antegrade diastolic pulmonary flow (Fig. 27.1), which is detected by pulsed Doppler interrogation of flow in the main pulmonary trunk, has been regarded as a qualitative surrogate of a poorly complaint (stiff) right ventricle. The antegrade flow occurs after the P wave on the electrocardiogram, suggesting that atrial contraction in responsible for the generation of the flow. It is believed that this phenomenon is caused by a stiff right ventricle that impairs filling in late diastole (at the time of atrial contraction) and acts only as a conduit for blood to flow from the right atrium to the pulmonary trunk during atrial systole.

Y.-f. Cheung, *Congenital and Paediatric Acquired Heart Disease in Practice*, https://doi.org/10.1007/978-981-99-2862-0_27

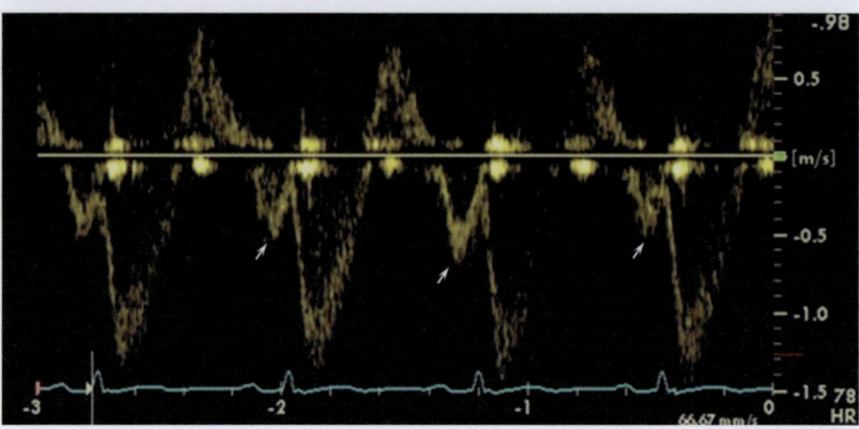

Fig. 27.1 Pulsed Doppler assessment of antegrade diastolic pulmonary flow. Antegrade diastolic pulmonary flow (arrows) occurs after the P wave and can be assessed by pulsed Doppler echocardiography with the sampling volume placed in the main pulmonary artery

27.2 Restrictive Right Ventricular Physiology Immediate After Surgery

Stiffening of the right ventricle after surgery limits right ventricular filling, increases systemic venous congestion, and reduces right ventricular output. Hence, the postoperative course of restrictive right ventricular physiology in patients with tetralogy of Fallot is characterized by low cardiac output syndrome, impaired renal function with oliguria, and fluid retention.

Development of right ventricular restrictive physiology immediate after surgery is thought to be related to myocardial damage during surgery. It is transient in nature and usually resolves over 48–72 h after surgery. Nonetheless, the low cardiac output syndrome can be significant. Doppler documentation of antegrade diastolic pulmonary flow has important implications on early postoperative management of these patients (Table 27.1).

Table 27.1 Implications of the presence of antegrade diastolic pulmonary flow (ADPF) on immediate postoperative management

Physiological implications	Management
Atrial contraction contributes to ADPF	Maintain a sinus rhythm to augment right ventricular output
ADPF contributes to cardiac output	Ensure adequate atrial preload to maintain the antegrade flow (judicious administration of fluid to avoid significant systemic venous congestion)
ADPF depends on the pressure gradient between the right atrium and pulmonary artery at late diastole	Minimize pulmonary vascular resistance
	Encourage spontaneous breathing with deep inspiration
	Optimize ventilation with low mean airway pressure and minimize the use of positive end-expiratory pressure
A stiff right ventricle promotes right-to-left interatrial shunting	Creation of an interatrial communication to augment cardiac output, albeit at the expense of cyanosis

27.3 Antegrade Diastolic Pulmonary Flow Late After Surgery

The phenomenon of antegrade diastolic pulmonary flow has also been documented in patients late after repair of tetralogy of Fallot. While it has been speculated that the presence of this phenomenon, which reflects a stiff right ventricle, may limit the severity of pulmonary regurgitation and right ventricular dilation and benefit patient outcomes, data on the long-term outcomes in patients after repair of tetralogy of Fallot with this phenomenon are conflicting.

Some studies have shown that antegrade diastolic pulmonary flow in patients late after repair of tetralogy of Fallot is associated with less pulmonary regurgitation, lesser right ventricular dilation, shorter QRS duration, better exercise capacity, and lower risk of ventricular arrhythmias. On the other hand, other studies have shown its associations with more severe pulmonary regurgitation, larger right ventricles, and worse exercise capacity. These observations beg the question of whether the presence of antegrade diastolic pulmonary flow is always suggestive of right ventricular restrictive physiology in these patients late after surgery.

It has been speculated that antegrade diastolic pulmonary flow might be a manifestation of two different phenotypes late after operation: (1) a genuine restrictive right ventricular physiology that develops early after surgery (related to myocardial damage and cardiopulmonary bypass) and persists on follow-up (due to myocardial fibrosis and non-functional patches used for repair), which limits pulmonary regurgitation and right ventricular dilation, and (2) progressive dilation of the right ventricle late after repair with rightward shifting of the pressure-volume curve and stiffening of the right ventricle (hence explaining the association with more severe pulmonary regurgitation and worse exercise capacity), but with no genuine restrictive right ventricular filling. More data are required to substantiate these speculations.

28 Ventricular-Ventricular Interaction

Ventricular-ventricular interaction describes the intricate link between the right and left ventricles and explains the influence of function, geometry, and timing of cardiac events of one ventricle on the other ventricle.

The bases for ventricular-ventricular interaction are (1) geometry of the common ventricular septum, (2) shared subepicardial myocardial fibres that encircle both ventricles (myocardial crosstalk), and (3) sharing of a common pericardial cavity (Table 28.1).

Table 28.1 Bases for ventricular-ventricular interaction

Basis	Pathophysiology	Examples
Septal geometry	Shifting of septum reduces volume, distorts geometry, alters timing of cardiac events, and reduces filling of contralateral ventricle	Shifting of septum to the left ventricle in the presence of right ventricular volume or pressure overloading
Myocardial crosstalk	Influence of myocardial contraction of one ventricle on the other via shared subepicardial myocardial fibres	Augmentation of right ventricular contractility with afterload-induced increase in left ventricular contractility (Anrep effect)
Sharing of pericardial cavity	Constraint of the pericardial sac limits ventricular distension and promotes septal displacement	Pericardial tamponade and constrictive pericarditis

Y.-f. Cheung, *Congenital and Paediatric Acquired Heart Disease in Practice*, https://doi.org/10.1007/978-981-99-2862-0_28

28.1 Ventricular-Ventricular Interaction in Paediatric Heart Disease

Systolic and diastolic ventricular-ventricular interaction is found in congenital and acquired heart disease in children. Commonly, adverse interactions are due to the impact of right ventricular volume or pressure overloading on left ventricular performance (Table 28.2). Knowledge on adverse ventricular-ventricular interaction enables better understanding of the pathophysiologic consequences and provides the basis for therapeutic interventions.

Table 28.2 Ventricular-ventricular interaction in paediatric cardiac conditions

Condition	Interaction	Comments
Repaired tetralogy of Fallot with severe pulmonary regurgitation	Correlation between systolic indices (ejection fraction, systolic strain) between the two ventricles	Left ventricular ejection fraction is an independent risk factor for adverse cardiovascular outcomes (functional class and mortality)
	Association between larger right ventricles and worse left ventricular dyssynchrony	
	Inverse relationship between right ventricular volume overloading and indices of left ventricular diastolic function (end-diastolic pressure and untwisting mechanics)	
Transposition of the great arteries post atrial switch operation	Correlation between systolic and diastolic indices between the systemic right ventricle and subpulmonary left ventricle	Basis for pulmonary arterial banding as a therapeutic intervention for a dilated systemic right ventricle with significant tricuspid regurgitation
	Systemic right ventricular dilation worsens left ventricular eccentricity and diastolic indices	
Congenitally corrected transposition of the great arteries	Correlation between systolic indices between the systemic right ventricle and subpulmonary left ventricle	Basis for pulmonary arterial banding as a therapeutic intervention for a dilated systemic right ventricle with significant tricuspid regurgitation
Right ventricle-to-pulmonary artery conduit obstruction	Right ventricular pressure overloading alters septal curvature and worsens left ventricular diastolic filling	Left ventricular diastolic filling improves with relief of the right ventricular outflow
Pulmonary arterial hypertension	Prolongation of right ventricular contraction when the left ventricle is beginning to relax causes leftward shifting of the septum and impairs left ventricular early diastolic filling	Assessment of left ventricular eccentricity provides an assessment of severity of pulmonary hypertension and its impact on left ventricular filling

28.2 Left Ventricular Eccentricity

Assessment of the septal geometry provides information on ventricular-ventricular interaction in the conditions as highlighted in Table 28.2. Septal geometry is altered by pressure and/or volume overloading of the right ventricle. Leftward shifting of the ventricular septum results in compression of the left ventricle and can be quantified echocardiographically by determination of the left ventricular eccentricity index.

The left ventricular eccentricity index is calculated during systole and diastole as the ratio of two left orthogonal ventricular axes (D2/D1): (1) D2 is the distance between the endocardial surfaces of the anterior and inferior walls) and (2) D1 is the distance from the endocardial surface of the mid-ventricular septum to that of the posterolateral left ventricular free wall (Fig. 28.1). Systolic and diastolic eccentricity indices of >1 suggest compression of the LV by the pressure- and volume-loaded right ventricle, respectively.

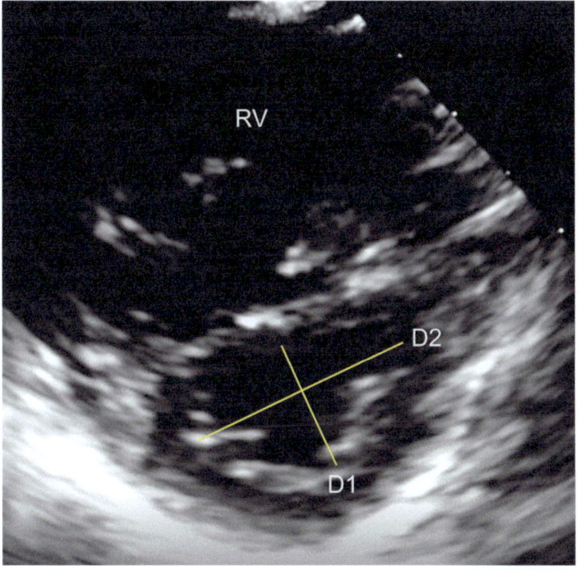

Fig. 28.1 Left ventricular eccentricity index. The left ventricular systolic eccentricity (D2/D1) is >1 in this patient with idiopathic pulmonary arterial hypertension (*RV* right ventricle)

28.3 Harnessing the Therapeutic Potentials of Ventricular-Ventricular Interaction

The elements of ventricular-ventricular interaction including the geometry of the ventricular septum and shared subepicardial myocardial fibres provide substrates for therapeutic manipulation (Table 28.3).

Table 28.3 Therapeutic translation of ventricular-ventricular interaction

Condition	Therapeutic intervention
Systemic right ventricular dysfunction with severe tricuspid regurgitation	Pulmonary arterial banding partially restores septal geometry, reduces tricuspid regurgitation, remodels the right ventricle, and may possibly increase its contractility
Subpulmonary right ventricular dysfunction	Systemic vasoconstrictors may augment right ventricular contractility through afterload-induced increase in left ventricular contractility (Anrep effect) and myocardial crosstalk
Dilated cardiomyopathy	Pulmonary arterial banding partially restores septal geometry, reduces mitral regurgitation, remodels the left ventricle, and may possibly increase left ventricular contractility through myocardial crosstalk

Shunt Physiology

29

29.1 Systemic-to-Pulmonary Arterial Shunt

Insertion of a systemic-to-pulmonary arterial shunt is an important palliative surgical intervention in cyanotic patients with inadequate pulmonary flow. The ascending aorta-to-right pulmonary artery shunt (Waterston shunt) and the descending aorta-to-left pulmonary artery shunt (Potts shunt) are no longer performed for this indication due to the complications of pulmonary arterial hypertension and distortion of pulmonary arterial anatomy. The reverse Potts shunt, however, is performed nowadays for the management of systemic pulmonary arterial hypertension (Chap. 35).

The modified Blalock-Taussig shunt is currently the most performed systemic-to-pulmonary arterial shunt. In its original form, first described by Dr. Alfred Blalock and Dr. Helen Taussig in 1944, the cut end of the subclavian artery is anastomosed to the side of the ipsilateral pulmonary artery. The current modified version utilizes an artificial tube that is sewn between the subclavian artery and the ipsilateral pulmonary artery (Fig. 29.1).

Stenting of the arterial duct is increasingly performed as an alternative to insertion of a systemic-to-pulmonary arterial shunt and shares similar physiology.

In patients with absence of atrioventricular valvar regurgitation, the output from the heart is distributed to two compartments: (1) pulmonary circulation (Qp) and (2) systemic circulation (Qs). An optimal Qp:Qs ratio of 1 has been suggested based on in vitro studies. Balancing the systemic and pulmonary perfusion therefore assumes major importance in early postoperative management of patients with a shunt-dependent circulation or after stenting of the arterial duct.

In patients after insertion of systemic-to-pulmonary arterial shunt, it is usual to aim for SaO2 between 70 and 85%, which reflects the so-called 'balance between pulmonary (Qp) and systemic (Qs) arterial flow' (i.e. Qp:Qs approximating 1) (Box 29.1). This is true to a certain extent only in the presence of an adequate cardiac

Y.-f. Cheung, *Congenital and Paediatric Acquired Heart Disease in Practice*, https://doi.org/10.1007/978-981-99-2862-0_29

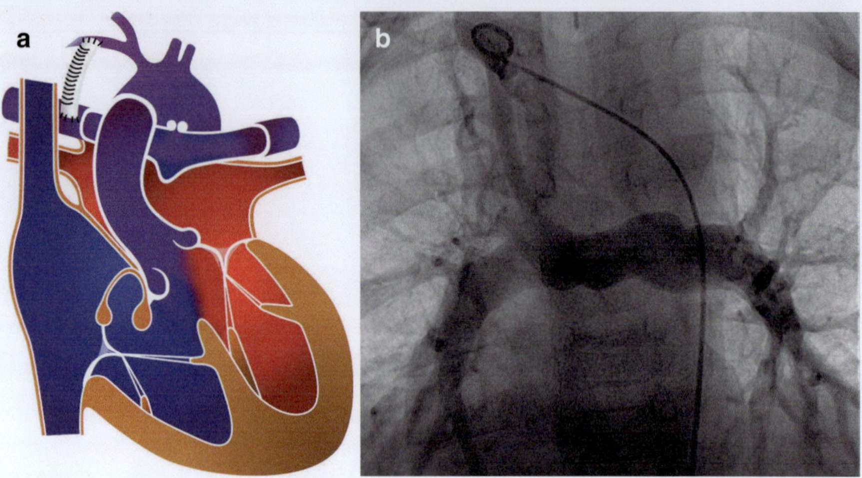

Fig. 29.1 Modified Blalock-Taussig shunt. (**a**) Drawing and (**b**) angiographic illustration of a modified Blalock-Taussig shunt

output and normal lung condition. However, in the presence of reduced cardiac output and/or impaired gaseous exchange due to pulmonary abnormalities, the Qp may have already exceeded Qs significantly to achieve a similar range of SaO2. Hence, the so-called optimal SaO2 needs to be interpreted in the context of cardiac and pulmonary function, and Qp:Qs is not always balanced in this range of SaO2.

Box 29.1 SaO2 (SA O2sat) and Qp:Qs in Shunted Patients

$$\mathbf{Qp / Qs = (SA\,O2sat - SV\,O2sat) / (PV\,O2sat - PA\,O2sat)}$$

O2sat is oxygen saturation, PA is pulmonary arterial, PV is pulmonary venous, SA is systemic arterial, and SV is systemic venous

In a shunted patient, SA O2sat = PA O2sat

$$\mathbf{Qp / Qs = (SA\,O2sat - SV\,O2sat) / (PV\,O2sat - SA\,O2sat)}$$

Assuming an adequate cardiac output, normal ventilation (PV O2sat about 95–100%), and usual oxygen extraction (SA O2sat – SV O2sat = 20%)

$$\mathbf{Qp / Qs = 20\% / (95\% - SA\,O2sat)}$$

If SA O2sat = 75%, then Qp:Qs = 1
If SA O2sat = 85%, then Qp:Qs = 2
If SA O2sat = 95%, then Qp:Qs = 4

With inadequate cardiac output and increased oxygen extraction (e.g. 40%)
If SA O2sat = 75%, then Qp:Qs = 2
In poor lung conditions, the PV O2sat drops (e.g. 85%)
If SA O2sat = 75%, then Qp:Qs = 2

The approach to low or high SaO2 after systemic-to-pulmonary arterial shunting is discussed in Chap. 54. While it is common to describe an imbalance of Qp:Qs as 'pulmonary under-circulation' or 'pulmonary over-circulation with systemic hypoperfusion' to explain respectively a low or a high SaO2, there are situations when these may not be true.

A low SaO2 can be due to respiratory condition or cardiac dysfunction (with increased oxygen extraction) in some patients rather reduced pulmonary flow. On the other hand, a high SaO2, while suggestive of more than adequate pulmonary flow, may not always imply systemic hypoperfusion and impending cardiovascular collapse. There are patients with a high SaO2 who remain relatively asymptomatic or only have mild respiratory distress if the cardiac output is adequate.

29.2 Bidirectional Glenn Shunt

The original Glenn shunt is an anastomosis between the divided distal right pulmonary artery to the side of the superior caval vein, with ligation of the superior caval vein at its entrance into the right atrium. It was first described by Dr. William Glenn is 1958 when the operation was performed in a 7-year-old boy with a single ventricle, transposition of the great vessels, and pulmonary stenosis. The limitations of this procedure include development of unilateral pulmonary arteriovenous malformations in the right lung and superior vena cava syndrome.

The bidirectional Glenn shunt (superior cavopulmonary connection) is a modification in which the divided superior caval vein is anastomosed end-to-side to the right pulmonary artery, thereby permitting blood to flow from the superior caval vein into both the right and left pulmonary arteries (Fig. 29.2). This procedure is performed as part of the staged procedure in the management of patients with

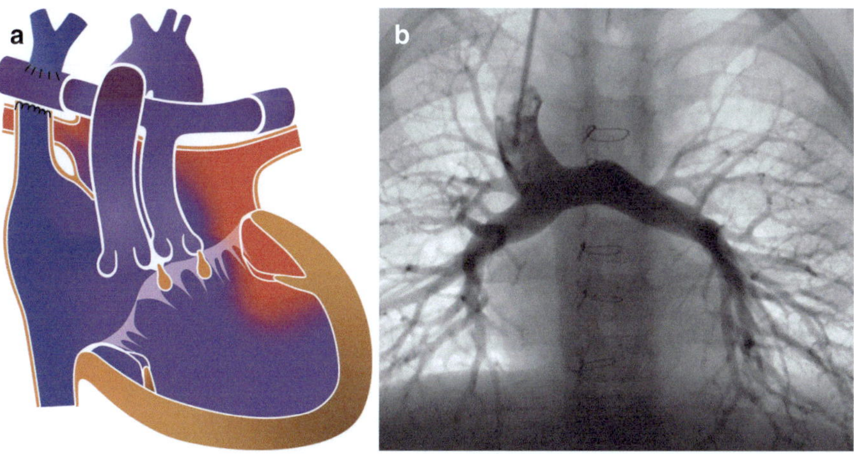

Fig. 29.2 Bidirectional Glenn shunt. (**a**) Drawing and (**b**) angiographic illustration of a bidirectional Glenn shunt

functional single ventricles (Chap. 19) and patients who require one-and-a-half ventricular repair (Chap. 32). In patients with heterotaxy syndrome (Chap. 20) and bilateral superior caval veins, bilateral bidirectional Glenn shunt is required.

Functioning of the bidirectional Glenn shunt requires the presence of a low pulmonary vascular resistance. While a cutoff has not been defined, a pulmonary vascular resistance index of <3 Wood unit·m^2 is probably required. The calculation of Qp:Qs ratio after bidirectional Glenn shunt is shown in Box 29.2. A Qp:Qs of 0.6 derived from cardiac catheterization has been reported in children after bidirectional Glenn shunt. Reported higher values based on noninvasive cardiac magnetic resonance assessment of flow and measurement of SVC O2sat during the same setting can be explained by the presence of aortopulmonary collaterals and questionable validity of the assumption of SVC O2sat being equal to IVC O2sat in some of the patients.

Box 29.2 Qp:Qs in Patients After Bidirectional Glenn Shunt

After bidirectional Glenn shunt

$$\mathbf{Qs = Qp + Qivc}$$

Qs is systemic flow
Qp is pulmonary flow
Qivc is inferior caval venous flow

For systemic oxygen delivery

$$\mathbf{Qs \times Ca = Qp \times Cpv + Qivc \times Civc}$$

$$\mathbf{Qs \times Ca = Qp \times Cpv + (Qs - Qp) \times Civc}$$

Ca, Cpv and Civs are respectively oxygen content in systemic artery, pulmonary vein, and inferior caval vein

Assuming minimal dissolved oxygen, oxygen saturation can substitute oxygen content

$$\mathbf{Qs \times SA\,O2sat = Qp \times PV\,O2sat + (Qs - Qp) \times IVC\,O2sat}$$

Rearranging the equation, and assuming SVC O2sat = IVC O2sat

$$\mathbf{Qp / Qs = (SA\,O2sat - IVC\,O2sat) / (PV\,O2sat - IVC\,O2sat)}$$

$$\mathbf{Qp / Qs = (SA\,O2sat - SVC\,O2sat) / (PV\,O2sat - SVC\,O2sat)}$$

SA O2sat, IVC O2sat, PV O2sat, and SVC O2sat are respectively oxygen saturation in systemic artery, inferior caval vein, pulmonary vein, and superior caval vein

29.3 Circular Shunt

A circular shunt is created when the following conditions are met: (1) large arterial duct with left to right shunting of blood, (2) significant pulmonary regurgitation, (3) significant tricuspid regurgitation, and (4) an unrestricted right-to-left atrial shunt. A low cardiac output syndrome develops as blood in the aorta flows in a retrograde manner through the arterial duct into the main pulmonary artery, from which the blood is emptied into the right ventricle, the right atrium, then the left atrium, and then back to the systemic circulation (Fig. 29.3). There can be rapid cardiac decompensation and development of multiorgan failure. A circular shunt may be encountered in two situations: (1) Ebstein anomaly, and (2) after opening of the right ventricular outflow in pulmonary atresia with intact ventricular septum.

In Ebstein anomaly (Chap. 22), concomitant pulmonary regurgitation is rare. However, the presence of a large arterial duct at birth with significant pulmonary regurgitation, and in the presence of a severely malformed tricuspid valve with significant tricuspid regurgitation and right-to-left atrial shunt, a circular shunt can easily be established. This phenomenon may even be present in utero and result in hydrops fetalis. Postnatally, a staged management approach is usually adopted. The first stage involves elimination of the circular shunt by one of the several options: (1) ligation of the arterial duct with insertion of a systemic-to-pulmonary arterial

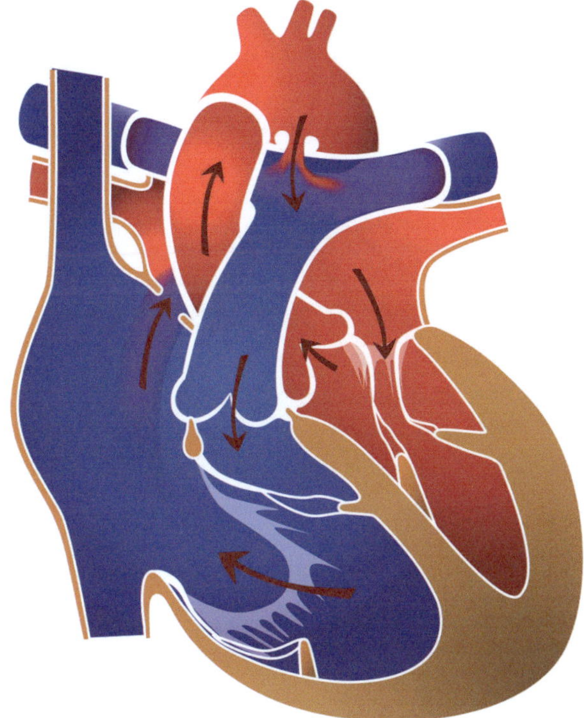

Fig. 29.3 Circular shunt in Ebstein anomaly. Illustration of a circular shunt in the setting of Ebstein anomaly with a large arterial duct and significant pulmonary regurgitation

shunt, (2) ligation of the arterial duct with pulmonary vasodilator therapy and a short duration of extracorporeal membranous oxygenation support, (3) ligation of the main pulmonary trunk and arterial duct with systemic-to-pulmonary arterial shunt insertion, or (4) ligation of the main pulmonary trunk with bilateral pulmonary arterial banding (while maintaining ductal patency by prostaglandin E or ductal stenting). The second stage is usually a Starnes procedure, but in suitable patients after ductal ligation, a biventricular repair may still be feasible.

In pulmonary atresia with intact ventricular septum (Chap. 16), a circular shunt may develop early after transcatheter perforation of the atretic pulmonary valve, especially when the arterial duct is large as a result of the pre-procedural infusion of prostaglandin E or when ductal stenting is concurrently performed. In the presence of severe low cardiac output syndrome, emergency ligation of the large arterial duct is lifesaving.

30 Fontan Physiology

The Fontan procedure represents the final stage of univentricular repair by which the entire systemic venous return is channelled to the pulmonary circulation without the need for a subpulmonary ventricular chamber. The operation, initially performed in two patients with tricuspid atresia, was first reported by Dr. Francis Fontan in 1971.

The operation is performed based on the premise that an elevation of central venous pressure can drive the systemic venous return across the pulmonary circulation to fill the functional single systemic ventricle. It becomes apparent that other driving factors are also in play, and these include the change in intrathoracic pressure during inspiration, suction force generated by relaxation of the systemic ventricle, and the peripheral skeletal muscle pump.

30.1 Evolution of the Fontan Procedure

In the original 1971 report, Dr. Fontan described an end-to-end anastomosis of the superior caval vein to the right pulmonary artery (Glenn shunt), inclusion of a homograft valve at the orifice of the inferior caval vein, and a connection between the right atrium and the bifurcation of the pulmonary arteries. At about the same time, Dr. Kreutzer and colleagues performed an atriopulmonary anastomosis with neither a valve in the inferior caval vein nor a Glenn shunt in a child with tricuspid atresia.

The Fontan procedure has since then undergone several modifications. It becomes evident that valves in the venous circuit and the incorporation of the right atrium are not necessary. Furthermore, flow energetics have been shown to be poor in atriopulmonary connection especially with progressive dilation of the atrium. This has led to the concept of total cavopulmonary connection.

Total cavopulmonary connection is achieved with a bidirectional Glenn shunt (to channel superior caval venous blood to the pulmonary artery) and either (1) a lateral

Y.-f. Cheung, *Congenital and Paediatric Acquired Heart Disease in Practice*, https://doi.org/10.1007/978-981-99-2862-0_30

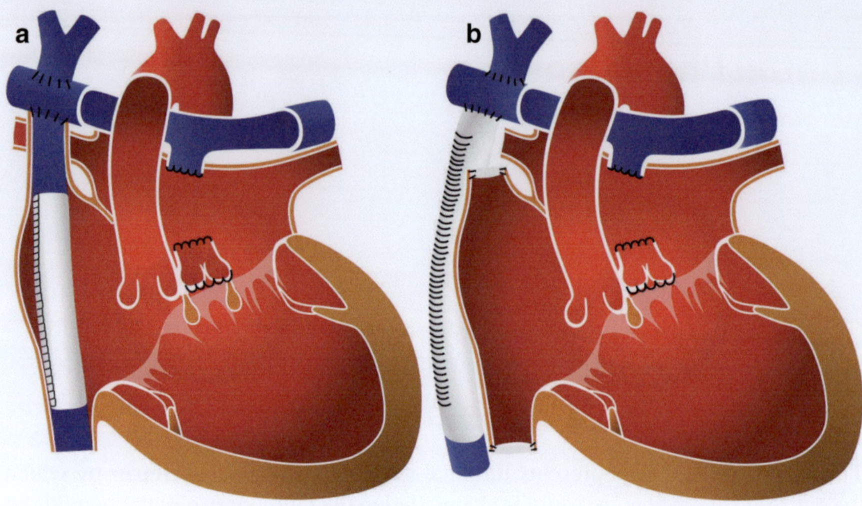

Fig. 30.1 Fontan procedure. (**a**) Lateral atrial tunnel (**b**) Extracardiac conduit

atrial tunnel that channels inferior caval venous blood to the anastomosis between the transected superior caval vein and the pulmonary artery (Fig. 30.1a) or (2) the use of an extracardiac prosthetic conduit interposed between the inferior caval vein and the pulmonary artery (Fig. 30.1b).

While total cavopulmonary connection can be performed as a one stage procedure, it is usually performed in stages with an initial bidirectional Glenn shunt and followed by completion later with a lateral atrial tunnel or an extracardiac conduit. This staged completion ameliorates the impact of significant acute volume unloading of the systemic ventricle that may have untoward consequences as described below.

Some centres routinely create a fenestration in the intraatrial baffle or the extracardiac conduit during total cavopulmonary connection, while others adopted this only in high-risk patients. The creation of a fenestration, which allows right-to-left shunting of blood, can increase ventricular preload and cardiac output and reduce systemic venous pressure after Fontan procedure.

30.2 Volume Unloading of the Systemic Ventricle

The functional single ventricle is volume overloaded before and after the first stage of palliative repair as its supports both the pulmonary and systemic circulation (Chap. 19) and atrioventricular regurgitant flow when present (Box 30.1). Consequences of significant volume overloading on the functional significant ventricle include ventricular dilation and remodelling, stretching of the atrioventricular valvar annulus causing atrioventricular valvar regurgitation, and increased wall stress that predisposes to subendocardial ischaemia.

With the bidirectional Glenn shunt (which accounts for about 50% of the total venous return in infants), the ventricular stroke volume decreases by 40–60%. Following the Fontan procedure, the entire systemic venous return needs to pass through the high resistance circuit to fill the systemic ventricle. Further volume unloading of the systemic ventricle occurs both acutely after surgery and in the long term. Although volume unloading may benefit by reducing atrioventricular valvar regurgitation and wall stress, it may also have pathophysiological consequences as described below.

Box 30.1 Volume Unloading After Bidirectional Glenn Shunt and Fontan Procedure

Before and after stage 1 palliation of functional single ventricle

$$\text{CO} = \text{Qivc} + \text{Qsvc} + \text{Qp}\left(\pm\text{Qregurgitant}\right)$$

After bidirectional Glenn shunt

$$\text{CO} = \text{Qivc} + \text{Qp}\left(\pm\text{Qregurgitant}\right)$$

After Fontan procedure

$$\text{CO} = \text{Qp}\left(\pm\text{Qregurgitant} \pm \text{Qfenestration}\right)$$

Qs is systemic flow
Qivc and Qscvc are respectively inferior and superior caval venous flow
Qregurgitant is atrioventricular and/or aortic regurgitant flow
Qfenestration is flow contributed by the Fontan fenestration

30.3 Pathophysiologic Consequences on Different Elements of the Fontan Circulation

The Fontan circuit, with the systemic ventricle providing the driving force, consists of different elements (or resistors) that result in progressive energy loss and pressure drop. Functioning of the Fontan circuit is based on the premise that an elevation of central venous pressure can drive the systemic venous return across the pulmonary circulation to fill the functional single systemic ventricle.

Important elements in the circuit include: (1) functional single ventricle, (2) systemic arterial circulation, (3), systemic venous return, (4) Fontan pathway (previously atriopulmonary connection, currently total cavopulmonary connection), (5) pulmonary arterial circulation, and (6) pulmonary venous circulation and pulmonary venous atrium. Each of these elements have distinct physiologic (or pathophysiologic in the long term) characteristics (Table 30.1).

Table 30.1 Physiologic (Pathophysiologic) characteristics of the elements in the Fontan circuit

Circuit elements	Physiologic and long-term pathophysiologic characteristics
Functional single ventricle	1. Diastolic dysfunction with incoordinate relaxation due to volume unloading (conservation of myocardial mass predicts acquired hypertrophy with increased mass-to-volume ratio), worsening of ventricular compliance with myocardial fibrosis
	2. Systolic dysfunction in the longer term related to altered myocardial substrate, surgery, progressive atrioventricular valvar regurgitation, and adverse ventriculo-arterial interaction
	3. Reduced cardiac output due to chronic underfilling of the ventricle and diastolic ventricular dysfunction (and late systolic dysfunction)
Systemic arterial circulation	Increased arterial resistance and impedance increase afterload and lead to adverse ventriculo-arterial interaction
Systemic venous system	Increased central venous pressure with reduced venous capacitance
Fontan pathway	Significant energy loss in atriopulmonary connection, driving force through the Fontan pathway requires an elevated central venous pressure, changes in intrathoracic pressure during inspiration, suction force generated by relaxation of the systemic ventricle, and the peripheral skeletal muscle pump
Pulmonary arterial circulation	1. Transpulmonary flow, which depends on pulmonary vascular resistance and transpulmonary pressure gradient, is the main determinant of cardiac output after Fontan procedure (as it determines systemic ventricular preload)
	2. Progressive increase in pulmonary vascular resistance may occur as a result of impaired endothelium-dependent vasodilation (due to low velocity non-pulsatile pulmonary flow with reduced vascular shear stress) and subclinical microthrombi
Pulmonary venous circulation and pulmonary venous atrium	1. Progressive atrial dilation after atriopulmonary connection may compress on the right pulmonary veins and cause pulmonary vein stenosis
	2. Fontan operation in the setting of heterotaxy syndrome (right atrial isomerism) can be associated with pulmonary vein stenosis
	3. Pulmonary venous and atrial hypertension occurs in the presence of significant systemic ventricular diastolic dysfunction and atrioventricular valvar regurgitation

30.4 Optimization of the Fontan Circulation

Haemodynamics of the Fontan circulation are inherently abnormal as described above. Given that pulmonary vascular resistance is the main determinant of cardiac output in Fontan patients, pulmonary vasodilators have been shown to improve haemodynamics, exercise capacity, and functional status in Fontan patients. While

Table 30.2 Optimization of haemodynamics of the Fontan circulation

Circuit elements	Measures
Functional single ventricle and atrioventricular valve	Surgical repair or replacement of the atrioventricular valve in the presence of significant regurgitation
	No effective lusitropic medications to improve diastolic filling
	Standard medical treatment of systolic dysfunction that may occur in the longer term
Systemic arterial circulation	The use of systemic vasodilators is debatable (reduction of afterload does not increase cardiac output in the presence of limited preload reserve), although commonly prescribed to patients with significant atrioventricular valvar regurgitation and systolic ventricular dysfunction
Systemic venous system	Diuretics to reduce systemic venous congestion
	Nitrates to increase systemic venous capacitance
	Warfarin or aspirin to reduce the risk of thrombosis and formation of microthrombi
Fontan pathway	Creation or enlargement of fenestration (at the expense of increased cyanosis and risk of thromboembolism)
	Conversion of atriopulmonary connection to total cavopulmonary connection
Pulmonary arterial and venous circulation	Pulmonary vasodilators to minimize pulmonary vascular resistance
	Transcatheter interventions to tackle pulmonary arterial and venous stenosis
	Embolization of arterial- and veno-venous collaterals

pulmonary vasodilators have increasingly been advocated for use in Fontan patients, the indications and timing of initiation remain debatable and vary among centres. Measures to optimize the different elements of the Fontan circulation are also important (Table 30.2).

The pathophysiologic abnormalities inherent to the Fontan circulation as highlighted in Table 30.1 may progress and lead to what is termed failure of the Fontan circulation. Although the concept of failure of Fontan circulation has not been very clearly defined, long-term complications due to maladaptive changes in the heart and other body systems are well recognized in adult Fontan patients. In the current era, premature occurrence of these complications is uncommon during childhood.

Progressive increase in pulmonary vascular resistance with elevated central pressure and chronically reduced cardiac output (with chronic underfilling and diastolic dysfunction of the functional single ventricle) are believed to be primarily responsible for the majority of the long-term complications in post Fontan patients (Table 30.3).

Table 30.3 Long-term complications after Fontan operation

Organ/body system	Complications
Cardiovascular system	1. Heart failure: Systolic and diastolic dysfunction, chronic ventricular underfilling, atrioventricular valvar regurgitation, and cardiac arrhythmias
	2. Cardiac arrhythmias: Sinus node dysfunction, supraventricular tachycardia, and less commonly ventricular tachycardia
	3. Systemic venous congestion: Dependent oedema, ascites, systemic venous thrombosis
Liver	Fontan-associated liver disease: Elevation of liver enzymes, liver fibrosis and cirrhosis, hepatocellular carcinoma
Lymphatic system	Protein-losing enteropathy and plastic bronchitis
Kidney	Decreased glomerular filtration rate, proteinuria, and albuminuria
Central nervous system	Cognitive, neurodevelopmental, and behavioural abnormalities
Body growth	Abnormal bone growth and somatic growth due to unknown mechanisms

30.5 Long-Term Monitoring

Apart from the regular clinical assessment, regular surveillance of the various organ function is required in children and adolescents after the Fontan procedure (Box 30.2).

Box 30.2 Long-Term Monitoring of Fontan Patients

Cardiovascular system

- history and physical assessment
- chest radiograph
- electrocardiogram and Holter monitoring
- echocardiography
- exercise testing
- serum brain natriuretic peptide (BNP) or N-terminal proBNP level
- cardiac magnetic resonance and cardiac catheterization

Other organ systems

- liver: liver function test, alpha-fetal protein level, ultrasound liver for parenchymal change, stiffness, and hepatocellular carcinoma
- lymphatic system: lymphocyte count, serum albumin, total protein, and immunoglobulin levels, faecal alpha-1 antitrypsin level, lymphatic imaging (Chap. 63)
- kidney: renal function test, renal ultrasound
- central nervous system: cognitive testing and neurodevelopmental assessment
- body growth: bone scan, serum calcium, vitamin D, and parathyroid hormone levels

31 Borderline Left Ventricle

Borderline left ventricle represents a spectrum of hypoplasia of the left ventricle. At either end of the spectrum, hypoplastic left heart syndrome with aortic and mitral atresia (Chap. 21) at one end and mild hypoplasia of the left ventricle with aortic stenosis or coarctation of the aorta at the other, adoption of respectively univentricular and biventricular repair is usually obvious. In the middle of this spectrum, however, the best management approach is less clear and may vary among centres.

Hypoplasia of the left ventricle is believed to result from reduced blood flow into the ventricular cavity (flow theory) due to left ventricular inflow and/or outflow obstruction. Hence, associated cardiac anomalies include mitral stenosis, aortic stenosis, coarctation of the aorta with arch hypoplasia, Shone complex with multi-level left sided obstruction, and unbalanced atrioventricular septal defect with right ventricular dominance. Endocardial fibroelastosis may occur in addition to hypoplastic growth of the left ventricle and impair left ventricular diastolic function.

31.1 Associated Cardiac Malformations

31.1.1 Critical Aortic Stenosis

The pathophysiology and management of critical aortic stenosis with relatively normal-sized left ventricle is discussed in Chap. 13. In the presence of left ventricular hypoplasia, which reflects possible impairment or cessation of ventricular growth in utero, prediction of ability of the left ventricle to support a biventricular circulation after relief of the stenosis is challenging.

An indexed left ventricular end-diastolic volume less than 20 mL/m^2 is usually considered unsuitable for biventricular repair. Several scores that take into account of the dimensions of cardiac structures (mitral and aortic valves, left ventricle, and aortic root) and left ventricular endocardial fibroelastosis have been developed to provide guidance to decision making (Box 31.1).

Y.-f. Cheung, *Congenital and Paediatric Acquired Heart Disease in Practice*, https://doi.org/10.1007/978-981-99-2862-0_31

These scoring systems apply mostly to infants with critical aortic stenosis with varying degrees of left ventricular hypoplasia and may not, however, apply in the presence of multilevel left heart hypoplasia. Another caveat is possible underestimation of the left ventricular measurements due to compression of the left ventricle by a dilated and pressure-overloaded right ventricle. Furthermore, left ventricular volume parameters based on 3D echocardiography have not yet been incorporated.

Box 31.1 Scores for Assessment of Borderline Left Ventricles (Values Favouring Biventricular Repair)

Rhodes score (cutoff ≥ 0.35)
14 (body surface area) + 0.943 (indexed aortic root diameter) + 4.78 (left ventricular to heart long-axis ratio) + 0.157 (indexed mitral valve area) – 12.03

Discriminant score (cutoff ≥ –0.65)
10.98 (body surface area) + 0.56 (aortic annulus z score) + 5.89 (left ventricular to heart long-axis ratio) – 0.79 (grade 2 or 3 endocardial fibroelastosis) – 6.78

CHSS (Congenital Heart Surgeons Society) 1 score (cutoff < 0)
30.55 (inverse of age at study entry [d] + 1) – 6.20 (aortic root z-score) + 12.14 (echocardiographic grade of endocardial fibroelastosis) + 23.33 (logarithm of ascending aorta size in mm) – 28.30 (presence of moderate or severe tricuspid regurgitation) – 0.70 (LV long-axis length z score) – 86.47

CHSS 2 score (cutoff <0)
Multivariable regression equation using body surface area, mitral valve z score, indexed heart long axis, minimum left ventricular outflow tract diameter, and indexed mid aortic arch

2V-score (cutoff ≤16.2)
[(mitral valve annulus in 4C/aortic valve annulus in PSLA)/(left ventricular length in 4C/right ventricular length in 4C) + main pulmonary artery diameter]/body surface area
(4C, 4-chamber, PSLA, parasternal long axis; the score has been used to assess borderline left ventricle in association with aortic arch hypoplasia)

31.1.2 Hypoplastic Aortic Arch

Aortic arch hypoplasia, usually in the presence of coarctation of the aorta, can also be associated with left ventricular hypoplasia. Studies have shown that satisfactory growth of the left ventricle and aortic arch can usually be achieved after repair of aortic coarctation.

31.1.3 Shone Complex

Shone complex or Shone syndrome, described by Dr. John Shone in 1963, comprises four left-sided cardiac lesions: (1) supravalvar mitral membrane, (2) parachute mitral valve, (3) subaortic stenosis (muscular or membranous), and (4) and coarctation of the aorta. The clinical setting is which the condition is currently recognized and reported is commonly based on the presence of congenital mitral valve stenosis with at least one additional level of left heart obstruction. Other associated cardiac lesions include atrial and ventricular septal defects.

The criteria for univentricular versus biventricular repair in patients with Shone complex and hypoplasia of the left ventricle vary among centres. Nonetheless, hypoplasia of the mitral valve and left ventricle (z scores <-2) and the presence of a moderate to large ventricular septal defect have been shown to be associated with high risk of failure of biventricular repair in infants with multiple left heart obstructive lesions. For patients undergoing biventricular repair, repeated surgical or transcatheter interventions for residual left heart lesions (mitral and aortic valve stenosis, subaortic stenosis, coarctation of the aorta) are to be expected.

31.2 Management Strategy

Selection of the appropriate management strategy of borderline left ventricle is challenging and requires preoperative echocardiographic evaluation of (1) the dimensions of the left-sided structures as described above (Box 31.1), (2) levels and nature of left ventricular outflow obstruction, and (3) associated cardiac malformations. The findings on intraoperative evaluation of mitral valve pathology and adequacy, left ventricular endocardial fibroelastosis, and size of the left ventricular cavity also influence the final decision making.

The types of interventions depend on patients and include repair of coarctation of the aorta, reconstruction of aortic arch, aortic and mitral valvoplasty, subaortic resection, and closure of associated septal defects for patients considered candidates for biventricular repair.

There is also emergence of different strategies that aim to promote left ventricular growth (the concept of left ventricular rehabilitation):

1. endocardial fibroelastosis resection during a Ross with or without Konno procedure for critical aortic stenosis with borderline left ventricle,

2. staged left ventricular recruitment with an initial Norwood operation (but with a restrictive atrial communication to enhance flow into the hypoplastic left ventricle), followed by endocardial fibroelastosis resection, mitral valvoplasty, and repair of the left ventricular outflow tract, and
3. staged hybrid left ventricular recruitment with initial bilateral pulmonary artery banding and ductal stenting leaving also a restrictive atrial communication, followed by endocardial fibroelastosis resection, mitral valvoplasty, and repair of left ventricular outflow tract and aortic arch obstruction.

31.3 Postoperative Considerations and Long-Term Monitoring

Given the long-term issues of single ventricular palliation (Chap. 30), a biventricular repair for borderline ventricle is thought to be preferable when possible. Nonetheless, there exist important postoperative issues related to biventricular repair for borderline left ventricles: (1) the growth and functional performance (especially diastolic function) of the left ventricle, (2) left atrial hypertension due to mitral valve pathology, endocardial fibroelastosis, and left ventricular diastolic dysfunction, (3) pulmonary hypertension, and (4) progressive, recurrent, or newly developed left-sided obstructive lesions. Multiple reinterventions are therefore expected in patients who have undergone recruitment and rehabilitation of the borderline left ventricle with multi-level left-sided obstruction. Patients with a failed biventricular circulation requires conversion to univentricular palliation or heart transplantation.

Borderline Right Ventricle

32

The right ventricle may be borderline from a morphologic (small-sized) or a functional (dysfunctional) perspective and leads to inadequacy of handling of the entire systemic venous return.

By contrast to borderline left ventricles, borderline right ventricles can be supported initially with alternative sources of pulmonary blood flow (systemic-to-pulmonary arterial shunt and ductal stenting) and subsequently either excluded from the circulation (univentricular palliation) or incorporated in the circulation as part of a biventricular or one-and-a-half ventricular repair.

32.1 Associated Cardiac Malformations

32.1.1 Pulmonary Atresia with Intact Ventricular Septum

Varying degree of right ventricular hypoplasia is characteristic of pulmonary atresia with intact ventricular septum. The management algorithm of patients in either end of the spectrum is discussed in Chap. 16.

In patients with borderline right ventricles, maintenance of an additional source of pulmonary flow (systemic-to-pulmonary arterial shunt or ductal stenting) even after establishment of right ventricular-pulmonary arterial continuity is often required. In patients with poor growth of the hypoplastic borderline right ventricle, a one-and-a-half ventricular repair as described below may be indicated. Morphologic factors that many indicate the adoption of this approach are listed in Box 32.1.

Y.-f. Cheung, *Congenital and Paediatric Acquired Heart Disease in Practice*, https://doi.org/10.1007/978-981-99-2862-0_32

Box 32.1 Morphologic Factors in Pulmonary Atresia with Intact Ventricular Septum That May Indicate One-and-a-Half Ventricular Repair

- bipartite right ventricle
- tricuspid valve z score between −2 and −5
- tricuspid annulus / mitral annulus 0.5–0.8
- absence of right ventricular-dependent coronary circulation

32.1.2 Ebstein Anomaly

Despite surgical restoration of the competence of the tricuspid valve, right ventricular dysfunction may persist and even progress given the abnormal right ventricular myocardium in Ebstein anomaly. The right ventricle may hence be borderline from the functional perspective and may benefit from partial unloading of the right ventricle by one-and-a-half ventricular repair.

32.1.3 Other Congenital Heart Disease

Unbalanced atrioventricular septal defect with left ventricular dominance (Chap. 11) and, less commonly, ventricular septal defect, tetralogy of Fallot, valvar tricuspid stenosis, transposition of the great arteries, and double-inlet left ventricle can be associated with right ventricular hypoplasia. Incorporation of one-and-a-half ventricular repair in the management algorithms of these conditions may also be appropriate.

32.2 Management Strategy

The concept of partial unloading of a morphologically or functionally borderline right ventricle with a superior cavopulmonary anastomosis (bidirectional Glenn shunt) is based on the premise that (1) the borderline right ventricle may still handle part of the systemic venous return, (2) univentricular palliation with Fontan operation is best avoided if possible, (3) this one-and-a-half ventricular physiology is better than a univentricular palliation, and (4) this repair can be performed with similar or less mortality compared with biventricular repair or Fontan procedure.

32.2.1 One-and-a-Half Ventricular Repair

One-and-a-half ventricular repair involves the establishment of a patent right ventricular outflow, partial closure of the interatrial communication, and a superior cavopulmonary anastomosis (bidirectional Glenn shunt). Studies have shown that one-and-a-half ventricular repair can be performed relatively safely in patients with borderline small right ventricles and in those with chronic right ventricular dysfunction.

Potential advantages of a bidirectional Glenn shunt in the setting of a borderline (morphologically or functionally) right ventricle include (1) volume unloading of the right ventricle, and (2) provision of a defined amount of pulmonary flow (from the superior caval vein) and left ventricular preload independent of right ventricular size and function. A low pulmonary arterial pressure and resistance is required for the one-and-a-half ventricular repair.

There are patients with borderline right ventricular ventricles in whom biventricular repair is initially contemplated but require subsequent conversion to one-and-a-half ventricular repair due to inadequate right ventricular cardiac output and significant systemic venous congestion.

32.3 Long-Term Monitoring

It remains unclear of the long-term results of the borderline right ventricle to handle even only part of the systemic venous return. Strong evidence of the hypothesized benefits of one-and-a-half ventricular repair over Fontan procedure is lacking at this moment. The right ventricular systolic and diastolic function remains fundamentally important in one-and-a-half ventricular repair. Long-term monitoring of the haemodynamic consequences, notably right atrial dilation and hypertension and systemic venous congestion, of a small and stiff right ventricle or a dilated and dysfunctional right ventricle in the context of a one-and-a-half ventricular physiology is warranted.

Part VI

Systemic and Pulmonary Arterial Anomalies

Aortopathies

33

Aortopathies are characterized by dilation of the aorta and aortic aneurysms. In children, aortopathies occur in association with inherited disorders of connective tissue disease and congenital heart disease. The most common genetic syndrome associated with aortopathy is Marfan syndrome, while the most comment congenital anomaly is bicuspid aortic valve.

33.1 Inherited Disorders of Connective Tissue Disease

33.1.1 Marfan Syndrome

First described by Antoine-Bernard Marfan in 1896, Marfan syndrome is an inherited disorder of connective tissue disease due to mutations in the *FBN1* gene. *FBN1* gene encodes a member of the fibrillin family of proteins. Fibrillin-1 is an extracellular matrix glycoprotein that serves as a structural component of microfibrils, the latter providing structural support in connective tissues. Marfan syndrome therefore affects tissues in multiple systems including the skeletal, ocular, cardiovascular, and respiratory systems, the dura, and the skin.

33.1.1.1 Diagnosis

The diagnosis of Marfan syndrome is based on the revised Ghent criteria (Box 33.1). The scoring of systemic features is shown in Table 33.1 (based on Loeys et al. J Med Genet 2010;47:476–485). The revised criteria have put more weight on aortic root dilation as defined by a z score ≥ 2.

Y.-f. Cheung, *Congenital and Paediatric Acquired Heart Disease in Practice*, https://doi.org/10.1007/978-981-99-2862-0_33

Table 33.1 Scoring of systemic features

Score	Features
3 (1)	Wrist and thumb sign (wrist or thumb sign)
2 (1)	Pectus carinatum deformity (pectus excavatum or chest asymmetry)
2 (1)	Hindfoot deformity (plain pes planus)
2	Pneumothorax
2	Dural ectasia
2	Protrusio acetabuli
1	Reduced upper segment/lower segment and increased arm/height and no severe scoliosis
1	Scoliosis or thoracolumbar kyphosis
1	Reduced elbow extension
1	Facial features (3/5) (dolichocephaly, enophthalmos, downslanting palpebral fissures, malar hypoplasia, retrognathia)
1	Skin striae
1	Myopia >3 diopters
1	Mitral valve prolapse

Box 33.1 Revised Ghent Criteria

In the absence of family history

- aortic root z score ≥ 2 and ectopia lentis
- aortic root z score ≥ 2 and fibrillin-1 mutation
- aortic root z score ≥ 2 and systemic score ≥ 7
- ectopia lentis and fibrillin-1 mutation

In the presence of family history

- ectopia lentis
- systemic score ≥ 7
- aortic root z score ≥ 2 (>20 years) or ≥ 3 (<20 years)

33.1.1.2 Cardiovascular Involvements

Cardiovascular involvements are the leading causes of morbidity and mortality. The characteristic cardiovascular manifestations are mitral valve prolapse (due to fibromyxomatous changes in the leaflets) and aortic root dilation (most prominent at the level of sinus of Valsalva). Dilation of the proximal aorta causes incomplete coaptation of the aortic cusps with development of aortic regurgitation. Tricuspid valve prolapse and dilation of the main pulmonary trunk are also commonly found. These complications are more commonly seen in older children and adolescents. An infantile type of Marfan syndrome is also recognized and is typically associated with severe cardiovascular and skeletal involvements.

33.1.1.3 Cardiovascular Management Strategy

Imaging: Echocardiography at the time of diagnosis and at 6 months later aims to assess aortic root (in particular the sinus of Valsalva) dimensions, mitral and tricuspid valve prolapse and regurgitation, and their rate of progression. The z scores of aortic root dimensions should be calculated for the purpose of serial monitoring and comparisons.

Annual echocardiographic assessment is recommended if the aortic root is not markedly enlarged and show no evidence of rapid enlargement. However, aortic dimensions that prompt more frequent evaluation in adults (aortic root diameter > 45 mm or rate of aortic dilation > 5 mm per year) are not available for children.

As aortic dilation can also involve the descending aorta, regular surveillance of the entire aorta with computed tomography or magnetic resonance angiography is indicated from late adolescence onwards (Fig. 33.1).

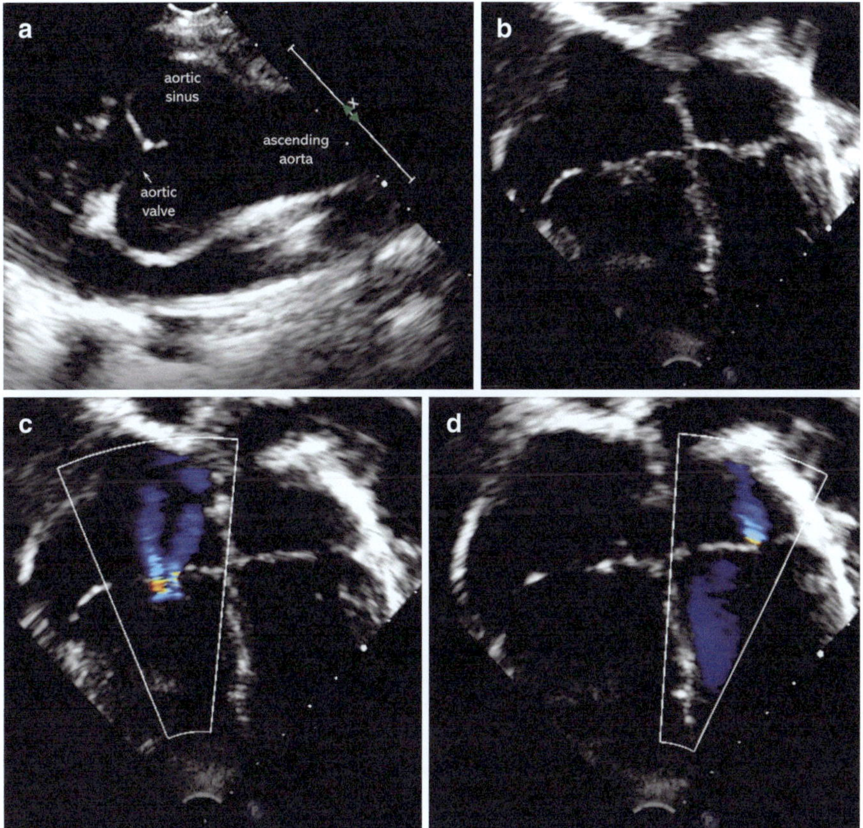

Fig. 33.1 Echocardiographic assessment of Marfan syndrome. (**a**) Dilation of the aortic root and effacement of the sinotubular junction (**b**) Mild tricuspid and mitral valve prolapse (**c**) Mild tricuspid regurgitation and (**d**) mitral regurgitation as shown by Doppler colour flow mapping

Medical treatments: For patients with aortic aneurysm, medical therapies include the use of (1) a beta-blocker for reduction of haemodynamic stress on the aortic wall (a long-acting beta-blocker, for example atenolol, may improve drug compliance), (2) an angiotensin receptor blocker for afterload reduction and blockade of the transforming growth factor-beta signalling that plays a pathogenetic role in aortic dilation and other connective tissue abnormalities in Marfan syndrome, or (3) in combination if tolerated.

For patients without aortic aneurysm, a beta-blocker or an angiotensin receptor blocker is also recommended when risk factors of aneurysm formation are present (positive genotype, evidence of aortic root dilation, and a family history of aortic root enlargement).

Surgical interventions: Aortic dissection is rare in children. While the optimal timing of elective aortic root replacement in children is unclear, the indications are similar to those recommended for adults (Box 33.2).

Aortic root replacement can be accomplished by (1) the use of a composite valve graft that consists of the aortic root and a prosthetic aortic valve with reimplantation of the coronary arteries (Bentall procedure) or (2) a valve sparing procedure (e.g. modified David operation that preserves the aortic valve and recreates neo-sinuses and a neo-sinotubular junction with excision of the sinus tissues), which spares the need for long-term anticoagulation.

Exercise restriction: Patients should be advised against participation in contact sports and isometric exercise.

Box 33.2 Indications for Aortic Root Replacement in Adults with Marfan Syndrome

- external aortic diameter ≥ 50 mm
- rapid increase of >5 mm per year
- external aortic diameter < 50 mm if
    - family history of aortic dissection at a diameter < 50 mm
    - presence of progressive aortic regurgitation
    - cardiac surgery for other reasons (e.g. mitral valve repair)

33.1.2 Loeys-Dietz Syndrome

Loeys–Dietz syndrome is an autosomal dominant connective tissue disorder first described by Dr. Bart Loeys and Dr. Harry (Hal) Dietz in 2005. It is caused by a heterozygous pathogenic variant in one of the following genes: *TGFBR1 and TGFBR2 (*transforming growth factor-β receptors), *TGFB2 and TGFB3 (*TGF-β ligands), and *SMAD2* and *SMAD3* (intracellular downstream effectors of the TGF-β pathway). Hence, disturbance of the transforming growth factor-β signalling plays an important role in its pathogenesis. Clinically, Loeys–Dietz syndrome is characterized by the constellation of vascular, skeletal, craniofacial, and cutaneous findings (Box 33.3).

Box 33.3 Systemic Findings in Loeys-Dietz Ayndrome

- vascular: cerebral, thoracic, and abdominal arterial aneurysms and/or dissection
- skeletal: pectus excavatum or pectus carinatum, scoliosis, joint laxity, arachnodactyly, talipes equinovarus, cervical spine malformation and/or instability
- craniofacial: widely spaced eyes, strabismus, bifid uvula, cleft palate, craniosynostosis
- cutaneous: velvety and translucent skin, easy bruising, dystrophic scars

33.1.2.1 Diagnosis

Diagnosis of Loeys-Dietz syndrome is established by the findings of (1) a heterozygous pathogenic variant in one of the six genes as mentioned earlier, and (2) either aortic root enlargement (aortic root z-score $\geq$ 2)/type A dissection or compatible systemic features as highlighted in Box 33.3 (in particular the vascular findings).

33.1.2.2 Cardiovascular Involvements

Cardiovascular involvements are the leading causes of morbidity and mortality in Loeys-Dietz syndrome and run a more aggressive course than Marfan syndrome. Dissection occurs at smaller aortic diameters than those observed in Marfan syndrome. Histologically, diffuse aortic medial degeneration with fragmentation of elastic fibres, increased collagen content, and accumulation of matrix components are found. Characteristic cardiovascular manifestations include aortic root dilation, arterial aneurysms (involving different aortic branches including subclavian, renal, superior mesenteric, hepatic, and coronary arteries), arterial tortuosity (especially involving the head and neck arteries), early aortic dissection (even in infants and young children), and mitral valve prolapse with or without mitral regurgitation.

33.1.2.3 Cardiovascular Management Strategy

Imaging: Echocardiography aims to assess aortic root dimensions (in particular diameter at the sinuses of Valsalva), the rate of progression of aortic root dilation, and mitral valve prolapse and regurgitation (Fig. 33.2). Aortic root dimensions should be interpreted based on age and body size, with conversion to z scores, for serial monitoring and comparisons. Computed tomography or magnetic resonance angiography to image the entire arterial tree is indicated.

Medical treatments: Medical therapies include the use of a beta-blocker or an angiotensin receptor blocker for reduction hemodynamic stress on the aortic wall.

Surgical interventions: The aggressive course of cardiovascular complications necessitates early aortic surgery (Box 33.4).

Exercise restriction: Patients should be advised against participation in contact sports and isometric exercise.

Box 33.4 Indications for Aortic Root Replacement in Loeys-Dietz Syndrome

- young children: aortic diameter > 99th centile for age and aortic annulus at least 18–20 mm
- older children and adolescents: when maximal aortic dimension approaches 40 mm
- other factors that influence the timing of surgery: disease subtype (with severe craniofacial features), family history of aortic dissection, rapid increase in aortic size (0.5 cm over 1 year), aortic regurgitation

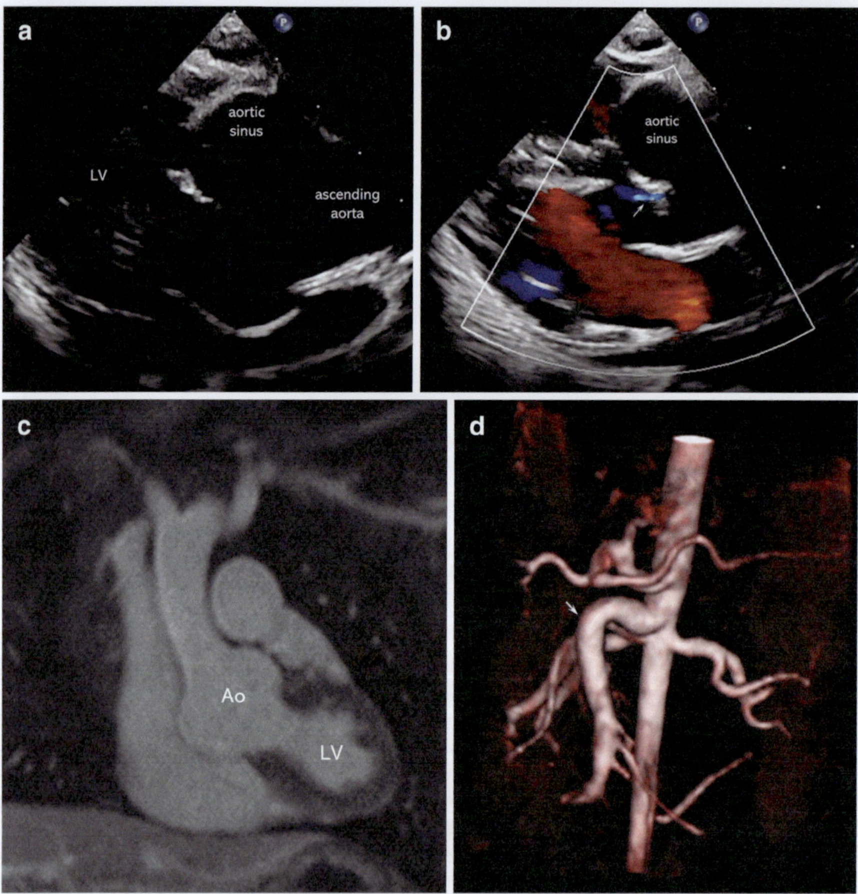

Fig. 33.2 Dilation of the aorta and other arteries in Loeys-Dietz syndrome. (**a**) Echocardiographic demonstration of severe dilation of the aortic root with effacement of the sinotubular junction (**b**) Doppler colour flow mapping showing trivial degree of aortic regurgitation (**c**) CMR showing dilation of aorta root (**d**) Abdominal magnetic resonance angiography showing dilation of the superior mesenteric artery (arrow) (*Ao* aorta, *LV* left ventricle)

33.1.3 Ehlers-Danlos Syndrome

Ehlers Danlos syndrome comprises genetic disorders of connective disease that is characterized by joint hypermobility, skin hyperextensibility, and tissue fragility.

33.1.3.1 Diagnosis

Based on the 2017 revised classification of the International Ehlers Danlos syndrome Consortium, 13 subtypes are recognized based on the phenotypes with a set of major (of high diagnostic specificity) and minor (of lower diagnostic specificity) clinical criteria for each of the subtypes.

33.1.3.2 Cardiovascular Involvements

Cardiovascular manifestations of Ehlers Danlos syndrome include aortic root dilation, mitral and aortic valve prolapse, aortic regurgitation, and aneurysms of the sinus of Valsalva and other blood vessels.

The following subtypes are known to have cardiovascular associations: (1) the cardiac-valvular subtype is associated with progressive severe dysfunction of the aortic and mitral valves, (2) the vascular subtype is associated with arterial aneurysms involving different parts of the arterial tree, spontaneous arterial rupture and dissection at a young age, and formation of carotid-cavernous sinus fistula in the absence of trauma, (3) the kyphoscoliotic subtype is associated with arterial fragility, spontaneous arterial rupture and dissection, and (4) classical and hypermobile subtypes are associated with usually mild and haemodynamically insignificant aortic root dilation and aortic valve prolapse.

33.1.3.3 Cardiovascular Management Strategy

Regular cardiovascular imaging (echocardiography, computed tomography and magnetic resonance angiography) for monitoring of arterial and valvar complications is required. For patients with arterial aneurysms, medical therapies include the use of a beta-blocker or an angiotensin receptor blocker. Vascular fragility results in high postoperative morbidity and mortality. Hence, surgical intervention is usually reserved for life-threatening situations.

33.2 Congenital Heart Disease

33.2.1 Bicuspid Aortic Valve

Bicuspid aortic valve is a common cause of congenital valvar aortic stenosis (Chap. 13). It can be isolated or can occur in association with coarctation of the aorta or interrupted aortic arch. Furthermore, bicuspid aortic valve is associated with dilation of the aortic root and ascending aortic aneurysm disproportionate to the degree of aortic stenosis.

The prevalence of dilated aortic root in children with bicuspid aortic valve has been reported to be about 50%. The cause of aortic dilation is, however, unclear.

Contributing factors include an intrinsic aortopathy with inherent structural abnormalities of the ascending aorta, abnormal flow dynamics, valvar morphology and stenosis, and genetic influence. Genetic variants associated with familial nonsyndromic bicuspid aortopathy include *NOTCH-1*, *SMAD6*, and *MAT2A*.

The occurrence of aortic root dilation in the absence of significance valvar aortic stenosis or regurgitation suggests an intrinsic developmental abnormality of the aortic wall (bicuspid aortopathy). Histological examination of the aortic media shows cystic medial degeneration and elastic fibre fragmentation. Mechanics of the aorta are altered with decreased elasticity and distensibility. Alteration of arterial haemodynamics, aortic mechanics, wall shear stress, and flow pattern (depending on the pattern of fusion of valve leaflets) possibly act in concert to cause bicuspid aortopathy. Bicuspid aortopathy increases the risk of aortic dissection during adulthood, especially in patients with Turner syndrome (Chap. 62).

33.2.1.1 Cardiovascular Management Strategy

Imaging: Regular echocardiography to assess valvar aortic stenosis and/or regurgitation and aortic root dimensions is indicated (Fig. 33.3). Aortic root dimensions should be interpreted based on age and body size, with conversion to z scores, for serial monitoring and comparisons.

Medical treatments: No medical therapies have been shown to alter the progression of aortic root dilation or the risk of aortic dissection in adults. Medical management focuses on the control of blood pressure in patients with hypertension (e.g. patients with repaired coarctation of the aorta or interrupted aortic arch).

Interventions: In the paediatric population, interventions are primarily targeted at the relief of significant valvar aortic stenosis in association with bicuspid aortic valve by either surgical or transcatheter intervention (Chap. 13). In adults, the threshold of ascending aortic diameter for prophylactic surgery is controversial but the usual recommendations are shown in Box 33.5.

Box 33.5 Indications for Aortic Root Surgery in Adults with Bicuspid Aortic Valve

- aortic root or ascending aorta diameter $\geq$ 55 mm
- aortic root or ascending aorta diameter $\geq$ 50 mm in the presence of
  - coarctation of the aorta
  - hypertension
  - family history of aortic dissection
  - progressive aortic regurgitation
  - rapid increase in size of >3 mm per year

33.2.2 Other Congenital Cardiac Malformations

Conotruncal congenital heart defects including tetralogy of Fallot, pulmonary atresia with ventricular septal defect, transposition of the great arteries, and truncus

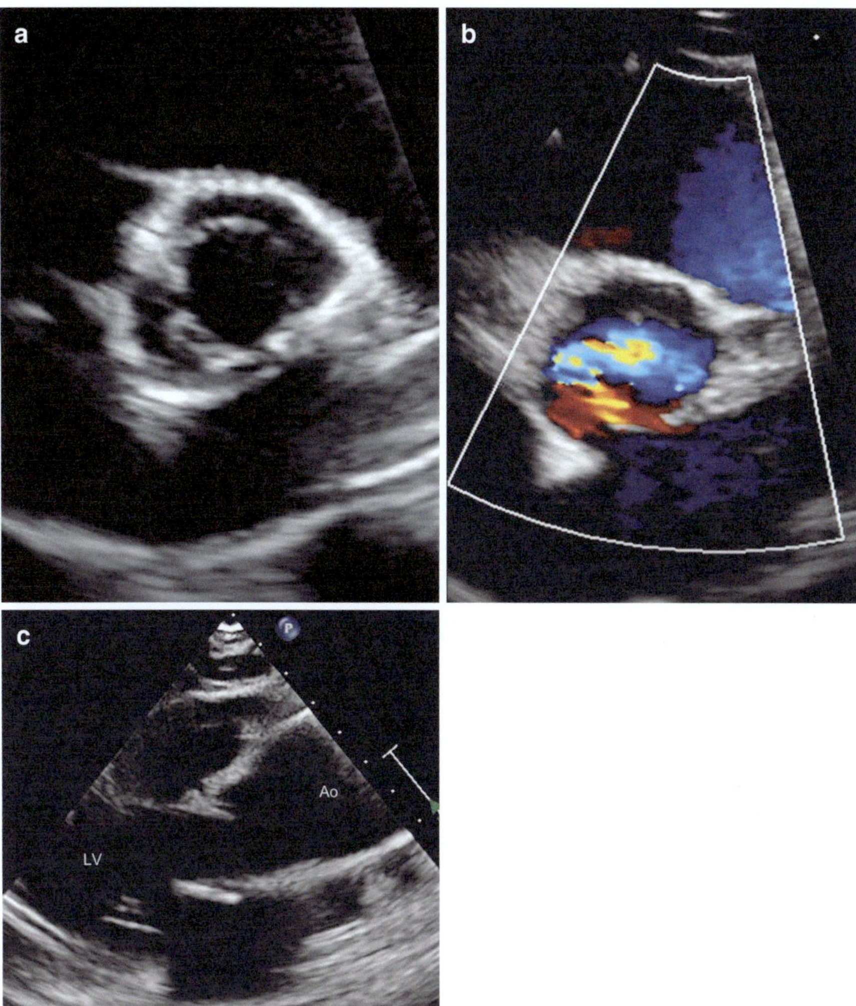

Fig. 33.3 Echocardiographic assessment of bicuspid aortopathy. (**a**) 2D and (**b**) Doppler colour echocardiographic findings of stenotic bicuspid aortic valve (**c**) Dilation of the ascending aorta is shown in the parasternal long-axis view (*Ao* aorta, *LV* left ventricle)

arteriosus are associated with dilated aortic root (or neoaorta after arterial switch operation for transposition of the great arteries). Proposed mechanisms include significant right-to-left shunt before surgery (increased aortic volume loading) and aortic medial abnormalities with elastic fibre fragmentation and reduced elasticity. Albeit rare, aortic dissection has been reported, mostly in patients after repair of tetralogy of Fallot.

33.2.2.1 Cardiovascular Management Strategy

Imaging: Regular echocardiography to assess aortic root dimensions and aortic regurgitation is indicated. Aortic root dimensions should be interpreted based on age and body size, with conversion to z scores, for serial monitoring and comparisons.

Medical treatments: No medical therapies have been shown to alter the progression of aortic root dilation or development of aortic complications in patients with conotruncal congenital heart defects.

Interventions: Given the limited data and the rarity of aortic dissection, prophylactic aortic root surgery based solely on the aortic diameter is not usually recommended. Some recommend aortic root surgery if the aortic diameter is >55 mm or even earlier if additional cardiac surgery is required.

34 Vascular Ring and Sling

The aorta, branch pulmonary arteries, and arterial duct are in close proximities to the tracheobronchial tree and the esophagus. Congenital anomalies of these vascular structures, in the form of a vascular ring or sling, can cause obstruction to the airways and/or esophagus.

34.1 Anatomy and Pathophysiology

Abnormal development of the components of the aortic arch may result in the formation of a vascular ring that completely or partially encircles the airway and esophagus. The most common causes of complete vascular rings are a double aortic arch and a right aortic arch with an aberrant left subclavian artery and a left persistent arterial duct (or ligamentum arteriosum). Complete vascular rings can cause extrinsic compression of the airways and esophagus and tracheobronchomalacia. Pulmonary artery sling, although not completely encircling the tracheobronchial tree, can also cause extrinsic compression of the trachea. Complete tracheal rings causing intrinsic tracheal stenosis also commonly occur in association with pulmonary artery sling.

Associated congenital cardiac anomalies include ventricular septal defect, coarctation of the aorta, and tetralogy of Fallot. Noncardiac associations include tracheoesophageal fistula, cleft lip, cleft palate, and syndromic disorders (DiGeorge syndrome and Down syndrome).

34.1.1 Double Aortic Arch

In double aortic arch, the two aortic arches bifurcate from the ascending aorta and rejoin to form the descending aorta. The two arches encircle and may compress on the trachea and esophagus. The right common carotid and right subclavian arteries

Y.-f. Cheung, *Congenital and Paediatric Acquired Heart Disease in Practice*, https://doi.org/10.1007/978-981-99-2862-0_34

arise from the usually larger right-sided arch, while the left common carotid and left subclavian arteries arise from the left-sided arch. The left arch is usually smaller or may be atretic.

34.1.2 Right Aortic Arch with an Aberrant Left Subclavian Artery and a Left Persistent Arterial Duct (or Arterial Ligament)

In this condition, the arterial duct (or ligamentum arteriosum) courses from its posterior origin (from the aberrant left subclavian artery that arises from the diverticulum of Kommerell at the descending aorta) to the anteriorly located pulmonary artery. The complete vascular ring is formed (a) anteriorly and rightward by the right-sided aortic arch, (b) posteriorly by the origin of the aberrant left subclavian artery and Kommerell diverticulum, and (c) leftward by the left arterial duct (or ligamentum arteriosum).

34.1.3 Pulmonary Artery Sling

Pulmonary artery sling is characterized by distal bifurcation of the branch pulmonary arteries, which result in the left pulmonary artery arising from the right pulmonary artery. The left pulmonary artery courses posterior to the distal trachea and anterior to the esophagus, which may lead to extrinsic compression of the trachea and/or esophagus. The ring-sling complex describes the common association between pulmonary artery sling and tracheal stenosis with complete tracheal rings. Airway obstruction in the ring-sling complex can be attributed to extrinsic compression by the left pulmonary artery, tracheal stenosis with complete tracheal rings, and tracheobronchomalacia.

34.2 Clinical Presentation and Findings

The timing of clinical presentation in infants and children with vascular ring and pulmonary artery sling depends on the severity of airway obstruction. Neonates and infants with significant airway obstruction due to pulmonary artery sling or double aortic arch present early with respiratory symptoms including shortness of breath, stridor, wheezing, cough, and episodes of respiratory infection that worsens respiratory distress. Noisy breath and signs of respiratory distress are obvious in these patients.

In the presence of significant esophageal compression, difficulties in feeding of solid food and vomiting may occur in infants and toddlers. Dysphagia is a more common complaint in older children and adolescents.

Some patients, especially those with incomplete vascular rings, can remain asymptomatic with no abnormal signs and the diagnosis is made incidentally when cardiovascular imaging is performed for investigations of associated congenital cardiac malformations or other reasons.

34.3 Investigations

Initial investigations are usually directed to unravel the cause of respiratory symptoms and signs in neonates and infants.

CXR: The chest radiograph may show the sidedness of the aortic arch and narrowing of the distal trachea due to compression by the double aortic arch or left pulmonary artery sling. Hyperinflation of the lungs may be present.

CT and CMR: Both imaging modalities enable three-dimensional visualization of the vascular anomalies. Computed tomography has the advantages of allowing better delineation of the airways, understanding of the relationship between the vascular structures and the airway, and faster acquisition without the need for general anaesthesia (Fig. 34.1).

Bronchoscopy: Bronchoscopic assessment is performed as part of the workup for the clinical presentation of upper airway obstruction. It can locate the level of compression and may suggest the possibility of pulsatile extrinsic compression of the airway. This invasive procedure can, however, induce airway oedema and worsen the severity of airway obstruction. It does not provide information of vascular anomalies. Postoperatively, bronchoscopic assessment permits the evaluation of the severity of tracheobronchomalacia.

Echocardiography: Echocardiography is usually prompted by clues of a vascular ring based on fetal ultrasound imaging, clinical findings of associated congenital cardiac malformations, or a high clinical suspicion of vascular ring or sling as a diagnosis of early onset respiratory distress after birth. Echocardiography can image the sidedness of the aortic arch, demonstrate the presence of a right arch in association with a left arterial duct, and diagnose a double aortic arch.

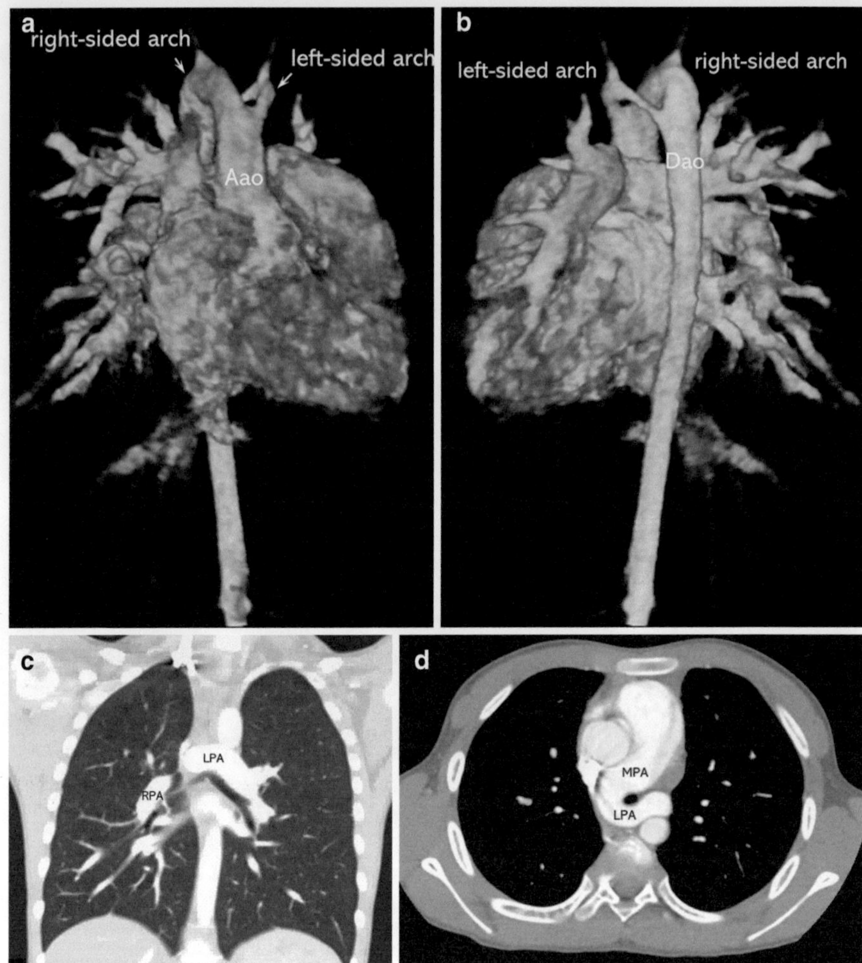

Fig. 34.1 Computed tomography findings of double aortic arch and pulmonary artery sling. (**a**) Anterior and (**b**) posterior views of double aortic arch (**c**) coronal and (**d**) axial computed tomographic views of pulmonary artery sling (Abbreviations: *Aao* ascending aorta, *Dao* descending aorta, *MPA* main pulmonary artery, *LPA* left pulmonary artery, *RPA* right pulmonary artery)

34.4 Management Strategy

Surgical intervention is the only definitive treatment of vascular ring and sling.

34.4.1 Double Aortic Arch

For the repair of double artic arch, the smaller of the two arches and the ligamentum arteriosum are divided.

34.4.2 Right Aortic Arch with an Aberrant Left Subclavian Artery and a Left Persistent Arterial Duct (or Arterial Ligament)

Division of the left persistent arterial duct (or ligamentum arteriosum) is performed. In some centres, resection of the Kommerell diverticulum (to reduce the risk of recurrent symptoms) with reimplantation of the left subclavian artery to the left common carotid artery is performed.

34.4.3 Pulmonary Artery Sling

In the absence of tracheal compression or stenosis, relocation of the left pulmonary artery to the main pulmonary artery anterior to the trachea is performed. In neonates and infants with associated severe tracheal stenosis and complete tracheal rings, slide tracheoplasty is performed to relief the stenosis.

34.5 Post Operative Considerations

Potential complications include damage to the recurrent laryngeal nerve and phrenic nerve. The postoperative haemodynamics are usually stable. Patients with several tracheobronchomalacia are at risk of recurrent lung collapse, hyperinflation, and infection. In these patients, longer term noninvasive ventilation with tracheostomy and effective clearance of airway secretions are required.

34.6 Long-Term Monitoring

The outcome after surgery is good with improvement of symptoms of airway and esophageal compression. Balloon dilation for restenosis of airway due to granulation tissue and scarring may be required. For patients with severe tracheobronchomalacia, stent implantation and aortopexy can be considered.

Pulmonary Hypertension

35

Pulmonary hypertension is characterized by an increase in pulmonary arterial pressure. Idiopathic including hereditary pulmonary arterial hypertension and pulmonary arterial hypertension associated with congenital heart disease are the most common causes of pulmonary hypertension in paediatric patients.

35.1 Definition

Pulmonary hypertension in children was previously defined as an increase in mean pulmonary arterial pressure to ≥25 mmHg in children aged >3 months. During the recent World Symposium on Pulmonary Hypertension in 2018, the threshold for the definition has been changed to >20 mmHg in both children and adults.

Definitions based on the updates in the World Symposium on Pulmonary Hypertension in 2018 are shown in Table 35.1. In paediatric pulmonary hypertension, the indexed pulmonary vascular resistance (PVRI) of ≥3 Wood units·m^2 has also been used to define pulmonary arterial hypertension or pulmonary hypertensive vascular disease. An elevated pulmonary arterial wedge pressure (PAWP) or left ventricular end-diastolic pressure (LVEDP) is suggestive of postcapillary pulmonary hypertension.

The original version of the chapter has been revised. A correction to this chapter can be found at https://doi.org/10.1007/978-981-99-2862-0_65

Y.-f. Cheung, *Congenital and Paediatric Acquired Heart Disease in Practice*, https://doi.org/10.1007/978-981-99-2862-0_35

Table 35.1 Definitions of pulmonary hypertension (PH) in children and adolescents

Type of PH	Mean PAP	PAWP or LVEDP	PVRI
Pulmonary arterial hypertension (precapillary PH)	>20 mmHg	≤15 mmHg	≥3 Wood units·m^2
Isolated postcapillary PH	>20 mmHg	>15 mmHg	<3 Wood units·m^2
Combined pre- and postcapillary PH	>20 mmHg	>15 mmHg	≥3 Wood units·m^2
Pulmonary hypertensive vascular disease (in congenital heart disease)	>20 mmHg for biventricular circulation Mean transpulmonary gradient >6 mmHg for univentricular circulation		≥3 Wood units·m^2 for biventricular circulation >3 Wood units·m^2 for univentricular circulation

Adapted with modifications from Hansmann et al. J Heart Lung Transplant 2019;38:879–901

Table 35.2 Causes of persistent pulmonary hypertension in children

Pulmonary arterial hypertension (PAH)	Other causes of pulmonary hypertension

PAH with no associated congenital heart disease
  Idiopathic PAH
  Hereditary PAH
  PAH with pulmonary veno-occlusive disease
  PAH associated with portal hypertension
  PAH associated with HIV infection (rare in children)
PAH with left-to-right shunts
  Unrepaired large shunts
  Late repair of large shunts
PAH with complex heart disease
  Unilateral absence of pulmonary artery
  One pulmonary artery arising from the aorta (previously referred to as hemitruncus)
  Functional single ventricle before and after Fontan procedure
	Respiratory disease or chronic hypoxaemic conditions
	  Bronchopulmonary dysplasia
	  Alveolar capillary dysplasia
	  Interstitial lung disease
	  Cystic fibrosis
	  Obstructive sleep apnoea
	Postcapillary pulmonary hypertension
	  Pulmonary vein stenosis
	  Cortriatriatum
	  Mitral stenosis
	  Hypoplasia of the left ventricle
	  Left ventricular systolic and/or diastolic dysfunction
	  Cardiomyopathies
	Pulmonary hypertension associated with systemic disorders
	  Connective tissue disease
	  Haemoglobinopathies
	  Metabolic disorders (glycogen storage disease, Gaucher disease, hypo- and hyperthyroidism)

35.2 Aetiology

Transient pulmonary hypertension occurs in neonates with pulmonary hypertension of the newborn, most premature babies with bronchopulmonary dysplasia, and infants with large left-to-right shunts who undergo timely repair of the congenital heart defects.

Causes of persistent and progressive pulmonary hypertension in children are shown in Table 35.2.

Table 35.3 Genetic mutations in pulmonary arterial hypertension

Gene	Inheritance	Comments
Genes related to transforming growth factor-beta receptor superfamily or related downstream signalling molecules		
BMPR2	AD	
ALK1	AD	Also causes hereditary haemorrhagic telangiectasia
ENG	AD	Also causes hereditary haemorrhagic telangiectasia
SMAD 4	AD	
SMAD 9	AD	
Genes not related to the transforming growth factor-beta receptor superfamily		
KCN3	AD	Encodes potassium channel
CAV1	AD	Encodes a membrane protein required for the formation of caveolae that mediate signaling pathways in pulmonary hypertension
EIF2AK4	AR	Encodes a kinase that modulates angiogenesis in response to cellular stress, causes pulmonary venoocclusive disease/pulmonary capillary haemangiomatosis
TBX4	AD	Encodes T-box transcription factor
Recently identified genes		
ABCC8		Encodes a regulatory subunit of potassium channel
GDF2		Encodes the ligand for the BMPR2/ALK1 receptor complex
AQP1		Encodes aquaporin-1 that promotes endothelial cell migration and angiogenesis
SOX17		Encodes transcription factor that promotes angiogenesis and arteriovenous differentiation

35.3 Genetics of Pulmonary Hypertension

Patients with an identifiable genetic cause are regarded as having hereditary pulmonary arterial hypertension. About 25–30% of patients diagnosed with idiopathic pulmonary arterial hypertension have an identifiable genetic cause with a Mendelian inheritance (Table 35.3). Mutation in *BMPR2* accounts for the majority (about 70%) of cases of hereditary pulmonary arterial hypertension.

35.4 Pathophysiology

Factors that lead to an increase in pulmonary arterial pressure are governed by the Ohm's law (Box 35.1). An increase in pulmonary arterial pressure can therefore be due to (a) an increase in pulmonary flow (as in large left-to-right shunts), (b) an increase in pulmonary vascular resistance (due to increased arteriolar constriction, decreased luminal diameter, or reduced number of pulmonary vessels), and/or (c) increase in pulmonary arterial wedge or left atrial pressure (as in pulmonary venous obstruction, mitral stenosis, or left ventricular diastolic dysfunction).

Box 35.1 Ohm's Law and Pulmonary Arterial Pressure

$$\textbf{voltage} = \textbf{flow} \times \textbf{resistance}$$

Applied to the pulmonary circulation

$$\textbf{transpulmonary gradient} = \textbf{Qp} \times \textbf{PVRI}$$

$$\textbf{mean PAP} - \textbf{LAP}\left(\textbf{or PAWP}\right) = \textbf{Qp} \times \textbf{PVRI}$$

Hence

$$\textbf{mean PAP} = \textbf{Qp} \times \textbf{PVRI} + \textbf{LA pressure}\left(\textbf{or PAWP}\right)$$

LAP is left atrial pressure, PAP is pulmonary arterial pressure, PAWP is pulmonary arterial wedge pressure, PVRI is pulmonary vascular resistance index, Qp is pulmonary flow

The underlying pathophysiologic processes in the pulmonary vasculature include (a) pulmonary arteriolar endothelial dysfunction, (b) smooth muscle hypertrophy with remodelling, (c) paucity of arterioles due to failure of development or postnatal destruction, (d) formation of microthrombi, and (e) increased arteriolar constriction. Pulmonary hypertension increases the afterload to the right ventricle and can lead to right ventricular failure. Left ventricular dysfunction develops as a result of adverse ventricular-ventricular interaction (Chap. 28).

Disruption of the three key signalling pathways, namely nitric oxide, prostaglandin, and endothelin pathways, plays a key role in the pathogenesis of progressive pulmonary arterial hypertension (Fig. 35.1). The understanding of the mechanisms of impaired pulmonary vasodilation and augmented pulmonary vasoconstriction has facilitated the development of targeted therapies for pulmonary arterial hypertension.

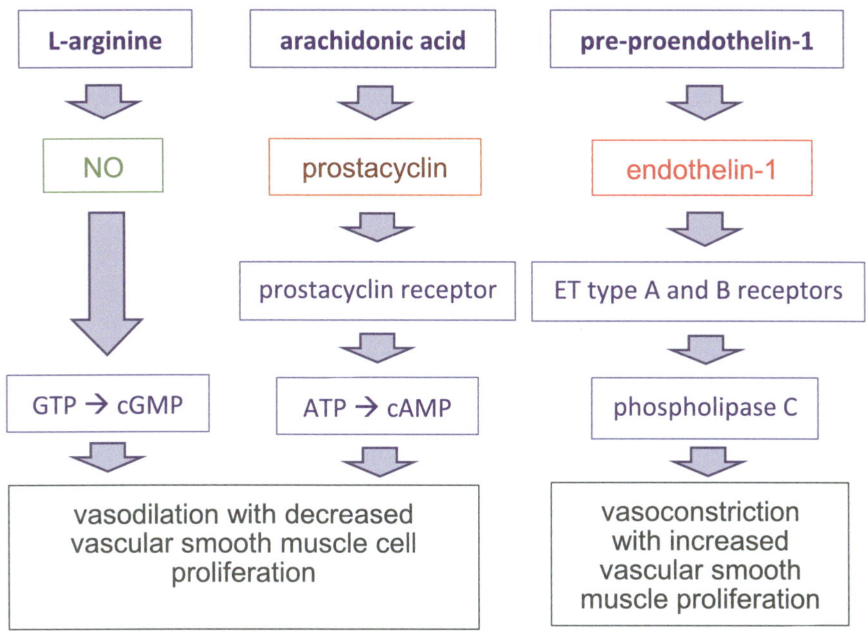

Fig. 35.1 Signalling pathways that are disrupted in pulmonary arterial hypertension. Abbreviations: *ATP* adenosine triphosphate, *cAMP* cyclic adenosine monophosphate, *AMP cGMP* cyclic guanosine monophosphate, *ET* endothelin, *GTP* guanosine triphosphate, *NO* nitric oxide

35.5 Clinical Presentation and Findings

Children with respiratory conditions, congenital cardiac malformations, systemic disease (e.g. connective tissue disease, haematologic disorders), and hereditary haemorrhagic telangiectasia (Chap. 36) present with symptoms of the underlying disorders. Diagnosis of pulmonary hypertension is made as part of the assessment and workup.

Children with mild or even moderate degree of idiopathic or hereditary pulmonary arterial hypertension may remain relatively asymptomatic. There is often a delay from the onset of symptoms to diagnosis. The most common symptoms, when present, are dyspnoea on exertion, fatigue, and syncope on exertion. Other symptoms, which can be non-specific, include failure to thrive, cough, and cyanosis at rest or on exertion. Symptoms of right heart failure are rare.

Signs of underlying associated conditions may be found. In children with moderate to severe idiopathic or hereditary pulmonary arterial hypertension, the signs are those of increased right ventricular afterload and increased pulmonary arterial pressure (Table 35.4). Signs of right heart failure due to systolic right ventricular failure are uncommon in children.

Table 35.4 Signs of moderate to severe idiopathic pulmonary hypertension

Signs	Origins
Cyanosis at rest or on exertion	Uncommon, due to right-to-left atrial shunt or associated pulmonary parenchymal disease
Left parasternal impulse	Increased right ventricular afterload
S2 narrowly split with loud P2	Loud closure sound of the pulmonary valve due to increased pulmonary diastolic pressure
An early diastolic murmur at the left sternal border	Related to pulmonary regurgitation
Right heart failure (increased jugular venous pressure, hepatomegaly, and ankle oedema)	Signs of right heart failure are uncommon and indicate severe pulmonary hypertension with right ventricular systolic dysfunction

35.6 Investigations

CXR: Chest radiograph may show cardiomegaly due to right ventricular enlargement and dilation of the main pulmonary trunk and proximal branch pulmonary arteries. Haziness of the lung fields suggests interstitial lung disease or pulmonary venous obstruction.

ECG: Electrocardiogram shows right axis deviation and right ventricular hypertrophy.

Echocardiography: Echocardiography identifies underlying cardiac anomalies that cause pulmonary hypertension. Severity of pulmonary hypertension can be quantified by (a) estimation of the pulmonary arterial systolic and diastolic pressure by Doppler interrogation of respectively the tricuspid and pulmonary regurgitant jet, (b) interrogation of pressure gradient or right to left shunting across the ventricular and atrial septal defects and arterial duct if present, and (c) septal geometry and eccentricity (Chap. 28) of the left ventricle (Fig. 35.2). Right ventricular systolic function can be assessed by measuring fractional area change, tricuspid annular plane systolic excursion, and right ventricular free wall myocardial tissue velocities.

Cardiac catheterization: Cardiac catheterization is a high-risk procedure for children with severe pulmonary hypertension and may not be required for initial diagnosis. Pulmonary hypertensive crisis and cardiac arrest are possible complications. It is indicated for (a) the confirmation of diagnosis when noninvasive investigations are nondiagnostic, (b) defining intracardiac or transductal shunting and pulmonary vascular resistance index, (c) assessment of pulmonary vasoreactivity prior to initiation of targeted medical therapies, (d) transcatheter interventions (e.g. atrioseptostomy), and (e) evaluation of potential candidacy for heart or heart-lung transplantation.

CT angiography: This is useful when pulmonary thromboembolism, pulmonary veno-obstruction, or pulmonary veno-occlusive disease is suspected.

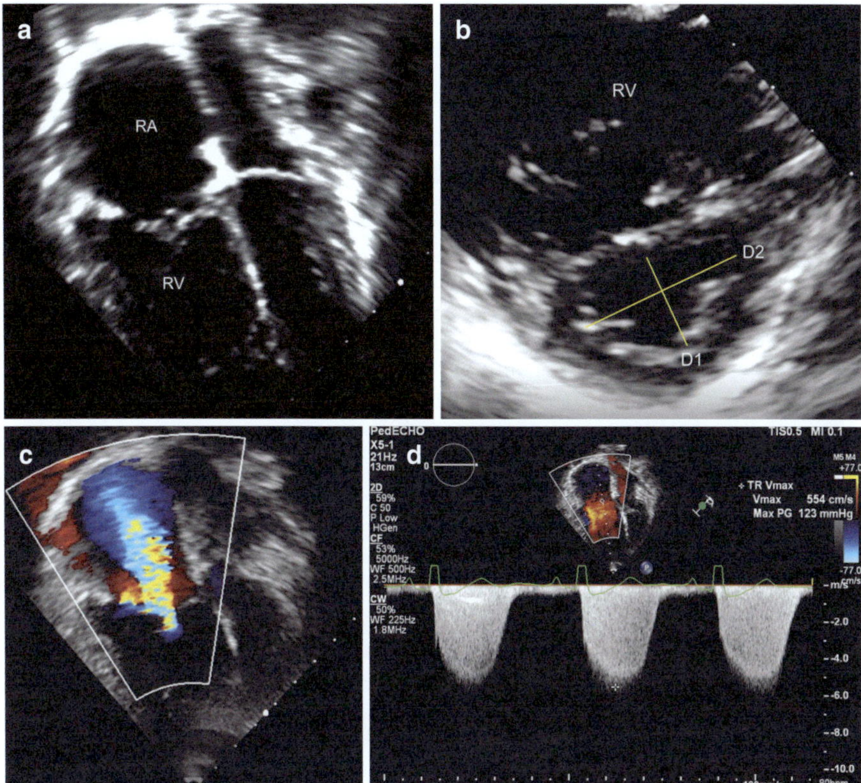

Fig. 35.2 Echocardiographic assessment of pulmonary hypertension. (**a**) Dilation of the right atrium and right ventricle (**b**) Compression of the left ventricle by the pressure-overloaded right ventricle is quantified by calculation of the eccentricity index (D2/D1) (**c**) Colour flow mapping showing severe functional tricuspid regurgitation secondary to right ventricular dilation (**d**) Continuous wave Doppler echocardiography for the estimation of the systolic pulmonary arterial pressure from the peak velocity of the tricuspid regurgitant jet (Abbreviations: *RA* right atrium, *RV* right ventricle)

Respiratory investigations: Additional respiratory investigations including polysomnography, lung function test, and computed tomography scan of the lungs may unveil respiratory cause of pulmonary hypertension.

Investigations for conditions associated with pulmonary hypertension: These include investigations for autoimmune connective tissue disease (ESR, CRP, antinuclear antibodies, rheumatoid factor), portal hypertension (liver function test, ultrasound), thyroid disorders, thrombophilia screening, and HIV testing.

Genetic evaluation: Genetic testing for mutation of genes associated with pulmonary hypertension (Table 35.3) is indicated in children with idiopathic pulmonary hypertension and in those with a positive family history.

35.7 Acute Vasoreactivity Testing

Cardiac catheterization with acute vasoreactivity testing is the next important investigation, which provides prognostic information and guides medical treatment. Acute vasoreactivity testing is an assessment of the haemodynamic response to the administration of a pulmonary vasodilator. Protocols on how to conduct the testing differ, however, among centres in terms of the followings: (a) the use of sedation and general anaesthesia, (b) the use of pulmonary vasodilators (inhaled nitric oxide with oxygen, inhaled nitric oxide only, or 100% oxygen only), and (c) criteria used to define pulmonary vasoreactivity (Box 35.2).

Box 35.2 Criteria Used to Define Pulmonary Vasoreactivity

Sitbon Criteria

- Decrease in mean pulmonary arterial pressure ≥10 mmHg to a value of ≤40 mmHg with an increased or unchanged cardiac output
- Recommended for use by the Paediatric Task Force of the 2018 World Symposium on Pulmonary Hypertension

Barst Criteria

- Decrease in mean pulmonary arterial pressure of ≥20%, unchanged or increased cardiac index, and decreased or unchanged pulmonary vascular resistance to systemic vascular resistance ratio

35.8 Management Strategy for Idiopathic Pulmonary Arterial Hypertension

Findings of acute vasoreactivity testing inform the choice of pulmonary vasodilator therapy in children with idiopathic (including hereditary) pulmonary arterial hypertension (Fig. 35.3).

35.8.1 Positive Vasoreactivity Testing

Patients showing vasoreactivity are treated with calcium channel blockers (nifedipine, amlodipine, or diltiazem). However, calcium channel blockers are contraindicated in patients with right ventricular dysfunction.

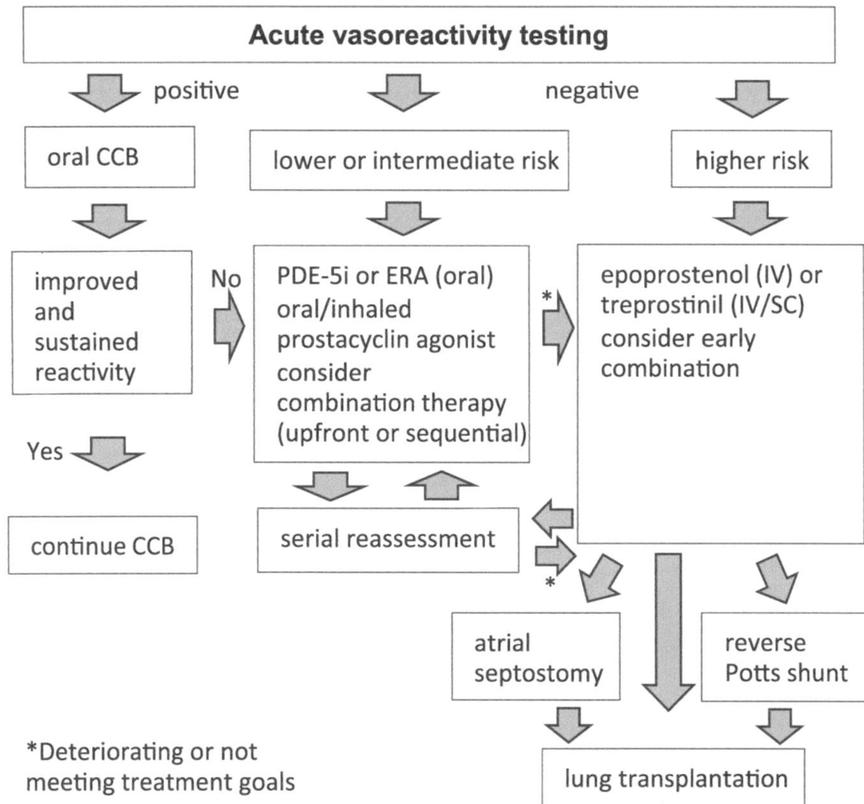

Fig. 35.3 Acute vasoreactivity testing. Abbreviations: *CCB* calcium channel blocker, *ERA* endothelin receptor antagonist IV, intravenous, *PDE-5i* phosphodiesterase 5 inhibitor, *SC* subcutaneous. (Reproduced with permission of the © ERS 2023. Rosenzweig et al. Eur Respir J 2019;53:1801916. DOI: 10.1183/13993003.01916-2018)

35.8.2 Negative Vasoreactivity Testing

Patients with negative vasoreactivity testing do not respond to calcium channel blockers. The drug of choice in these patients depends on an initial risk assessment (Table 35.5).

35.8.3 Drug Therapies

Based on the risk assessment, initial treatment options are (a) oral phosphodiesterase 5 inhibitors, oral endothelin receptor antagonists, and inhaled prostanoids for low-risk patients, and (b) intravenous or subcutaneous prostanoids for high-risk patients (Table 35.6). In high-risk patients, combination therapy is commonly used (Fig. 35.3).

Table 35.5 Risk assessment of pulmonary hypertension

Determinants of risk	Lower risk	Higher risk
Clinical evidence of RV failure	No	Yes
Progression of symptoms	No	Yes
Syncope	No	Yes
Growth	Normal	Failure to thrive
WHO functional class	I, II	III, IV
Serum N-terminal proBNP	Minimally elevated for age or not elevated	Greatly elevated for age > 1200 pg/mL (>1 year old) Rising NT-proBNP level
Echocardiography, CMR	Minimal RA/RV enlargement No RV systolic dysfunction RV/LV e.s. ratio < 1 (PSAX) TAPSE normal ($z > -2$) S/D ratio < 1.0 (TR jet) PAAT >100 ms (>1 year old)	Severe RA/RV enlargement RV systolic dysfunction RV/LV e.s. ratio > 1.5 (PSAX) TAPSE ↓ ↓ ($z < -3$) S/D ratio > 1.4 (TR jet) PAAT <70 ms (>1 year old) Pericardial effusion
Invasive haemodynamics	CI >3.0 l/min/m^2 Mean RAP <10 mm Hg mPAP/mSAP <0.5 Acute vasoreactivity +	CI <2.5 l/min/m^2 Mean RAP >15 mm Hg mPAP/mSAP >0.75 PVRi >15 WU·m^2

Adapted with modifications from Hansmann et al. J Heart Lung Transplant 2019;38:879–901
Abbreviations: *BNP* brain natriuretic peptide, *CI* cardiac index, *e.s.* end-systolic, *LV* left ventricular, *mPAP* mean pulmonary arterial pressure, *mSAP* mean systolic arterial pressure, *PAAT* pulmonary artery acceleration time, *PVRi* pulmonary vascular resistance index, *RA* right atrial, *RV* right ventricular, *S/D* systolic to diastolic duration, *TAPSE* tricuspid annular plane systolic excursion, *TR* tricuspid regurgitant

35.8.4 Pulmonary Hypertension Refractory to Medical Therapy

The management options include (a) an atrioseptostomy (with or without stenting of the atrial septum defect or implantation of a custom-made fenestrated atrial septal defect occluder or an arial flow regulator) to unload the right ventricle and to improve the filling of the left ventricle and cardiac output, (b) performance of a Potts shunt (anastomosis of the descending aorta to the left pulmonary artery) to allow right-to-left shunting of blood for decompressing the hypertensive right ventricle and increasing systemic flow (hence also referred to as a 'reverse' Potts shunt), and (c) stenting of the arterial duct if still patent. Mechanical circulatory support may be required to for patients who deteriorate during infection or due to other reversible conditions. Lung transplantation is indicated in children with severe pulmonary hypertension refractory to all of the treatment modalities.

Table 35.6 Medical therapies for idiopathic pulmonary arterial hypertension

Medication	Pharmacology
Phosphodiesterase type 5 inhibitors	
Sildenafil	Route: Oral Mechanism: Reduces the breakdown of cyclic GMP to cause pulmonary vasodilation and may inhibit vascular remodelling Side effects: Headache, flushing, diarrhoea, dyspepsia, epistaxis, priapism
Tadalafil	Route: Oral, longer acting With limited paediatric data
Endothelin receptor antagonists	
Bosentan	Route: Oral Mechanism: Blocks the vasoconstrictive and mitogenic actions of endothelin-1 Side effects: Headache, flushing, nasal congestion, abdominal pain, swelling of extremities, increased liver enzymes
Ambrisentan	Limited paediatric data
Macitentan	Limited paediatric data
Prostacyclin analogues	
Iloprost	Route: Inhaled with the use of a nebulizer Mechanism: Prostacyclin analogue that increases intracellular cyclic AMP and phosphorylation of other proteins to cause vasodilation and inhibits smooth muscle cell proliferation, inflammation, and platelet aggregation Side effects: Headache, dizziness, flushing, cough, wheeze, chest discomfort, throat irritation, jaw pain, diarrhoea
Selexipag	Route: Oral Mechanism: Non-prostanoid prostacyclin receptor agonist Limited paediatric data
Epoprostenol	Route: Continuous intravenous infusion Mechanism: Prostacyclin analogue as described above Side effects: Headache, dizziness, flushing, cough, wheeze, chest discomfort, throat irritation, jaw pain, nausea, diarrhoea, hypotension, complications related to central venous catheter Limited paediatric data on long-term use, usually for short-term use to stabilize critically ill patients
Treprostinil	Route: Oral, subcutaneous, intravenous, inhaled Mechanism and side effects as described above Limited paediatric data

35.9 Management Strategy for Severe Pulmonary Arterial Hypertension in Patients with Congenital Shunt Lesions

Acute vasoreactivity testing should be performed in patients with shunt lesions (ventricular and atrial septal defects, atrioventricular septal defect, persistent arterial duct, aortopulmonary windows) exhibiting evidence of pulmonary hypertension and increased pulmonary vascular resistance (especially in older patients and those with associated syndromic disorders) to distinguish between reversible pulmonary hypertension, which suggests potential operability, and irreversible pulmonary hypertension that contraindicates surgical repair (Table 35.7).

Table 35.7 Assessment of operability congenital shunt lesions with increased pulmonary vascular resistance

Pulmonary vascular resistance index (Wood units•m^2)	Operability
<4	Yes
4–8	Individual patient evaluation in tertiary centres (the grey zone usually lies between 6 to 8 WU•m^2)
>8	No

In the grey zone with a pulmonary vascular resistance index 6 to 8 Wood units•m^2, a treat-and-repair approach is commonly adopted. The treatment is usually single or dual oral pulmonary vasodilator therapy. In patients with pulmonary vascular resistance index >8 Wood units•m^2, the result of a second acute pulmonary vasoreactivity testing after a trial of oral pulmonary vasodilator therapy would inform whether surgical repair is an option (Fig. 35.4).

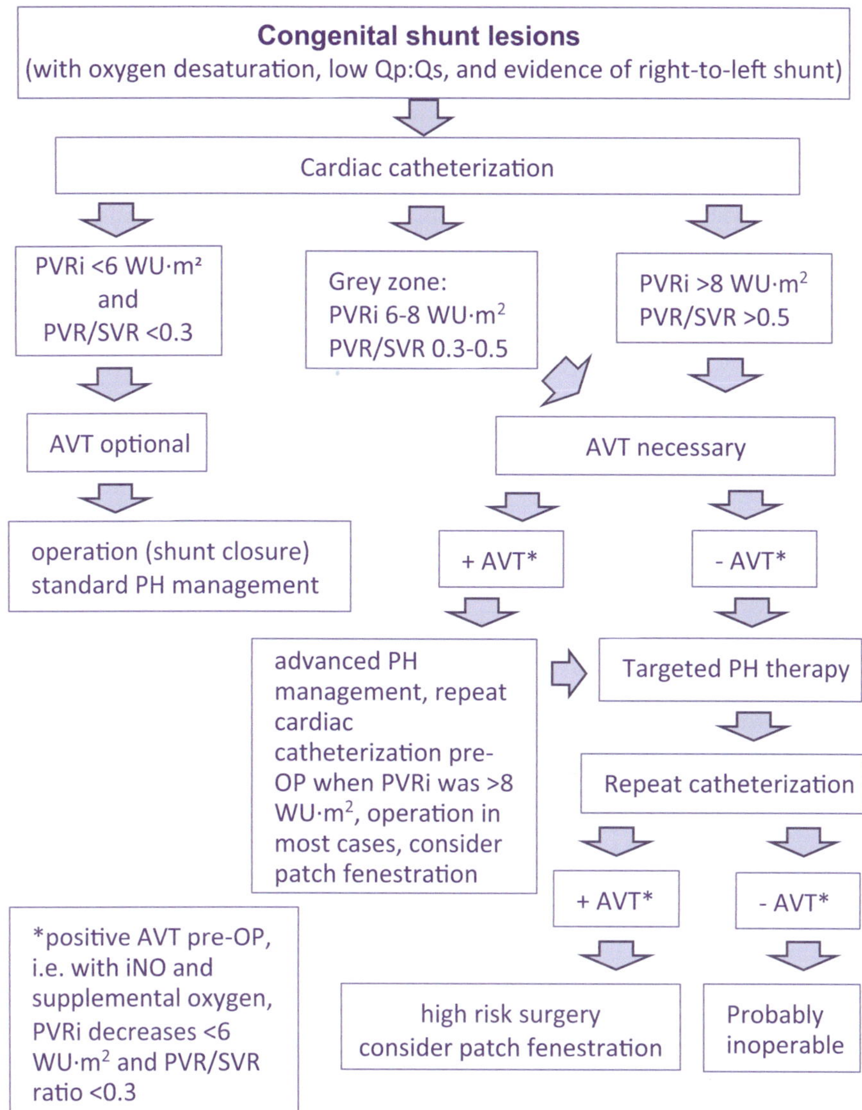

Fig. 35.4 Management of patients with congenital shunt lesions and pulmonary hypertension (Adapted from Hansmann et al. J Heart Lung Transplant 2019;38:879–901). Abbreviations: *AVT* acute vasoreactivity testing, *iNO* inhale nitric oxide, *OP* operation, *PH* pulmonary hypertension, *PVR* pulmonary vascular resistance, *PVRi* pulmonary vascular resistance index, *SVR* systemic vascular resistance

35.10 Long-Term Monitoring

The estimated five-year survival for children with idiopathic, hereditary, congenital heart disease-related pulmonary arterial hypertension is about 60–75%. Monitoring of growth, exercise capacity, symptoms and signs of right heart failure, echocardiographic assessment of pulmonary arterial pressure, right and left ventricular function, six-minute walk testing, and brain natriuretic peptide (or N-terminal pro-brain natriuretic peptide) level is required during follow up. Repeat cardiac catheterization is indicated for assessment of response to medical therapy or when clinical deterioration is evident.

Pulmonary Arteriovenous Malformations 36

Pulmonary arteriovenous malformations are abnormal blood vessels that bypass the pulmonary capillaries to allow direct communications between the pulmonary arterial and venous circulation.

36.1 Aetiology

36.1.1 Hereditary Haemorrhagic Telangiectasia

Most of the pulmonary arteriovenous malformations (80–95%) are associated with hereditary haemorrhagic telangiectasia (HHT) (Box 36.1) inherited as an autosomal dominant trait, while the remaining are sporadic in occurrence. The second International Guideline on HHT (2020) recommends its diagnosis to be based on the Curacao criteria and/or identification of the pathogenic variant in one of the HHT genes.

Box 36.1 Diagnosis of Hereditary Haemorrhagic Telangiectasia

Curacao Criteria

- Spontaneous and recurrent epistaxis
- Multiple mucocutaneous telangiectasia (characteristically over the lips, oral mucosa and fingertips)
- Involvement of other viscera (gastrointestinal telangiectasia, cerebral, pulmonary and hepatic arteriovenous malformations)
- A first degree relative with HHT
  (3–4 criteria: definite HHT, 2 criteria: suspected HHT)

Y.-f. Cheung, *Congenital and Paediatric Acquired Heart Disease in Practice*, https://doi.org/10.1007/978-981-99-2862-0_36

Major HHT Genes

- *ENG* (protein product is endoglin)
- *ALK1 (ACVRL1)* (protein product is activin receptor-like kinase 1)
- *SMAD4* (protein product is a member of the SMAD family of signal transduction proteins and its pathogenic variant is associated with both HHT and juvenile polyposis syndrome)

36.1.2 Hepatopulmonary Syndrome

Hepatopulmonary syndrome is associated with portal hypertension due to chronic liver disease or cirrhosis. Dilation of the pulmonary capillaries in hepatopulmonary syndrome results in rapid passage of blood through the pulmonary vasculature without adequate gaseous exchange, which results in ventilation-perfusion mismatch and hypoxaemia.

While the exact mechanism is unclear, dilation of the pulmonary vasculature is thought to be caused by an imbalance between pulmonary vasodilators and vasoconstrictors. Prominent pulmonary vasodilation at the lung base explains the features of platypnoea and orthodeoxia (dyspnoea and oxygen desaturation respectively occurring when changing from the recumbent position to sitting or standing), which may be present in adolescents and adults. Liver transplantation is the only therapeutic option.

36.1.3 Post Bidirectional Glenn Shunt

Pulmonary arteriovenous malformations may develop after Kawashima procedure in patients with left atrial isomerism (Chap. 20) and after bidirectional Glenn shunt (superior cavopulmonary connection) as a staged repair for functional univentricular hearts (Chap. 19) due to the lack of supply of 'hepatic factors' (nature remains unknown) to the pulmonary circulation. Completion of the Fontan circuit with inclusion of the hepatic venous return to the pulmonary arteries usually leads to regression of pulmonary arteriovenous malformations in both lungs (unless the flow is directed preferentially to one lung).

36.2 Anatomy

Pulmonary arteriovenous malformations may appear as a single vascular sac, a multi-lobated vascular sac, enlarged tortuous vessels, or a plexiform of dilated vessels. They are classified into two types: (a) simple pulmonary arteriovenous malformations being supplied by a single artery, and (b) complex pulmonary arteriovenous malformations being supplied by more than one artery.

36.3 Pathophysiology

Pulmonary vascular arteriovenous malformations are low resistance pathways that allow pulmonary arterial blood to bypass the pulmonary capillaries. These malformations allow right-to-left shunting of systemic venous blood to the systemic arterial circulation, impair gaseous exchange in the lungs, and reduce pulmonary filtration of microthrombi and bacteria. The consequences are systemic hypoxaemia, ventilation-perfusion mismatch, and paradoxical embolization with complications of stroke and formation of cerebral abscess.

Pulmonary hypertension can occur in patients with HHT via several mechanisms including high pulmonary arterial wedge pressure, a high flow state (especially in the presence of hepatic or gastrointestinal arteriovenous malformations), pulmonary vascular remodelling that increases pulmonary vascular resistance, and shared genetic mutations (Chap. 35).

36.4 Clinical Manifestations and Findings

The clinical manifestations depend on the size of the pulmonary arteriovenous malformations and the degree of right-to-left shunt. Most children with pulmonary arteriovenous malformations are asymptomatic, which may remain unrecognized until adulthood. Some children may present with incidental findings of mild cyanosis at rest with worsening of cyanosis during exercise and finger clubbing. It is uncommon for children to present with shortness of breath, platypnoea, or orthodeoxia. Less commonly, some may present with the complications of stroke and cerebral abscess, for which assessment of possible pulmonary arteriovenous malformations is required. Life-threatening complications including haemoptysis and haemothorax due to intra-bronchial rupture of pulmonary vascular arteriovenous malformations or endobronchial telangiectasia are unusual in children.

Physical signs include cyanosis, clubbing of fingers and mucocutaneous telangiectasia over the lips, oral mucosa and fingertips (although signs of HHT may not be obvious in young children). Occasionally, a soft systolic or continuous murmur due to superficially located pulmonary arteriovenous malformations is heard.

36.5 Investigations

CXR: Large pulmonary arteriovenous malformations may appear as round nodules on chest radiograph.

Transthoracic contrast echocardiography: Contrast echocardiography is imaging of choice for initial screening of possible pulmonary arteriovenous malformations. The diagnosis is suggested by echocardiographic visualization of microbubble contrast in the left atrium and left ventricle after intravenous administration of agitated saline. The appearance of microbubbles within three to four cardiac cycles suggests intrapulmonary shunting (as contrast to the appearance of microbubbles within two cardiac cycles in the presence of an intra-cardiac right-to-left shunt).

Imaging of pulmonary arteriovenous malformations: Computed tomography with 3D volume rendering enables the diagnosis of complex pulmonary arteriovenous malformations and facilitates transcatheter embolization of the malformations (Fig. 36.1).

Imaging of other arteriovenous malformations: Different imaging modalities are required for the imaging of arteriovenous malformations in the brain (MRI and digital subtraction angiography), spine (digital subtraction angiography) and liver (ultrasound, CT or MRI).

Genetic evaluation: Genetic testing assists in the diagnosis of HHT even in suspected cases by identification of pathogenic variants in *ENG*, *ALK1*, or *SMAD4*, provides information for counselling of the family, and informs the need for additional evaluation (e.g. performing colonoscopies in patients with pathogenic variants in *SMAD4*).

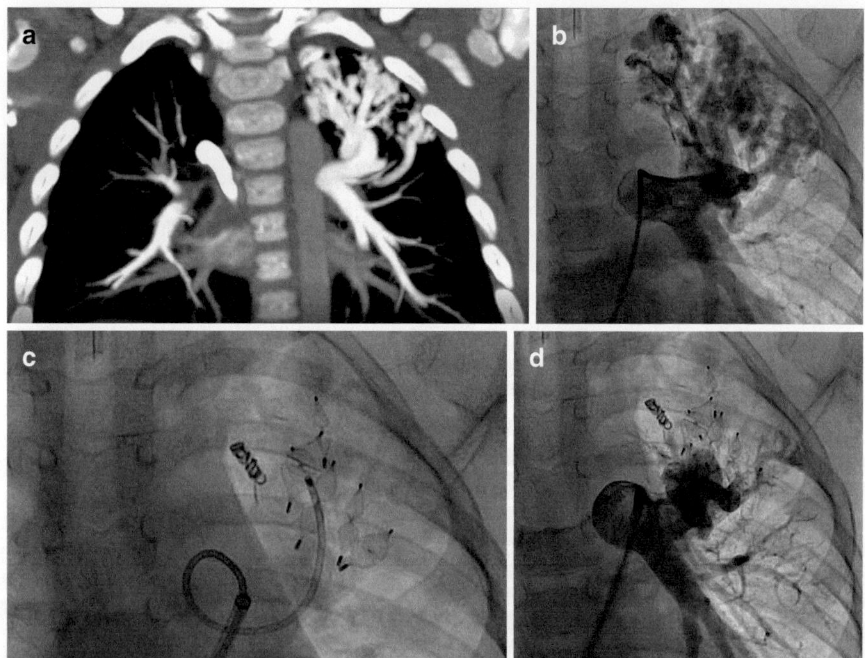

Fig. 36.1 Pulmonary arteriovenous malformations. (**a**) Computed tomography and (**b**) angiographic findings of complex arteriovenous malformations involving the left upper lobe (**c**) Transcatheter occlusion of the pulmonary arteriovenous malformations with coils and Amplatzer vascular plugs (**d**) Angiographic demonstration of occlusion of the large arteriovenous malformation after deployment of multiple coils and vascular plugs

36.6 Management Strategy

For pulmonary arteriovenous malformations <3 mm and without evidence of HHT, follow up by computed tomography every 1–5 years has been suggested. Definitive treatment should be provided in all patients with pulmonary arteriovenous malformations >3 mm regardless of symptoms for prevention of complications as described above.
Transcatheter intervention: Percutaneous transcatheter embolization of the pulmonary arteriovenous malformations is the treatment of choice. Coils and Amplatzer vascular plugs have been used for this purpose. The presence of pulmonary hypertension is, however, a relative contraindication.
Surgical intervention: Surgery is seldom performed nowadays as transcatheter intervention by device occlusion is usually feasible. Significant pulmonary haemorrhage may, however, require segmental lung resection, lobectomy, or rarely pneumonectomy.

36.7 Long-Term Monitoring

Recurrence of pulmonary arteriovenous malformations occurs in up to 20% of patients after device embolization due to recanalization of occluded vessels, collateralization of adjacent arteries, or opening of small vessels not tackled during intervention. Transthoracic contrast echocardiography is not useful after embolization due to its persistent positivity in about 90% of patients. Regular clinical assessment for oxygen desaturation at rest and during exercise with computed tomography imaging every 3–5 years are required for the monitoring of recurrence. Patients should be advised to receive antibiotic prophylaxis against bacterial endocarditis, to caution medical personnel against inadvertent intravenous administration of air bubbles, and to avoid scuba diving.

Part VII

Systemic and Pulmonary Venous Anomalies

Anomalous Pulmonary Venous Connection

37

Anomalous pulmonary venous connection refers to the condition when one or more of the pulmonary veins connect anomalously to sites other than the left atrium.

37.1 Total Anomalous Pulmonary Venous Connection

37.1.1 Anatomy

When all the pulmonary veins drain to sites other than the morphologic left atrium, this is described as total anomalous pulmonary venous connection (Fig. 37.1).

The four pulmonary veins usually join to form a pulmonary venous chamber, which then drains anomalously into either: (a) the innominate or superior caval vein via an ascending vertical vein (supracardiac type), (b) the right atrium directly or through the coronary sinus (cardiac type), or (c) the portal system or hepatic veins via a descending vertical vein (infracardiac type). Different pulmonary veins may also drain into different sites, a condition referred as mixed type of total anomalous pulmonary venous drainage.

Obstruction of the anomalous pulmonary venous pathway can be due to intrinsic stenosis, extrinsic compression (e.g. compression of the ascending vertical vein between the left pulmonary artery and left bronchus or between the right pulmonary artery and carina, or compression of the descending vertical vein as its passes through the diaphragm), or its emptying into a high resistance vasculature (e.g. drainage of the descending vein into the hepatic and portal circulation). Hence, obstruction of pulmonary venous return is more commonly encountered in infracardiac and supracardiac types but is unusual in cardiac type of anomalous pulmonary venous connection.

Y.-f. Cheung, *Congenital and Paediatric Acquired Heart Disease in Practice*, https://doi.org/10.1007/978-981-99-2862-0_37

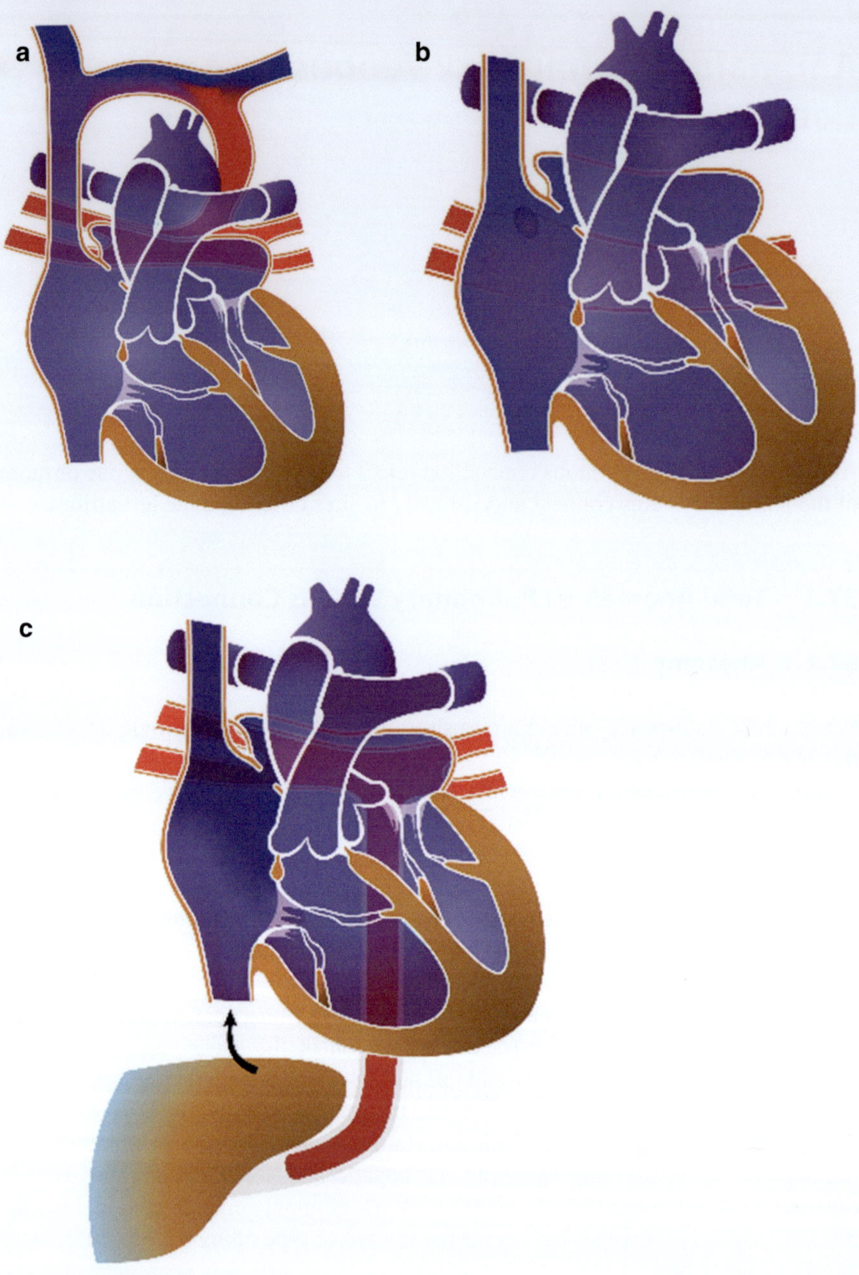

Fig. 37.1 Types of total anomalous pulmonary venous drainage. (**a**) Supracardiac type (**b**) Cardiac type (**c**) Infracardiac type

In total anomalous pulmonary venous connection, an interatrial communication exists to allow systemic venous blood to enter the left heart to maintain systemic circulation. Associated significant congenital abnormalities include right atrial isomerism (Chap. 20) and tetralogy of Fallot (Chap. 16).

37.1.2 Pathophysiology

Total anomalous pulmonary venous connection represents a common- mixing situation as the deoxygenated systemic venous blood mixes with the oxygenated pulmonary venous blood in the systemic veins or the right atrium. The right atrium and right ventricle are volume overloaded. Obligatory right-to-left shunting of blood occurs at the atrial level through either a patent oval foramen or an atrial septal defect. A small interatrial communication may therefore limit cardiac output.

The pathophysiology also depends on whether pulmonary venous obstruction is present or not. In the absence of pulmonary venous obstruction, the haemodynamics resemble those of a large atrial septal defect, with increased blood flow to the pulmonary circulation. When pulmonary venous obstruction is present, pulmonary venous hypertension leads to pulmonary oedema and lymphangiectasia, reflex pulmonary arteriolar constriction, secondary pulmonary arterial hypertension, and eventually right ventricular failure. Muscularization of the pulmonary venules and arterioles further contribute further to the increase in pulmonary vascular resistance.

37.1.3 Clinical Manifestations

In the absence of pulmonary venous obstruction, the cyanosis is mild and may be unnoticeable. Infants usually present with heart failure symptoms at 1–2 months of age. The signs are those of a large atrial septal defect and heart failure (Chap. 11).

In the presence of pulmonary venous obstruction, the patient presents early after birth with cyanosis and respiratory distress. The cardiac signs are subtle (Table 37.1).

Table 37.1 Signs of unobstructed and obstructed total anomalous pulmonary venous connection (TAPVC)

	TAPVC without pulmonary venous obstruction	TAPVC with pulmonary venous obstruction
Cyanosis	Mild	Moderate to severe
Respiratory distress	+ (increased pulmonary flow)	++ (pulmonary venous congestion and pulmonary oedema)
RV impulse	++	++
Wide splitting of S2	+	Not obvious
Increased P2	+	+
Murmur	A soft ejection systolic murmur at the left upper sternal border due to high pulmonary flow	–

This is one of the few congenital heart defects that present in the neonatal period with features mimicking those of pulmonary parenchymal disease (respiratory distress, cyanosis, hazy lung fields, and absence of cardiomegaly) or mistaken for persistent pulmonary hypertension of the newborn. Hence, obstructed total anomalous pulmonary venous return must be excluded in neonates with presumed pneumonia or persistent pulmonary hypertension but not responding to conventional therapy.

37.1.4 Investigations

CXR: (a) In the absence of pulmonary venous obstruction, the radiographic appearance is similar to that of a large atrial septal defect with cardiomegaly, increased convexity of the right cardiac border, prominent main pulmonary artery, and increased pulmonary vascular markings. In supracardiac total anomalous pulmonary venous connection, the dilated ascending vertical vein and superior caval vein forms the 'head' of the so-called 'snowman appearance' in the chest radiograph. (b) In the presence of pulmonary venous obstruction, the lung fields have a ground-glass appearance, with the pulmonary vascular markings having a reticular pattern and radiating from the hilar regions. The cardiac size, on the other hand, is usually normal.

ECG: The electrocardiogram shows right atrial and right ventricular dilation.

Echocardiography: The echocardiographic findings of volume-overloaded right atrium and right ventricles with pure right-to-left shunting at the atrial level provide important clues to diagnosing total anomalous pulmonary venous connection. Further echocardiographic evaluation enables the demonstration of the absence of normal pulmonary venous return to the left atrium, delineation of the site(s) of anomalous drainage, and definition of presence and aetiology or absence of pulmonary venous obstruction (Fig. 37.2a–c). The pulmonary arterial pressure should further be estimated and associated cardiac malformations should be defined.

CT: Computed tomography angiography is required if echocardiography cannot clearly define the pulmonary venous anatomy (Fig. 37.2d), especially when mixed anomalous pulmonary venous connection is suspected.

Fig. 37.2 Echocardiographic and CT assessment of total anomalous pulmonary venous drainage. (**a**) Echocardiographic demonstration of a pulmonary venous chamber with no connection to the left atrium (**b**) Supracardiac pulmonary venous drainage to the innominate vein via the ascending vein (**c**) Infracardiac pulmonary venous drainage to the hepatic vein via the descending vein (**d**) CT angiographic illustration of the descending vein (Abbreviations: *IVC* inferior caval vein, *LA* left atrium, *PV* pulmonary venous, *RA* right atrium, *SVC* superior caval vein)

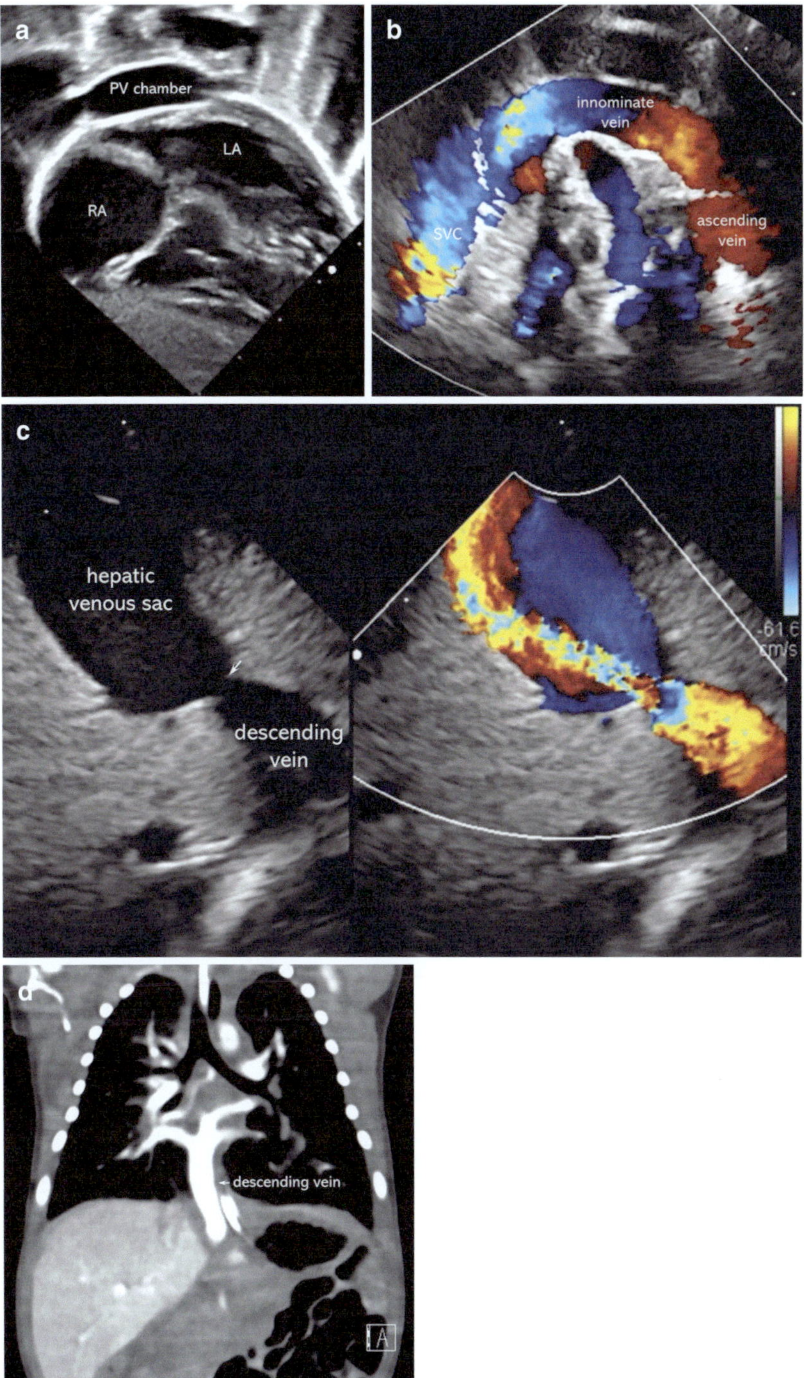
a
PV chamber
LA
RA
b
innominate vein
SVC
ascending vein
c
hepatic venous sac
descending vein
d
descending vein

37.1.5 Management

Stabilization: Critically ill neonates with severe pulmonary venous obstructive requires stabilization with intubation and ventilatory support, inotropic support, and correction of metabolic acidosis. Prostaglandin E is a double-edged sword. Enlargement of the arterial duct in the presence of left-to-right ductal shunt may worsen pulmonary oedema, while in the presence of right-to-left ductal shunt in neonates with high pulmonary vascular resistance, prostaglandin may provide temporary relief of the pulmonary venous congestion. Infants with non-obstructed pulmonary venous connection and heart failure are treated with diuretics.
Timing of surgery: Emergency surgical repair is indicated in neonates with obstructed total anomalous pulmonary venous connection. In patients with unobstructed total anomalous venous drainage, with diagnosis usually made beyond the neonatal period, surgery is commonly performed semi-electively at 3–6 months of age.
Surgery repair: For cardiac types of total anomalous pulmonary venous connection, surgical correction is performed by unroofing of the coronary sinus or diverting the pulmonary venous blood from the right atrium to the left atrium using a baffle depending on the site of drainage.

For supracardiac and infracardiac types of total anomalous pulmonary venous connection, surgery involves the anastomosis of the incision made in pulmonary venous confluence to the corresponding incision in the left atrium. Increasingly, the sutureless technique, introduced originally for postsurgical pulmonary venous stenosis, is adopted for use in primary repair. This involves direct suturing of the left atrium to the pericardium around the divided pulmonary venous confluence, thus avoiding direct trauma to pulmonary venous tissue. This technique may be associated with a lower rate of pulmonary venous stenosis post operation.

The vertical vein is usually ligated at the time of surgery. While some may argue that an unligated vertical vein may provide temporary decompression of the pulmonary venous pathways to prevent early postoperative compromise of cardiac output related to poor compliance of left atrium and left ventricle, the unloading function of the patent vertical vein is debatable. In the long term, the unligated vertical vein may constitute a sizable left-to-right shunt and requires surgical ligation or transcatheter device closure. The patent oval foramen or the atrial septal defect is closed at surgery.

37.1.6 Postoperative Considerations

Important postoperative complications in neonates with obstructed total anomalous pulmonary venous connection include pulmonary hypertensive crisis, low cardiac output syndrome, and supraventricular tachyarrhythmias.

Structural alteration with muscularization of the pulmonary arterioles and venules increases reactivity of the pulmonary vasculature and predisposes to development of pulmonary hypertensive crisis postoperatively. These crises usually subside within few days after surgery. There are situations, however, in which pulmonary hypertension and hypertensive crisis are refractory to treatment. These patients are often found to have diffuse hypoplasia of the pulmonary veins found at surgery or by postoperative imaging and/or lymphangiectasia confirmed by lung biopsy.

The left ventricle is poorly compliant and relatively small given the chronic volume unloading before surgery. Judicious fluid replacement is necessary to avoid significant increase in left atrial pressure (which can lead to pulmonary oedema and aggravate pulmonary hypertension) but, on the other hand, is required to maintain systemic cardiac output. Afterload reduction may be beneficial.

The postoperative course of infants with non-obstructed pulmonary venous connection is usually uneventful.

37.1.7 Long-Term Monitoring

Regular monitoring for development of pulmonary venous stenosis, usually detectable by echocardiography within 6 months of surgery, is required. The stenosis can be due to progressive constriction at the anastomotic site or, less commonly, related to intrinsic abnormalities of the pulmonary veins (Chap. 38). Computed tomography and magnetic resonance imaging are used to confirm the diagnosis and to plan subsequent surgical (sutureless repair for those who had conventional surgery) or transcatheter interventions (balloon angioplasty and/or stent implantation).

37.2 Partial Anomalous Pulmonary Venous Connection

37.2.1 Anatomy

Partial anomalous pulmonary venous connection occurs when one or more of the pulmonary veins connect to the systemic vein or right atrium while the others drain normally into the left atrium. This can occur in isolation or in association with sinus venosus atrial septal defect (Chap. 11) or scimitar syndrome.

37.2.1.1 Scimitar Syndrome

Scimitar syndrome is an association of congenital cardiac and pulmonary anomalies. It comprises (a) anomalous drainage of one or all of the right pulmonary veins into the upper part of the inferior caval vein, (b) hypoplasia of the right lung with or without pulmonary sequestration, and (c) systemic arterial supply from the descending aorta to the right lung (usually the right lower lobe).

The term ‘scimitar’ (a sword with a curve blade) describes the shape of the anomalous right pulmonary vein as it drains acutely into the inferior caval vein. The scimitar vein drains usually the right lower lobe, sometimes also the middle lobe, and less commonly the entire right lung. It may be stenotic and run a supra- or infra-diaphragmatic course.

Associated cardiac anomalies include commonly an atrial septal defect and, less commonly, other congenital cardiac anomalies (e.g. tetralogy of Fallot, ventricular septal defect, coarctation of the aorta, hypoplastic left heart syndrome).

37.2.2 Pathophysiology

The haemodynamic consequences of partial anomalous pulmonary venous connection are those of a left-to-right interatrial shunt. The right atrium and right ventricle are volume overloaded. However, when only one of the pulmonary veins is draining anomalously, there may be no significant haemodynamic disturbance. Pulmonary hypertension is unusual except in patients with scimitar syndrome.

37.2.3 Clinical Manifestations

The clinical presentation and findings are similar to those of an atrial septal defect. Patients are usually asymptomatic. The physical signs are those of an atrial septum defect although the wide splitting of the second heart sound may vary with respiration. Infants and children with scimitar syndrome may, on the other hand, present with symptoms of heart failure (due to aortopulmonary collaterals), recurrent pneumonia, haemoptysis, and signs of pulmonary hypertension.

37.2.4 Investigations

CXR: The radiographic appearance is similar to that of a large atrial septal defect with cardiomegaly. In scimitar syndrome, the scimitar vein may be seen and the chest radiograph shows hypoplasia of the right lung and secondary dextrocardia.
ECG: Electrocardiographic findings are similar to those found in atrial septal defect and include right axis deviation and right atrial and right ventricular dilation. With volume overloading of the right ventricle, an incomplete right bundle branch block (rsR') pattern in lead V1 is commonly observed.
Echocardiography: Important clues to the possibility of partial anomalous pulmonary venous connection include (a) findings of volume-overloaded right atrium and right ventricle, especially in the absence of an associated atrial septal defect, (b) increased flow in superior or inferior caval vein, and (c) the presence of associated cardiac or pulmonary anomalies (e.g. sinus venosus atrial septal defect, hypoplasia of the right lung). Further echocardiographic evaluation should aim to delineate the anomalous drainage. In infants with scimitar syndrome, the pulmonary arterial pressure should be estimated and associated cardiac malformations should be defined.
CT and cardiac catheterization: These may be required if echocardiography cannot clearly define the pulmonary venous anatomy. These modalities are useful for defining the pulmonary venous and arterial anatomy and aortopulmonary collaterals

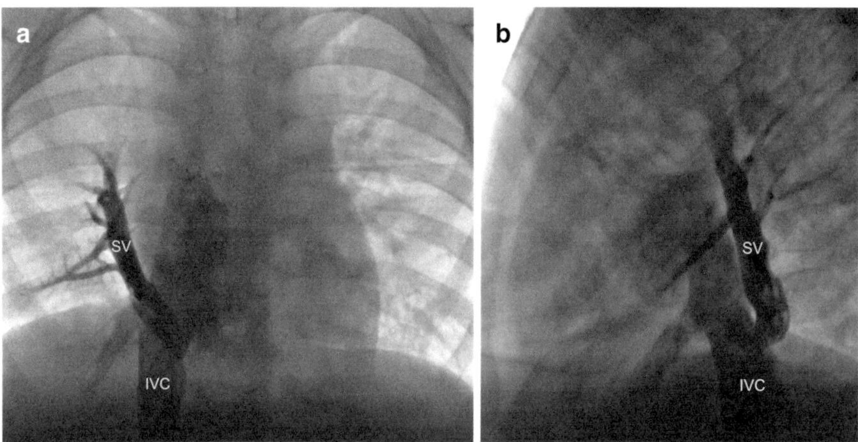

Fig. 37.3 Scimitar syndrome. (**a**) Anteroposterior and (**b**) lateral projection of the angiographic illustration of the partial anomalous drainage of the right pulmonary vein (scimitar vein) into the inferior caval vein (Abbreviations: *IVC* inferior caval vein, *SV* scimitar vein)

(Fig. 37.3). Pulmonary venous anomalies can also be defined by CT in infants with scimitar syndrome.

37.2.5 Management

Surgery repair: Repair of partial anomalous pulmonary venous connection can be performed on an elective basis. Repair of partial anomalous right-sided pulmonary venous connection in association with a sinus venosus septal defect involves patch closure of the defect with redirection of the anomalous pulmonary venous flow into the left atrium (Chap. 13). For partial anomalous left-sided pulmonary venous connection into a vertical vein, the vertical vein can be anastomosed to the left atrium. **Management of scimitar syndrome:** In patients with scimitar syndrome, the anomalous right pulmonary vein can be anastomosed directly or with the use of an interposition graft to the left atrium or baffled to the left atrium through an atrial septal defect. Device embolization of the aortopulmonary collaterals may be required to reduce the left-to-right shunt and pulmonary hypertension. Rarely, lobectomy or right pneumectomy is considered when there is severe right pulmonary hypoplasia with recurrent chest infection and haemoptysis.

37.2.6 Postoperative Considerations

The postoperative course of most of the patients with partial pulmonary venous connection is usually uneventful. In infants with scimitar syndrome, postoperative complications include pulmonary hypertensive crisis and pneumonia.

37.2.7 Long-Term Monitoring

Regular monitoring for development of pulmonary venous stenosis is required.

Pulmonary Vein Stenosis

38

Pulmonary vein stenosis is a rare and devastating disease that occurs in infants and children with heterogeneous associated conditions. There are significant challenges in its management given an unknown aetiology, the progressive nature, and suboptimal treatment outcomes.

38.1 Classification

Pulmonary vein stenosis is classified as primary or acquired. In children, pulmonary vein stenosis is usually acquired after previous repair of total anomalous pulmonary venous connection (Chap. 37) with or without associated heterotaxy syndrome (Chap. 20). Primary pulmonary vein stenosis occurs in the absence of previous interventions of the pulmonary veins and is associated with syndromic disorders, developmental conditions, and haemodynamic perturbation (Box 38.1).

Box 38.1 Conditions Associated with Primary Pulmonary Vein Stenosis

Syndromic Disorders

- Down syndrome.
- DiGeorge syndrome.
- Smith–Lemli–Opitz.
- VACTERYL association.

Developmental Conditions

- Bronchopulmonary dysplasia.
- Fetal growth restriction and twinning.
- Prematurity and related issues (bronchopulmonary dysplasia, necrotizing enterocolitis).

Y.-f. Cheung, *Congenital and Paediatric Acquired Heart Disease in Practice*,
https://doi.org/10.1007/978-981-99-2862-0_38

Haemodynamic Perturbation

- Congenital heart disease with left-to-right shunts.
- Angulation of pulmonary veins.
- Cardiomegaly causing displacement and compression of left pulmonary veins in functional single ventricle.
- Gross atrial dilation in atriopulmonary connection causing compression of right pulmonary veins in Fontan patients.

38.2 Pathology and Pathophysiology

Grossly, the stenosis may involve one or multiple pulmonary veins, may occur on one side (more common on the left) or both sides, and may be focal, diffuse or completely atretic. The pathologic findings in primary pulmonary vein stenosis are characterized by neointimal obstructive lesions. These lesions consist of myofibroblast-like cells and extracellular matrix, with characteristic paucity of inflammatory cells, and are progressive in nature. Progression of the neointimal lesions has been hypothesized to resemble a neoplastic-like process with altered cellular signalling involving the transforming growth factor-beta and mammalian target of rapamycin (mTOR) pathways.

Progressive obstruction of the pulmonary venous lumen, either as a local stenosis at where the pulmonary veins join the left atrium or diffuse involvement of the pulmonary veins with extension to those in the pulmonary parenchyma, leads to severe pulmonary hypertension, right ventricular failure, and death.

38.3 Clinical Presentation and Findings

In patients with previous repair of total anomalous pulmonary venous connection, pulmonary vein stenosis is diagnosed by echocardiographic assessment on follow up or based on clinical symptoms and signs of progressive respiratory distress.

Infants with primary pulmonary vein stenosis present usually with shortness of breath. The initial clinical diagnoses may be pneumonia or interstitial lung disease. Signs of respiratory distress and pulmonary hypertension with right ventricular impulse and increased intensity of the pulmonary heart sound may be found.

Infants born premature and with bronchopulmonary dysplasia may present with increasing respiratory distress, need for supplemental oxygen and respiratory support, lung haziness on chest radiograph, and evidence of worsening pulmonary hypertension.

38.4 Diagnosis

Initial investigations are usually initially directed to unravel the cause of respiratory symptoms and signs in neonates and infants.
CXR: The lung fields appear diffusely hazy with or without pulmonary oedema. The cardiac size is usually normal.
ECG: The electrocardiogram shows right atrial and right ventricular dilation.
Echocardiography: Echocardiography shows turbulent flow into the left atrium originating from one or more of the stenosed pulmonary veins, pulmonary hypertension, right ventricular dysfunction, and associated congenital cardiac malformations. Different criteria for diagnosing pulmonary vein stenosis based on Doppler echocardiography have been used. These include flow velocities >1.5–1.6 m/s or a mean pressure gradient of ≥3 mmHg, 4 mmHg, or 5 mmHg. Mean gradients of 5–7 mmHg and >7 mmHg have been used to define respectively moderate and severe pulmonary vein stenosis.
CT: Computed tomography angiography defines the pulmonary veins involved, severity of localized stenosis, and the diffuse nature with upstream involvement of pulmonary vein in the lung parenchyma (Fig. 38.1). It also provides road mapping for catheter and surgical interventions.

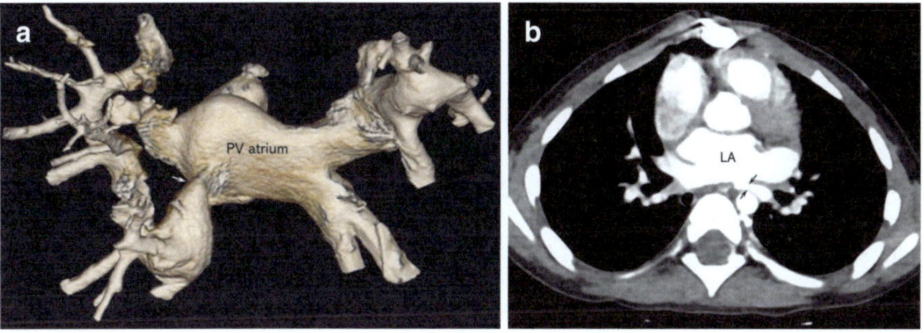

Fig. 38.1 Computed tomographic assessment of pulmonary vein stenosis. (**a**) Stenosis of the left pulmonary vein (white arrow) after Fontan procedure in a patient with left atrial isomerism and double-outlet right ventricle (**b**) Stenosis of the left lower pulmonary vein (black arrows) after repair of mixed total anomalous pulmonary venous connection (Abbreviation: *LA* left atrium, *PV* pulmonary venous)

38.5 Management Strategy

Management of this rare and devastating condition requires a multidisciplinary team with expertise in cardiac imaging, transcatheter intervention, paediatric cardiac surgery, pulmonary hypertension management, paediatric oncology, neonatology, and nutritional care.

Medical therapy: Diuretics may improve pulmonary venous congestion. Inotropic support is required in patients with right ventricular failure. To target at the altered cellular signalling, vinblastine, methotrexate, imatinib, bevacizumab, losartan, and sirolimus have been used with, however, inconclusive results. The use of pulmonary vasodilators is controversial due to the possibility of worsening pulmonary oedema in the presence of pulmonary venous obstruction.

Transcatheter intervention: Transcatheter procedures are indicated in patients with severe pulmonary vein stenosis that cause severe respiratory distress, pulmonary hypertension, and right ventricular dysfunction. The procedures require transseptal puncture and include balloon angioplasty with conventional and/or cutting balloon and metal or drug-eluted stent implantation.

Surgical intervention: The best result is obtained with the use of the sutureless technique for postsurgical pulmonary venous stenosis. However, with upstream pulmonary vein stenosis, the surgical outcomes are usually poor. Lung or heart-lung transplantation is an option for patients with severe pulmonary vein stenosis refractory to other treatments.

38.6 Long-Term Monitoring

Proactive surveillance with clinical assessment and imaging for early detection of recurrence or progression of pulmonary vein stenosis and timely reinterventions is necessary to improve the dismal outcomes. Reported survival of children with primary pulmonary vein stenosis despite active treatment remains disappointing at about 50–60% at 1–2 years of follow up. Collaborative effort, as the PVS network registry, is required to advance the clinical management and care of these patients and facilitate development of evidence-based management guidelines.

39 Anomalous Systemic Venous Return

Anomalous systemic venous return may occur in isolation or in association with congenital cardiac malformations. While many of these systemic venous anomalies are regarded as normal anatomic variants, some have clinical importance, and a few may have haemodynamic consequence. The commonly encountered anomalies involving the superior and inferior caval venous return are described.

39.1 Left Superior Caval Vein

39.1.1 Anatomy

Persistence of the left superior caval vein is the most common congenital anomaly of the systemic venous return. Among individuals with persistence of the left superior caval vein, 90% have bilateral superior caval veins with or without a bridging vein (left brachiocephalic vein) between the right and left superior caval veins.

The left superior caval vein usually drains into the right atrium (80–90%) through a dilated coronary sinus with no haemodynamic significance. In 10–20% of cases, the left superior caval vein drains into the left atrium directly or indirectly via the left pulmonary veins or the unroofed coronary sinus causing a small right-to-left shunt.

Associated congenital cardiac malformations include left-to-right shunts, conotruncal malformations, heterotaxy syndrome, coronary sinus ostial atresia, left-sided obstructive lesions (cortriatriatum, mitral stenosis, bicuspid aortic valve, and coarctation of the aorta) and right-sided aortic arch.

Y.-f. Cheung, *Congenital and Paediatric Acquired Heart Disease in Practice*, https://doi.org/10.1007/978-981-99-2862-0_39

39.1.2 Diagnosis

Isolated persistence of left superior caval vein is asymptomatic. This anomaly is usually detected incidentally as part of the echocardiographic assessment of associated congenital cardiac malformations or found during cardiac surgery.

On echocardiographic evaluation, the finding of a dilated coronary sinus should prompt further assessment of an associated persistent left superior caval vein and a bridging vein. Saline contrast echocardiography with intravenous administration of agitated saline through a vein in the left upper limb demonstrates right-to-left shunt if the left superior caval vein drains into the left atrium. Other diagnostic imaging modalities include computed tomography, magnetic resonance imaging, and catheter angiography (Fig. 39.1).

39.1.3 Clinical Implications

Persistence of the left superior caval vein, although usually haemodynamically insignificant, has the following clinical implications: (a) placement of central venous and Swan-Ganz catheters, (b) implantation of pacemaker and implantable cardioverter defibrillator, (c) catheter manipulation during diagnostic and interventional cardiac catheterization (especially in the presence of coronary sinus ostial stenosis), (d) surgical interventions involving the superior caval vein (Glenn shunt, Fontan operation, heart transplantation), (e) predisposition to cardiac arrhythmias

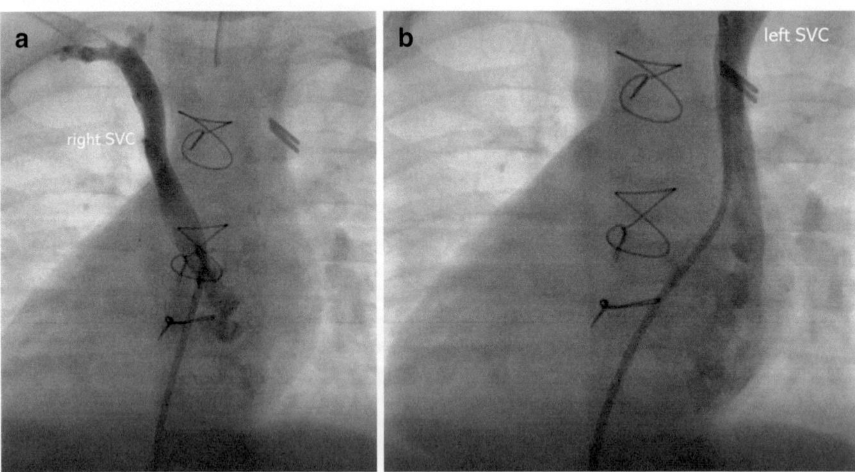

Fig. 39.1 Bilateral superior caval veins in right atrial isomerism. (**a**) Right superior caval vein draining into the right side of the common atrium (**b**) Left superior caval vein draining into the left side of the common atrium (Abbreviation: *SVC* superior caval vein)

(due to the dilated coronary sinus), and (f) rarely significant cyanosis and thromboembolism due to significant right-to-left shunt in the presence of an unroofed coronary sinus.

39.2 Interruption of Inferior Caval Vein with Azygous Continuation

Absence of the infra-hepatic portion of the inferior caval vein, commonly referred to as interruption of the inferior caval vein, is the most common congenital anomaly of the inferior caval vein. Blood from the lower part of the body is drained into either the right or the left superior caval vein by way of the azygous venous system. On the other hand, blood from the hepatic veins and the splanchnic circulation drains into the right atrium.

This congenital anomaly of the inferior caval vein occurs most commonly in the setting of left atrial isomerism, although it can also occur as an isolated anomaly. The management of left isomerism with interruption of inferior caval vein with azygous continuation and functional univentricular heart by Kawashima procedure and the need to include hepatic venous return to complete the Fontan circuit is discussed in Chap. 20.

Part VIII

Coronary Arterial Anomalies

Coronary Arterial Fistulas

40

Although rare, coronary arterial fistulas are the most common coronary arterial anomalies in children. These fistulas represent abnormal communications between the coronary arteries and the cardiac chambers or blood vessels. While most of the coronary arterial fistulas in children are congenital in origin, some fistulas may be acquired after congenital heart surgery or myocardial biopsy.

40.1 Anatomy

Congenital coronary arterial fistulas usually originate from one of the two main coronary arteries, occasionally from the coronary branches, and can drain into any of the cardiac chambers, pulmonary artery, pulmonary vein, coronary sinus, or superior caval vein (Fig. 40.1). Most of the fistulas originate from the right coronary artery, followed by the left anterior descending and left circumflex arteries, and occasionally from both coronary arteries.

Drainage of coronary fistulas into the right-sided structures (right ventricle, right atrium, and pulmonary artery, and less commonly superior caval vein and coronary sinus) is more common than drainage into the left-sided structures. The feeding artery of the fistula is usually dilated and tortuous.

Coronary artery fistulas are also found in pulmonary atresia with an intact ventricular septum in association with severe hypoplasia of the right ventricle. These right ventriculo-coronary sinusoidal communications differ from isolated congenital coronary arterial fistula in terms of the pathophysiologic significance and management (Chap. 16). Coronary arterial fistulas may also occur in association with atrial septal defect, ventricular septal defect, persistent arterial duct, and tetralogy of Fallot.

Y.-f. Cheung, *Congenital and Paediatric Acquired Heart Disease in Practice*, https://doi.org/10.1007/978-981-99-2862-0_40

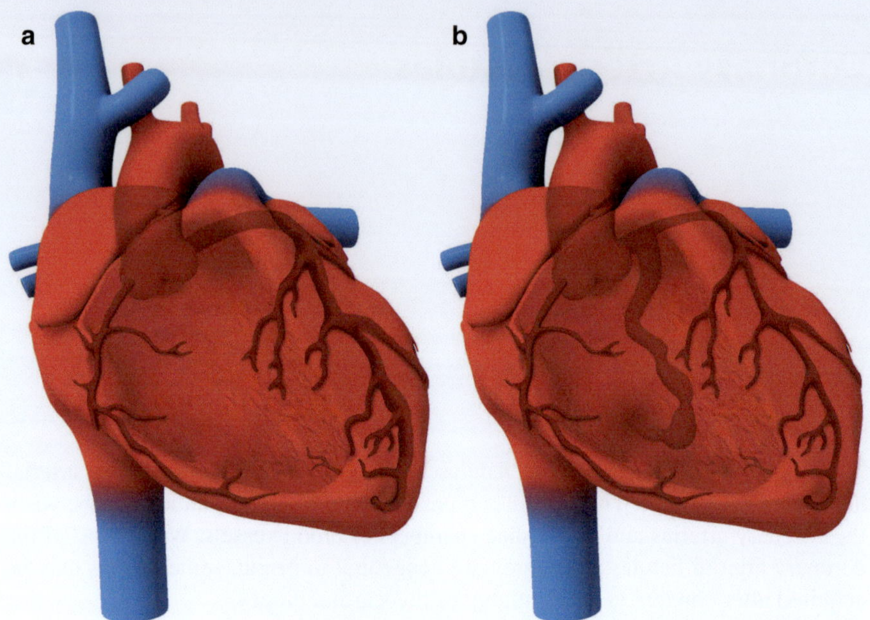

Fig. 40.1 Types of coronary arterial fistulas. (**a**) A distal fistula arising from the distal end of the left anterior descending artery with dilation of the left main coronary artery and proximal anterior descending artery (**b**) A proximal fistula arising from the left main coronary artery

40.2 Pathophysiology

The pressure gradient between the aorta and the cardiac chamber or blood vessel, in which the fistula empties into, drives blood to flow continuously through fistula throughout the cardiac cycle. Depending on the site of drainage, the fistula may constitute a left-to-right, which is more common, or a left-to-left shunt. The magnitude of the shunt is determined by the pressure gradient and the size of the fistula.

A large coronary arterial fistula that empties into a right-sided structure constitutes a large left-to-right shunt and leads to dilation of the right heart structures, increased pulmonary arterial flow and rarely pulmonary hypertension, and volume overloading of the left ventricle. If the fistula empties into the pulmonary artery, the pathophysiology mimics that of a large persistent arterial duct. If a large fistula empties into the left atrium or pulmonary vein, the left-to-left shunt causes volume overloading of the left heart. High cardiac output failure may occur with either type of fistulas.

Coronary arterial perfusion distal to the fistula may be diminished as the fistula offers a low resistance pathway for blood to bypass the high resistance arterioles and capillaries in the myocardium. The coronary steal phenomenon may lead to myocardial ischaemia during exertion as myocardial oxygen consumption increases.

40.3 Clinical Presentation and Findings

Most children with coronary arterial fistulas, even moderate-sized or large ones, are asymptomatic. They usually present with incidental finding of a cardiac murmur, which is best audible on the praecordium at where the fistula empties into the cardiac chamber or blood vessel. The murmur is continuous, but louder during diastole, in nature.

Neonates and infants with large coronary arterial fistulas, on the other hand, present with symptoms and signs of heart failure. A loud continuous murmur due to the systolic and diastolic flow in large fistula is characteristically audible. Older children and adults with large fistulas may present with symptoms of coronary steal phenomenon including angina, shortness on exertion, and syncope.

40.4 Investigations

CXR: The chest radiographic findings are usually normal. Cardiomegaly may be present in patients with significant left-to-right or left-to-left shunting through large fistulas.

ECG: The electrocardiogram is usually normal. Ischaemic changes in the resting electrocardiogram in children are uncommon.

Echocardiography: Echocardiography with Doppler colour mapping demonstrates the size and morphology (tortuosity and stenosis) of the fistula (Fig. 40.2), its origin and emptying site, continuous fistulous flow, dilation of the feeding coronary artery, and enables the assessment of ventricular function.

Cardiac catheterization: This has been the gold standard investigation for diagnosis and imaging of the fistula. In the present era, the diagnostic part is usually followed by transcatheter closure in the same setting.

CT: Computed tomography provides the diagnosis, facilitates surgical or transcatheter management by defining from a three-dimensional perspective the size and morphology, and origin, course, and drainage site of the fistula, and helps in the selection of suitable device for embolization.

Stress testing: Stress cardiovascular magnetic resonance imaging or thallium perfusion scan may identify myocardial ischaemia due to coronary steal phenomenon in older children.

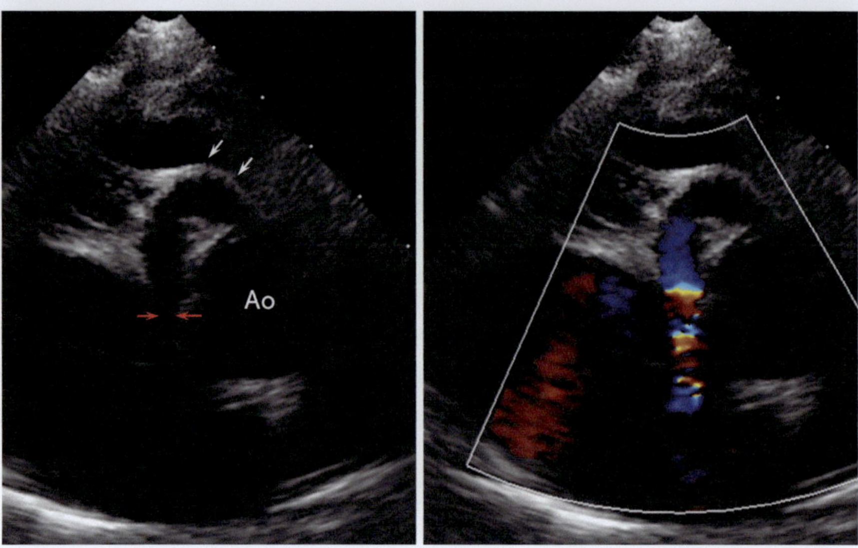

Fig. 40.2 Echocardiographic assessment of coronary arterial fistula. Two-dimensional (left) and Doppler colour (right) echocardiographic demonstration of a dilated right coronary artery (white arrows) feeding a tortuous and stenosed fistula that empties into the right atrium (Abbreviation: *Ao* aorta)

40.5 Management Strategy

The optimal timing and the approach to management of children with coronary arterial fistulas remain debatable. The following aspects should be considered when managing this rare condition: (a) indications for closure, (b) proximal versus distal fistulas, (c) surgical versus transcatheter closure, and (d) the use of antiplatelet and/or anticoagulation before and after closure.

Indications: The recent 2018 AHA/ACC guideline highlights the importance of a team approach in the evaluation of the appropriateness and feasibility of surgical or transcatheter closure of coronary arterial fistula, but without providing specific indications. The presence of symptoms or haemodynamic sequalae (e.g. cardiac ischaemia, volume loading of the cardiac chambers, cardiac dysfunction, heart failure), attributable to a medium or large-sized fistula, are usually considered to be reasonable indications for closure. In asymptomatic patients, the indications for closing medium or large-sized fistulas (possibly with stenosis along its tortuous course and/or restriction at the site of emptying) are less clear. As these fistulas may increase in size with growth of the child, elective closure has been considered reasonable. Small fistulas, which may close spontaneously during childhood, can be monitored without intervention.

Proximal versus distal fistulas: Proximal fistulas arise from the proximal coronary segment, while distal fistulas arise from the distal end of the native coronary artery.

Closure of distal fistula may predispose to myocardial infarction due to thrombus formation within the proximally dilated coronary artery that gives off branches to supply the myocardium. Hence, while closure of large proximal fistulas with or without symptoms have been recommended, a conservative approach with indefinite aspirin therapy has been suggested as an option for large asymptomatic distal fistulas.

Surgical versus transcatheter closure: The choice depends on institutional expertise. In the present era, transcatheter closure of fistulas with coils and vascular plugs has become the treatment of choice.

Antiplatelet and anticoagulation therapy: There is no standardized algorithm on the use of antiplatelet agents and warfarin. The use of these medications is not indicated for small fistulas. For large asymptomatic distal fistulas with conservative management, indefinite aspirin therapy has been recommended. After surgical or transcatheter closure of fistulas, 6–12 months of warfarin therapy followed by 1 year or indefinite use of antiplatelet agents is usually recommended.

40.6 Long-Term Monitoring

Small fistulas in children may have a chance of spontaneous closure. Unclosed moderate to large-size fistulas should be monitored for complications including thrombosis, rupture, myocardial ischaemia, and endocarditis. After surgically or device closure, especially of distal fistulas, monitoring for thrombus formation and myocardial ischaemia and infarction is warranted.

41 Anomalous Origin of the Left Coronary Artery from the Pulmonary Artery

In structurally normal hearts, the left coronary artery arises from the left sinus of Valsalva while the right coronary artery arises from the right sinus of Valsalva. However, one of the coronary arteries may arise from the pulmonary circulation, which is discussed in this Chapter, or it may also arise anonymously from the opposite sinus (Chap. 42).

41.1 Anatomy

Anomalous origin of the left coronary artery from the pulmonary artery (ALCAPA), also known as Bland-White-Garland syndrome, was described in a comprehensive fashion in 1933 by three American physicians Edward Bland, Paul Dudley White and Joseph Garland. While the left coronary artery may originate anomalously from anywhere of the pulmonary arterial circulation, it arises most commonly from the main pulmonary trunk.

41.2 Pathophysiology

With the postnatal drop in pulmonary vascular resistance, reduction of diastolic perfusion pressure reduces flow in the left coronary artery. As the pulmonary vascular resistance decreases further during the first few weeks of life, it becomes lower than the coronary arterial resistance and reversal of left coronary arterial flow occurs (with coronary blood emptying into the pulmonary artery during diastole). The steal of blood from the left coronary arterial circulation causes myocardial ischaemia and dysfunction. The clinical presentation mimics that of dilated cardiomyopathy and hence exclusion of ALCAPA is mandatory in infants suspected to have dilated cardiomyopathy.

Y.-f. Cheung, *Congenital and Paediatric Acquired Heart Disease in Practice*, https://doi.org/10.1007/978-981-99-2862-0_41

Extensive collaterals between the right and left coronary arteries may develop in some patients to maintain left coronary arterial perfusion. This constitutes a small left-to-right shunt (flow from the right coronary artery drains through collaterals into the left coronary arteries and then the pulmonary artery). These patients may present later in childhood or even during adulthood.

Mitral regurgitation occurs commonly in ALCAPA due to ischaemic papillary muscle dysfunction and annular dilation of the mitral valve secondary to left ventricular dilation.

41.3 Clinical Presentation and Findings

Infants present typically with symptoms of heart failure at 1 to 2 months of age. In older children and adolescents, chest pain on exertion and impaired exercise capacity may be the presenting symptoms. Signs of heart failure in infants are obvious. Characteristic findings are signs of respiratory distress, gross displacement of the cardiac apex, a gallop rhythm, an apical pansystolic murmur due to mitral regurgitation, and hepatomegaly.

41.4 Investigations

CXR: Chest radiograph shows cardiomegaly with or without pulmonary venous congestion and oedema (Fig. 41.1a).

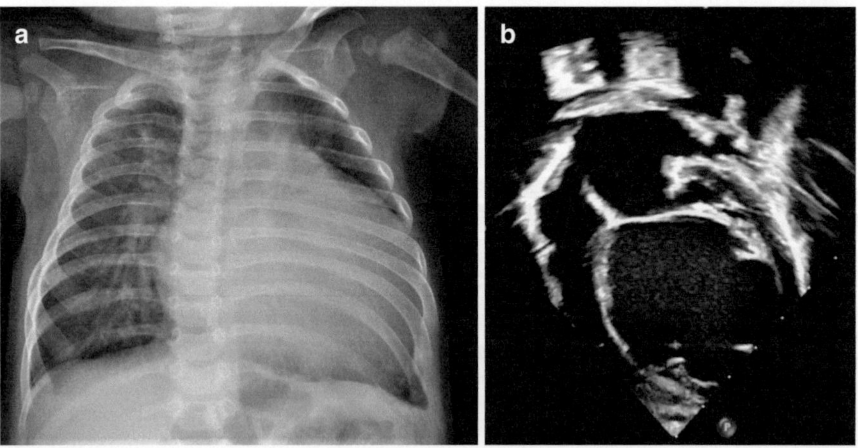

Fig. 41.1 Radiographic and echocardiographic assessment of ALCAPA. (**a**) Chest radiograph showing gross cardiomegaly due to left ventricular dilation and pulmonary venous congestion (**b**) Echocardiographic findings from the four-chamber view include dilation of the left atrium and echogenicity of the papillary muscles

ECG: The classic abnormal electrocardiographic findings are Q waves in leads I, aVL, V5, and V6 (suggestive of anterolateral infarct) (Fig. 41.2a). ST segment depression or inversion and non-specific T wave changes are also found in the inferior and lateral leads.

Echocardiography: Echocardiography shows a poorly contractile and dilated left ventricle, echogenicity of the left ventricular endocardium and papillary muscles, and varying degrees of mitral regurgitation (Fig. 41.1b). The demonstration of the left coronary artery arising from the main pulmonary artery or from the branch pulmonary arteries and reversal of flow into the pulmonary artery is diagnostic. In some infants, the left coronary artery appears to be in close proximity to and may seem to arise from the left sinus of Valsalva, although the direction of flow is reversed.

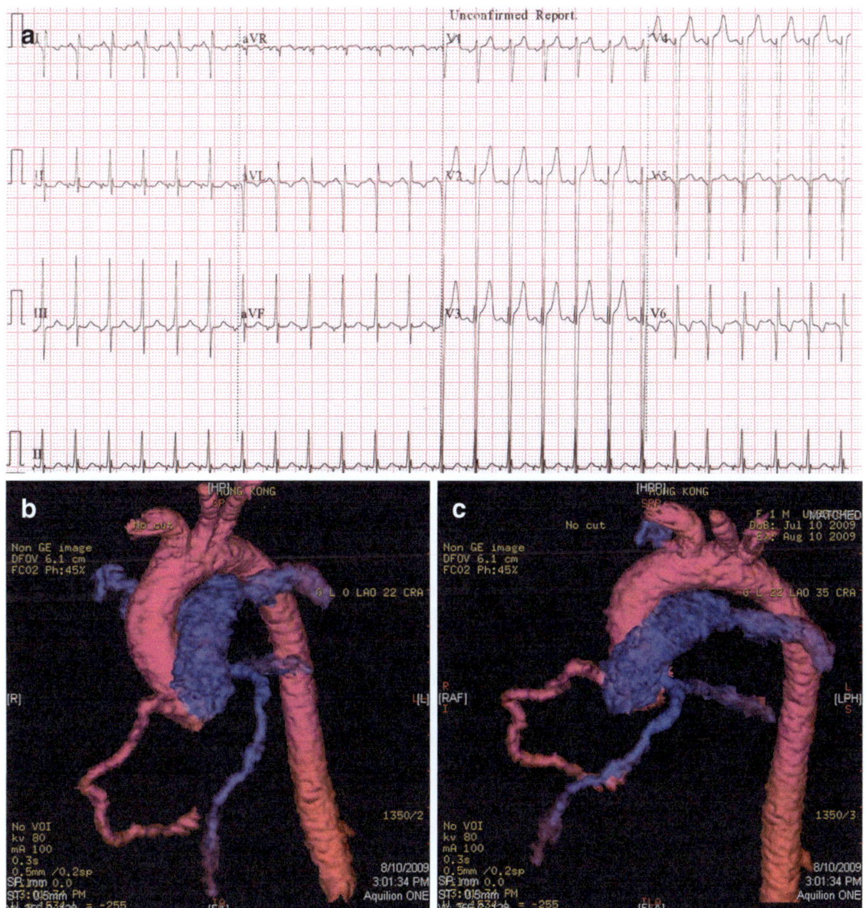

Fig. 41.2 ECG and CT findings in ALCAPA. (**a**) Characteristic ECG findings of Q waves in lead I, aVL, V5 and V6 and T wave inversion in V6 (**b** and **c**) Different CT angiographic projections showing anomalous origin of the left coronary artery from the main pulmonary artery

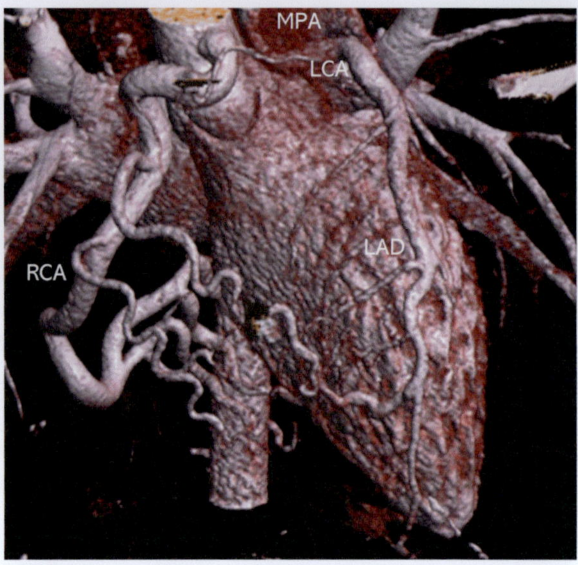

Fig. 41.3 CT angiography volume rendered image of ALCAPA. CT angiography volume rendered image showing a dilated and tortuous right coronary artery with extensive collaterals supplying the left coronary arterial system. *LCA* left coronary artery, *LAD* left anterior descending artery, *MPA* main pulmonary artery, *RCA* right coronary artery

CT angiogram: This may be required to delineate the coronary arteries in elusive situations (Figs. 41.2b, c and 41.3).

Cardiac catheterization: When echocardiographic assessment and CT angiogram are inconclusive, cardiac catheterization with angiography should be performed for diagnostic purpose. Selective coronary angiograms show dilation of right coronary artery, collateral supply to the left coronary arteries, and retrograde flow from the left coronary artery into the pulmonary artery. This investigation poses, however, an increased risk to infants with very poor ventricular function.

41.5 Management Strategy

Initial stabilization: The medical management aims at treating congestive heart failure and stabilizing infants with low cardiac output syndrome. For less symptomatic patients, diuretics and afterload reduction may help. Critically ill infants with severe myocardial dysfunction and mitral regurgitation require inotropic support, afterload reduction, and mechanical ventilation (avoid hyperventilation and high FiO_2 to prevent further drop in pulmonary vascular resistance). Systemic vasoconstrictors may worsen left ventricular function by increasing systemic afterload and should be avoided.

Surgical intervention: Surgical repair is the definitive treatment. Induction of an anaesthesia and intubation are high risk procedures that may precipitate cardiac arrest. Preparations must be made in the operation room for emergency institution of cardiopulmonary bypass. Direct reimplantation of the anomalous left coronary artery onto the aortic root is commonly performed. If reimplantation is not feasible, Takeuchi operation, which involves the creation of an aortopulmonary window and an intrapulmonary arterial tunnel to baffle the aorta to the origin of the anomalous left coronary artery is performed. Mitral valve repair is usually not required as mitral regurgitation usually improves with better left ventricular and papillary muscle function after surgery.

41.6 Postoperative Considerations

Potential complications immediately after surgery include low cardiac output syndrome and atrial or ventricular arrhythmias. Initial intensive care management includes fluid restriction, low dose milrinone and adrenaline infusion, diuretics, and use of antiarrhythmics when indicated. Mechanical circulatory support may be required for patients who cannot be weaned from cardiopulmonary bypass.

41.7 Long-Term Monitoring

Regular assessment for monitoring of recovery of left ventricular function, residual mitral regurgitation, and occurrence of stenosis of the reimplanted left coronary artery are necessary. While long-term survival and recovery of left ventricular function are usually expected after surgery, some of the patients require mitral valve repair or replacement during late childhood and some may continue to harbour the phenotype of dilated cardiomyopathy.

Anomalous Origin of a Coronary Artery from the Opposite Sinus

42

Anomalous aortic origin of a coronary artery from the opposite sinus has raised clinical concerns due to its reported association with sudden cardiac death. The estimated cumulative risk of death over a 20-year period in children and young adults aged 15 to 35 years with anomalous aortic origin of a coronary artery participating in competitive sports has been reported to be 6.3% for anomalous origin of the left coronary artery from the right sinus and 0.2% for anomalous origin of the right coronary artery from the left sinus.

The prevalence of this coronary arterial anomaly ranges from 0.1% to 0.3%, with anomalous origin of the right coronary artery from the left sinus of Valsalva being about 6 to 10 times more prevalent than anomalous origin of the left coronary artery rises from the right sinus of Valsalva. However, the latter is associated with 80% to 90% of sudden cardiac death related to anomalous aortic origin of a coronary artery.

42.1 Anatomy

The coronary artery that arises anomalously from the opposite sinus can run anterior to the pulmonary trunk or posterior to the aorta, and this is generally considered as benign. On the other hand, there are several anatomic features that are regarded as high-risk factors for sudden cardiac death (Box 42.1).

Box 42.1 High-Risk Anatomic Features of the Anomalous Coronary Artery

- inter-arterial course between the aorta and pulmonary trunk
- intramural course
- acute angle take-off of the coronary artery from the aorta
- slit-like coronary arterial orifice

Y.-f. Cheung, *Congenital and Paediatric Acquired Heart Disease in Practice*,
https://doi.org/10.1007/978-981-99-2862-0_42

42.2 Pathophysiology

Although anomalous origin of either the right or the left coronary artery from the opposite sinus has been associated with sudden death, the risk is significantly higher with anomalous origin of the left coronary artery from the right sinus of Valsalva. It is believed that inadequate myocardial oxygen delivery due to anomalous origin of the coronary artery may have resulted in myocardial ischaemia and sudden cardiac death.

Several mechanisms have been proposed: (1) dilation of the aorta during exercise stretches the anomalous coronary artery and worsens stenosis in the presence of risk factors (Box 42.1), (2) increased flow in the aorta and the pulmonary artery during exercise may compress on the coronary artery with an inter-arterial course, (3) areas of myocardial fibrosis due to intermittent ischaemia may become foci of ventricular arrhythmias, and (4) impaired coronary perfusion due to intussusception, vessel spasm, and noncompliant pericommissural area.

42.3 Clinical Presentation and Findings

Patients are typically asymptomatic, and the diagnosis is usually made incidentally during echocardiographic assessment for unrelated reasons (e.g. heart murmur). Occasionally, patients may complain of chest pain, syncope, dizziness, or palpitations on exertion. Rarely, the initial presentation may be an aborted sudden cardiac death or unexplained life-threatening cardiac arrhythmias, for which coronary anomalies including anomalous aortic origin of a coronary artery from the opposite sinus have to be evaluated. The physical findings are normal.

42.4 Investigations

ECG: The electrocardiogram is usually normal.
Echocardiography: Echocardiography demonstrates the anomalous origin of the coronary artery from the opposite sinus (Fig. 42.1a), identifies an intramural course with the use of Doppler colour flow mapping, and enables the evaluation of ventricular function.
CT angiography: This provides detailed information on the course and angle-takeoff of the coronary artery and anatomy of its orifice (Fig. 42.1b and 42.2).
CMR: Cardiac magnetic resonance provides information on the coronary arterial anatomy, cardiac function, and myocardial fibrosis.
Stress testing: Exercise stress testing is indicated after establishment of the diagnosis for the assessment of inducible cardiac ischaemia and arrhythmias. Further assessment with stress echocardiography, radionuclide perfusion scan, or cardiac magnetic resonance perfusion scan increases the sensitivity of detection of myocardial ischaemia.

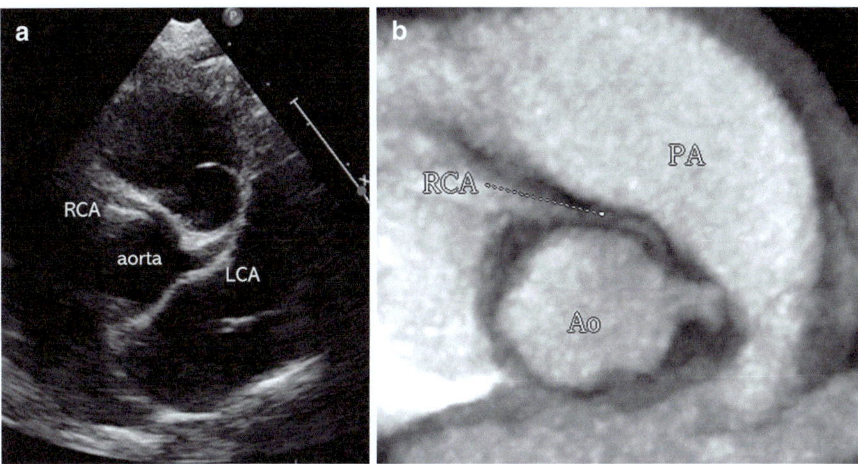

Fig. 42.1 Imaging of anomalous origin of right coronary artery from the left sinus of Valsalva. (**a**) Echocardiographic and (**b**) CT angiographic demonstration of anomalous origin of the right coronary artery from the left coronary sinus. *Ao* aorta, *LCA* left coronary artery, *PA* pulmonary artery, *RCA* right coronary artery

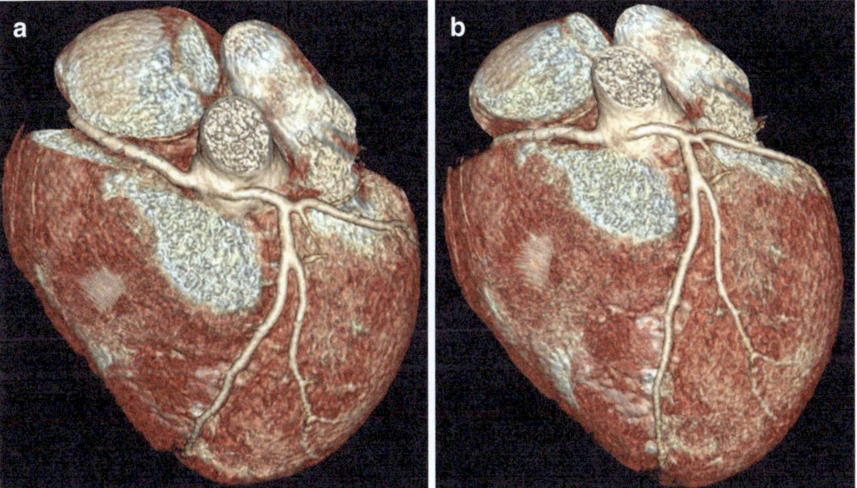

Fig. 42.2 Imaging of anomalous origin of left coronary artery from the right sinus of Valsalva. (**a** and **b**) CT angiographic demonstration of anomalous origin of the left coronary artery from the right coronary sinus with an intramural course from different projections in an adolescent presenting with ventricular fibrillation

42.5 Management Strategy

Surgical intervention: The previously reported high rates of sudden cardiac death based on autopsy data have favoured the management decision towards surgical intervention for patients with or without symptoms. However, taking into account of the prevalence of the condition in the general population, the actual risk of dying from anomalous aortic origin of a coronary artery from the opposite sinus is likely to be much lower. Hence, the current indications for intervention are based on a risk assessment of sudden cardiac death and balancing the benefits and risks of interventions after detailed discussion with the patient and the family (Box 42.2).

Box 42.2 Indications for Surgical Interventions for Anomalous Origin of Coronary Artery from the Opposite Sinus

Indications adopted by most

- cardiac symptoms suggestive of cardiac ischaemia or arrhythmias
- investigation findings of myocardial ischaemia at rest or during exertion
- history of an aborted cardiac arrest
- anomalous origin of the left coronary artery from the right sinus of Valsalva with high-risk anatomy even if asymptomatic (surgery usually performed at the age of 10 years or older)

Indication adopted by some

- anomalous origin of the left coronary artery from the right sinus of Valsalva even if asymptomatic and without high-risk anatomy

Controversial

- anomalous origin of the right coronary artery from the left sinus of Valsalva with no symptoms or evidence of myocardial ischaemia or arrhythmias

The surgical options, depending on the anatomic features and course of the anomalous coronary artery, include: (1) unroofing of the interatrial and intramural anomalous coronary artery, (2) pulmonary artery translocation to relief the compression of the anomalous coronary artery, (3) reimplantation of the anomalous coronary artery to its appropriate sinus, (4) ostioplasy, and (5) rarely coronary bypass with a graft (not favoured due to competitive flow causing early graft failure).

Exercise restriction: Evaluation and recommendations should be based on the type of coronary artery anomaly, presence of absence high-risk anatomic features, symptoms, findings of stress testing, and discussion and counselling with patients and their family. Recommendations based on the 2015 AHA/ACC Scientific Statement are shown in Box 42.3.

Box 42.3 Exercise Restrictions for Anomalous Origin of Coronary Artery from the Opposite Sinus

Anomalous origin of the right coronary artery from the left sinus

- restricted from participation in all competitive sports in the presence of symptoms, arrhythmias, or signs of ischaemia on exercise stress test
- permission to compete in sports can be considered after adequate counseling (and taking into consideration of the uncertainty of a negative stress test) in patients without symptoms or without positive exercise stress test

Anomalous origin of the left coronary artery from the right sinus

- restricted from participation in all competitive sports before surgical repair independent of symptoms

42.6 Postoperative Considerations

The postoperative course is usually uneventful. Non-specific diffuse ST segment changes suggestive of pericarditis may be evident. Echocardiographic demonstration of wall motion abnormalities and electrocardiographic finding of ST segment elevation should prompt further investigations for coronary insufficiency. Aspirin, ranging from 3 month to indefinite, is recommended after surgery. Recreational or competitive exercise may be allowed at least 3 months, or up to 12 months in patients presenting with aborted sudden cardiac death, after surgery in the absence of symptoms and evidence of myocardial ischaemia or cardiac arrhythmias on stress testing.

42.7 Long-Term Monitoring

Lifelong clinical follow up with clinical, electrocardiographic, and echocardiographic assessments and stress testing is required whether surgery is performed or not. There remains a gap in the understanding of the long-term outcomes after surgical intervention.

Part IX

Myocardial and Pericardial Diseases

43 Myocarditis

Myocarditis is an inflammatory condition of the myocardium. It may be difficult to recognize myocarditis in the early phase of the disease process in young infants and children due to the non-specific presentations. Confirmation of myocarditis can also be a diagnostic challenge.

43.1 Aetiology and Pathogenesis

Acute myocarditis in children is usually caused by an infection, with viral causes being most common. The most common viral causes of myocarditis are enterovirus (especially Coxsackie B virus), adenovirus, parvovirus B19 and human herpes virus 6. Non-infectious causes include autoimmune conditions, medications, and vaccines (Table 43.1). Recently, myocarditis is recognized as a complication of acute COVID-19 infection and after COVID-19 mRNA vaccination (Chap. 61).

Pathogenesis of myocarditis involves activation of the innate immune response as the virus enters into the cardiomyocytes and the adaptive immune response with activation of the T cells and B cells. Some cases of myocarditis are autoimmune in origin.

Y.-f. Cheung, *Congenital and Paediatric Acquired Heart Disease in Practice*,
https://doi.org/10.1007/978-981-99-2862-0_43

Table 43.1 Causes of myocarditis in children

Infectious causes	Non-infectious causes
Viral	Autoimmune
enterovirus (Coxsackie A and B)	idiopathic juvenile rheumatoid arthritis
adenovirus	systemic lupus erythematosus
parvovirus B19	other connective tissue disease
human herpes virus 6	Kawasaki disease
others (influenza, COVID-19, cytomegalovirus, Ebstein-Barr virus, etc.)	Drug hypersensitivity
Bacterial	antibiotics
Group A Streptococcus	anticonvulsants
Streptococcus pneumoniae	alcohol
others (Haemophilus influenzae, Mycobacterium tuberculosis, etc.)	cocaine
Fungal	Vaccines
candida	smallpox vaccine
others (actinomyces, aspergillus, etc.)	COVID-19 mRNA vaccine
Others	
rickettsial	
spirochaetal	
protozoal	

43.2 Clinical Presentation and Findings

The clinical presentation of acute myocarditis can be non-specific. There is usually a history of viral prodrome. Non-specific symptoms including fever, fatigue, and in particular gastrointestinal symptoms (abdominal pain and vomiting) are the prominent presenting features in infants and young children. This clinical presentation may to lead to an initial diagnosis of gastroenteritis or an acute surgical abdominal condition. Symptoms and signs of heart failure may be more obvious in some patients. Cardiac arrhythmias in association with myocarditis (supraventricular and ventricular arrhythmias and complete heart block) may lead to syncope or convulsion as a presenting symptom. Patients with fulminant myocarditis present with shock.

43.3 Initial Investigations

CXR: Findings on the chest radiograph are non-specific. There may be absence of cardiomegaly due to the acute nature of the presentation or cardiomegaly with pulmonary venous congestion (Fig. 43.1a).

ECG: Electrocardiographic changes may be non-specific. Abnormal findings include sinus tachycardia, generalized decrease in voltage, ST segment changes and T wave abnormalities (Fig. 43.1c). Cardiac arrhythmias include supraventricular and ventricular tachycardias and complete heart block,

Markers of inflammation: Erythrocyte sedimentation rate, C reactive protein, and leukocyte count are elevated.

Cardiac biomarkers: Troponin I and troponin T are elevated in children with acute myocarditis. Elevation of brain natriuretic peptide (BNP) or N-terminal proBNP reflects the severity of heart failure and is not specific for diagnosis of myocarditis.

Viral studies: Viral culture of the stool and viral serology are commonly performed, although the diagnostic yield is low. Viral genome in myocardial biopsy specimens may be identified using polymerase chain reaction.

Echocardiography: The echocardiogram shows varying degrees of impairment of left ventricular systolic function and global or regional hypokinesia of the myocardial segments. Functional mitral regurgitation and pericardial effusion may also be present (Fig. 43.1b).

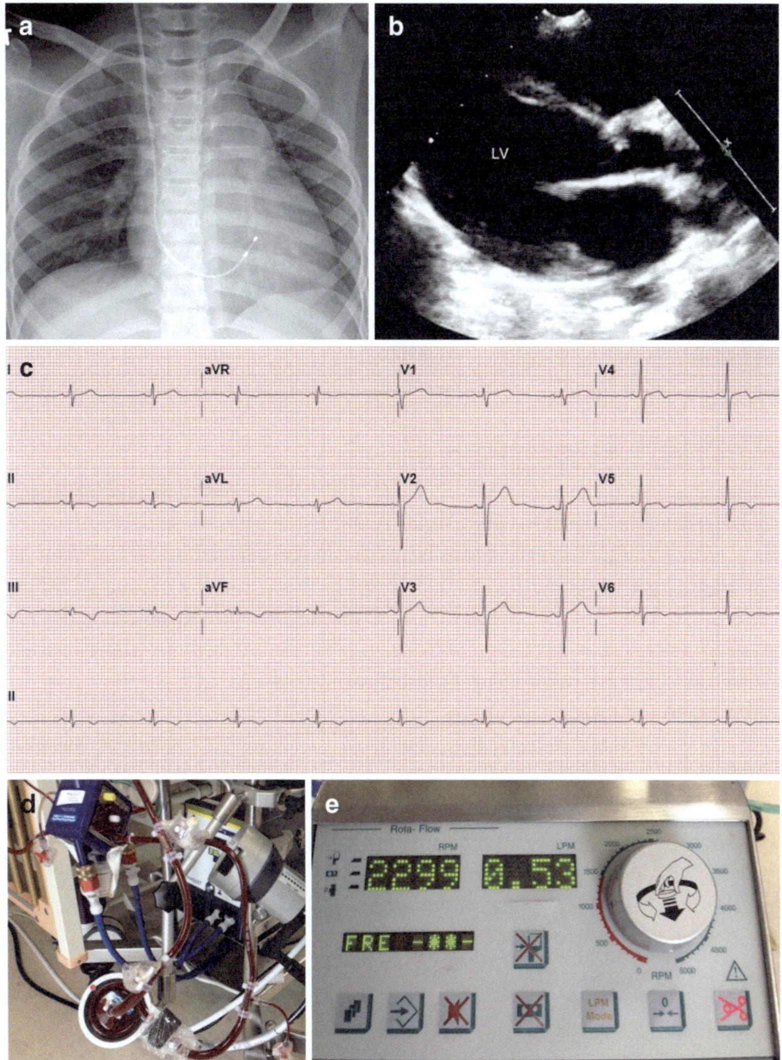

Fig. 43.1 Investigations and management of acute myocarditis (**a**) Chest radiograph showing mild cardiomegaly and pulmonary venous congestion in patient with myocarditis and complete heart block that requires pacing (**b**) Echocardiographic finding of left ventricular dilation (**c**) ECG showing sinus bradycardia and T wave inversion in multiple leads in another patient (**d** and **e**) Extracorporeal membrane oxygenation support. *LV* left ventricle

43.4 Further Investigations

The constellation of clinical manifestations and initial investigation findings enable the clinical diagnosis of myocarditis to be made (Box 43.1).

Box 43.1 Diagnosis of Myocarditis Based on Clinical and Initial Investigations Findings

Clinical manifestations
- history of viral prodrome
- symptoms of acute heart failure and arrhythmias: shortness of breath, chest pain, exercise incapacity, palpitation, syncope
- signs of heart failure: tachycardia, gallop rhythm, signs of cardiogenic shock, hepatomegaly

Initial investigations findings
- increased plasma troponin T or troponin I level
- echocardiographic finding of impaired ventricular systolic function
- ECG findings of heart block or supraventricular or ventricular tachycardia

Further investigations including cardiac magnetic resonance and endomyocardial biopsy may provide more confirmatory evidence of myocarditis.

CMR: Cardiac magnetic resonance is increasingly performed in children with a clinical diagnosis of myocarditis to define the location and the extend of inflammation (Chap. 8). The new 2018 Lake Louise criteria use a combination of T1- and T2-based imaging criteria for the CMR diagnosis of myocardial inflammation (Box 43.2, based on Ferreira et al. J Am Coll Cardiol 2018;72:3158–3176).

Endomyocardial biopsy: Although endomyocardial biopsy is considered the gold standard for diagnosing myocarditis, the focal and transient nature of the myocardial infiltrates and the randomness of biopsy sampling have led to a high false negative rate. Given these considerations and the procedural risk involved, endomyocardial biopsy is not routinely performed in most centres. If biopsy is performed, diagnosis of myocarditis can be made based on light microscopic findings according to the Dallas criteria (Box 43.3). Examination of the biopsies by the newer molecular and immunocytochemistry techniques may improve the diagnostic yield.

Box 43.2 The 2018 Lake Louise Criteria for CMR Diagnosis of Myocardial Inflammation

Main criteria

T2-based imaging

- regional high T2 signal intensity, or
- global T2 signal intensity ratio ≥ 2.0 in T2W CMR images, or
- regional or global increase of myocardial T2 relaxation time

T1-based imaging

- regional or global increase of native myocardial T1 relaxation time or extracellular volume or
- areas with high signal intensity in a nonischaemic distribution pattern in late gadolinium enhancement (LGE) images

Supportive criteria

- pericardial effusion in cine CMR images or high signal intensity of the pericardium in LGE images or T1-mapping or T2-mapping
- systolic LV wall motion abnormality in cine CMR images

Box 43.3 Dallas Criteria

Active myocarditis

- the presence of an inflammatory infiltrate with necrosis or degeneration or both of adjacent myocytes not typical of the ischaemic damage associated with coronary heart disease

Borderline myocarditis

- when myocardial lymphocytic infiltrate is present but without necrosis or degeneration of adjacent myocytes

43.5 Management Strategy

Close monitoring of haemodynamics in terms of the adequacy of the cardiac output and the cardiac rhythm is important.

Children with mildly impaired ventricular function and mild symptoms and signs of heart failure can be managed with diuretics and afterload reducing agents. Patients with low cardiac output syndrome require intravenous inotropic support with milrinone and adrenaline infusion and mechanical ventilation. Early institution of mechanical circulatory support in patients with fulminant myocarditis can be lifesaving (Fig. 43.1d, e).

For cardiac arrhythmias, temporary pacing is required for complete heart block and anti-arrhythmic medications with or without electrical conversion are required for the control of supraventricular and ventricular arrhythmias.

Data on the use immunomodulatory therapy including steroid and intravenous immunoglobulin therapy are inconclusive. When myocarditis occurs in relation to systemic autoimmune disease, immunosuppressive therapy should be targeted at the underlying condition. The indications for antiviral therapy are unclear, although it may be reasonable to treat if active viral infection is evident. The benefit of aspirin or anticoagulation therapy in patients with severe ventricular dysfunction is also uncertain.

Management of myocarditis in association with multisystem inflammatory syndrome in children after COVID-19 infection and COVID-19 mRNA vaccine is discussed in Chap. 61.

43.6 Long-Term Monitoring

Mortality during the acute illness is about 10%. In patients with resolved myocarditis, physical activities should be restricted for at least 6 months after the onset of the disease. Most survivors recover without long-term cardiac impairment. A subset of patients developed dilated cardiomyopathy, in whom long-term medical therapies (Chap. 44) are indicated. About 5% to 20% of children with acute myocarditis has been reported to require heart transplantation.

Cardiomyopathies

44

Cardiomyopathies are defined as abnormalities of the ventricular myocardium unexplained by abnormal loading conditions or congenital heart disease. While classification of cardiomyopathies based on different genetic mutations has been proposed, classification based on the phenotypic and functional characteristics remains to the most commonly used approach in paediatric cardiomyopathy registries.

The commonly encountered phenotypes in children are: (1) dilated cardiomyopathy, (2) hypertrophic cardiomyopathy, (3) restrictive cardiomyopathy, and (4) noncompaction cardiomyopathy. A rare type of cardiomyopathy with substrates for cardiac arrhythmias, the arrhythmogenic right ventricular cardiomyopathy, is rarely diagnosed in children.

Among the different types, dilated and hypertrophic cardiomyopathies are the most common types of cardiomyopathies in children (Table 44.1).

Table 44.1 Types of paediatric cardiomyopathies

Type	Proportion	Incidence
Dilated cardiomyopathy	>50%	0.6–0.7 cases per 100,000 children
Hypertrophic cardiomyopathy	40%	0.3–0.5 cases per 100,000 children
Restrictive cardiomyopathy	About 3–5%	0.03–0.04 cases per 100,000 children
Noncompaction cardiomyopathy	About 5%	≤0.81 and 0.12 per 100,000 infants and children, respectively

Based on Lee et al. Circ Res 2017;121:855–873

Y.-f. Cheung, *Congenital and Paediatric Acquired Heart Disease in Practice*, https://doi.org/10.1007/978-981-99-2862-0_44

44.1 Aetiology

44.1.1 Genetic Aetiologies

Mutations in sarcomeric genes constitute the important causes of paediatric cardiomyopathies (Table 44.2). Other causes include mutations in genes that encode proteins of the Z-disc, desmosome, cytoskeleton, and nuclear and plasma membrane. The mode of inheritance can be autosomal dominant (most common), autosomal recessive, or X-linked. Variants in the same gene can cause different phenotypes, while variants in different genes can cause the same type of cardiomyopathy. Incorporation of genetic evaluation in the diagnostic algorithm enables the identification of an underlying cause in about 75% of affected children with cardiomyopathies.

Paediatric cardiomyopathies may also be associated with genetic syndromes and conditions with systemic involvements (Table 44.3). These include syndromic disorders, inborn errors of metabolism, storage disorders, and neuromuscular or neurodegenerative disorders (Chap. 50).

44.1.2 Non-Genetic Aetiologies

Dilated cardiomyopathy in children can have non-genetic aetiologies. These include inflammatory causes (post viral myocarditis and autoimmune disease), endocrine disorders (e.g. thyrotoxicosis and catecholamine secreting tumours), and exposure to toxic substance (e.g. anthracycline, iron, and radiation).

Table 44.2 Common sarcomeric genes associated with cardiomyopathies in children

Gene (Inheritance)	Protein	Types of cardiomyopathy
Thin filament		
ACTC1 (AD)	Cardiac alpha-actin	Dilated, hypertrophic, restrictive, noncompaction
TNNC1 (AD)	Cardiac troponin C	Dilated, hypertrophic
TNNI3 (AD, AR)	Cardiac troponin I	Dilated, hypertrophic, restrictive
TNNT2 (AD)	Cardiac troponin T	Dilated, hypertrophic, restrictive, noncompaction
TPM1 (AD)	Tropomyosin alpha-1 chain	Dilated, hypertrophic, noncompaction
Thick filament		
MYBPC3 (AD)	Cardiac myosin binding protein C	Dilated, hypertrophic, restrictive, noncompaction
MYH7 (AD)	Beta-myosin heavy chain	Dilated, hypertrophic, restrictive, noncompaction
MYL2 (AD)	Myosin light chain-2	Hypertrophic
MYL3 (AD, AR)	Myosin light chain-3	Hypertrophic, restrictive

Adapted with modifications from Lee et al. Circ Res 2017;121:855–873

Table 44.3 Genetic syndromes and conditions associated with cardiomyopathies in children

Genetic syndromes and conditions (Inheritance)	Gene	Type of cardiomyopathy
Syndromic		
RASopathies (Noonan, Costello, craniofaciocutaneous syndromes) (AD)	*BRAF*, *HRAS*, *KRAS*, *PTP11*, *SOS1*, *SPRED1*	Hypertrophic
Metabolic		
Primary carnitine deficiency (AR)	*SLC22A5*	Dilated
Barth syndrome (X-linked)	*TAZ*	Dilated, noncompaction
Danon disease (X-linked)	*LAMP2*	Dilated, hypertrophic
Pompe disease (AR)	*GAA*	Hypertrophic
Cardiac glycogen storage disease (AD)	*PRKAG2*	Hypertrophic
Carnitine palmitoyltransferase II deficiency (AR)	*CPT2*	Dilated
MELAS syndrome (mitochondrial)	*MTlTL1*	Dilated
Neuromuscular or neurodegenerative		
Duchenne/Becker muscular dystrophy (X-linked)	*DMD*	Dilated
Friedreich ataxia	*FRDA1*	Hypertrophic

Adapted with modifications from Lee et al. Circ Res 2017;121:855–873

44.2 Types of Cardiomyopathies

44.2.1 Dilated Cardiomyopathy

44.2.1.1 Pathology and Pathophysiology

The heart is grossly dilated with thinning of myocardial wall. There is progressive loss of cardiomyocytes and increase in fibrous tissue. The enlarged left ventricle initially adapts by increasing the force of contraction to maintain ejection fraction in response to the increased preload (Frank-Starling mechanism). Late decompensation with systolic ventricular failure and low cardiac output leads to activation of the neurohormonal system.

44.2.1.2 Clinical Presentation and Findings

Majority of children are symptomatic at presentation. The symptoms and signs range from those of compensated and decompensated heart failure to those of cardiogenic shock. Hepatomegaly and ankle oedema are due to an increase in central venous pressure secondary to systolic dysfunction of the myocardium and fluid retention. In older children and adolescents, the increase in jugular venous pressure is noticeable.

44.2.1.3 Investigations

CXR: Cardiomegaly and pulmonary venous congestion are present (Fig. 44.1a).

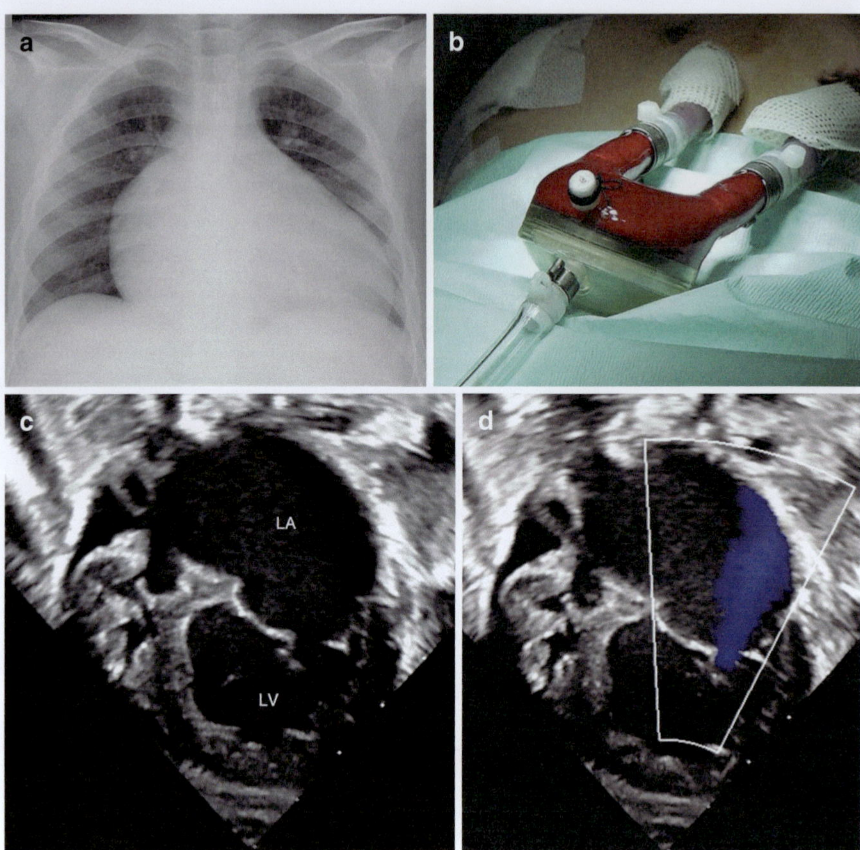

Fig. 44.1 Imaging and management of dilated cardiomyopathy. (**a**) Chest radiograph showing gross cardiomegaly and pulmonary venous congestion (**b**) Use of the Berlin heart as a bridge to heart transplantation (**c**) 2D echocardiographic findings of gross dilation of the left atrium and left ventricle (**d**) Colour flow mapping showing functional mitral regurgitation and a low-velocity mitral regurgitation jet suggestive of poor ventricular contractility. *LA* left atrium, *LV* left ventricle

ECG: Electrocardiogram may be normal or show nonspecific abnormalities of the ST segment and T wave. Repolarization abnormalities with T wave inversion especially in the lateral leads are common.

Echocardiography: Echocardiography shows dilation of the left ventricle and left ventricular systolic dysfunction with or without functional mitral regurgitation (Fig. 44.1c, d). Right ventricular dilation and dysfunction may also be present. Anomalous origin of the left coronary artery from the pulmonary artery (Chap. 41) must be excluded

44.2.1.4 Management Strategy

Medical treatment: Data on the usefulness of heart failure medications in children with dilated cardiomyopathy are limited. Medical therapies are based on data extrapolated from adults with dilated cardiomyopathy (Box 44.1), which may not necessarily apply to the paediatric patient population. New paediatric medical therapies that have attracted attention include ivabradine, a novel heart rate-lowering agent that inhibits the pacemaker channel (If or funny current), and sacubitril/valsartan, a combination of a neprilysin inhibitor and an angiotensin II receptor blocker (Chap. 64).

Surgical and device interventions: Pulmonary arterial banding (with shifting the ventricular septum to the left) and mitral valve repair in patients with significant functional mitral regurgitation may potentially improve left ventricular remodelling and function. In patients not responding adequately to medical therapy (with or without a trial of the above surgical procedures), ventricular assist devices are used to bridge the patient to heart transplantation (Fig. 44.1b).

Box 44.1 Medical Therapies

- loop diuretics: frusemide, bumetanide
- thiazide diuretics: hydrochlorothiazide, metolazone
- aldosterone antagonist: spironolactone
- angiotensin-converting enzyme inhibitors: captopril, enalapril
- angiotensin receptor blockers: losartan, valsartan
- beta-blockers: carvedilol, metoprolol
- digoxin

44.2.2 Hypertrophic Cardiomyopathy

44.2.2.1 Pathology and Pathophysiology

While asymmetric septal hypertrophy is classically described in hypertrophic cardiomyopathy, patterns of concentric, mid-cavity and apical hypertrophy are also found. Right ventricular hypertrophy may also be present. Histological findings include myocyte hypertrophy, myocardial fibre disarray, and fibrosis.

Systolic ventricular function is usually well preserved in the majority of patients. A small subset of patients, however, develop the so-called ‘burned-out’ phenotype with left ventricular thinning, dilation, and systolic dysfunction. Impairment of ventricular relaxation and worsening of ventricular compliance result in left ventricular diastolic dysfunction. Septal hypertrophy and systolic anterior motion of the mitral valve cause left ventricular outflow obstruction. Life-threatening ventricular arrhythmias are related to the altered myocardial substrate, while atrial fibrillation is uncommon in children.

44.2.2.2 Clinical Presentation and Findings

Asymptomatic patients with or without underlying syndromic and metabolic disorders are usually diagnosed when assessed for a cardiac murmur, associated cardiovascular disorders, or as part of the familial screening. Older patients may present with exercise incapacity, palpitation, and syncope.

Characteristic physical signs include pulsus bisferiens, double apical impulse (the second impulse is related to filling of the ventricle during atrial contraction), and an ejection systolic murmur when left ventricular outflow obstruction is present.

44.2.2.3 Investigations

ECG: Electrocardiogram is usually abnormal but nonspecific. Common findings are left axis deviation, increased left ventricular voltage, and ST segment and T wave abnormalities including T wave inversion. Ambulatory electrocardiography is useful for detection of asymptomatic atrial and ventricular arrhythmias.

Echocardiography: Echocardiographic assessment defines the severity and distribution of left ventricular hypertrophy (Fig. 44.2) and concurrent presence of right ventricular hypertrophy, enables the assessment of systolic anterior motion of the mitral valve, posteriorly direct mitral regurgitation, left ventricular outflow and

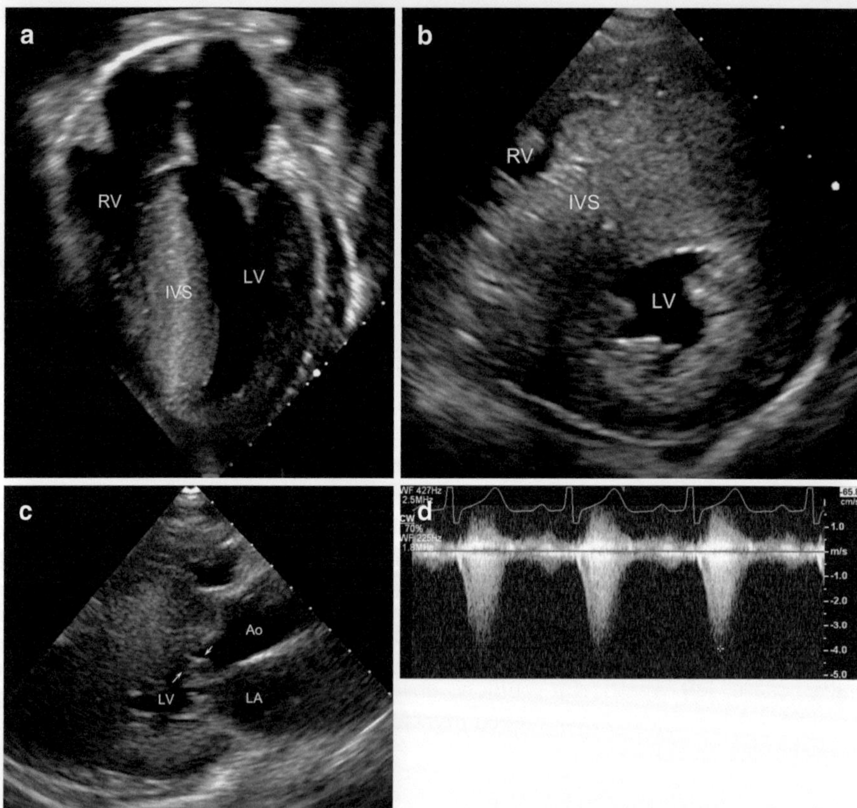

Fig. 44.2 Echocardiographic assessment of hypertrophic cardiomyopathy. (**a**) Four-chamber (**b**) parasternal long-axis and (**c**) parasternal short-axis views for assessment of asymmetric septal hypertrophy and systolic anterior motion of the mitral valve (arrows) (**d**) Continuous Doppler interrogation of left ventricle outflow obstruction. *Ao* aorta, *IVS* interventricular septum, *LA* left atrium, *LV* left ventricle, *RV* right ventricle

intracavitary systolic pressure gradients, and provides clues to distinguish pathologic hypertrophy from physiological hypertrophic response (e.g. athlete's heart) (Box 44.2). Tissue Doppler echocardiography and strain imaging provide further clues to differentiate hypertrophic cardiomyopathy from physiological causes of hypertrophy.

Box 44.2 Echocardiographic Clues Favouring Hypertrophic Cardiomyopathy Rather Than an Athlete's Heart

- asymmetric hypertrophy
- systolic anterior motion of mitral valve
- evidence of diastolic dysfunction with abnormal left ventricular filling
- decreased early diastolic mitral annular velocity
- decreased left ventricular systolic strain
- provocable gradient across left ventricular outflow on stress echocardiography
- lack of left ventricular dilation
- lack of response to detraining

Cardiopulmonary exercise testing: Identification of a blunted blood pressure response helps to stratify patients (adolescents and adults) at risk for sudden death. It also enables the evaluation of exercise-induced left ventricular outflow tract obstruction.

Cardiac resonance imaging: Although myocardial fibrosis as determined by late gadolinium enhancement cardiac magnetic resonance is a risk factor of adverse outcomes in adult patients, paediatric data are lacking.

44.2.2.4 Management Strategy

The treatment goals of medical, surgical, and device therapy are to reduce symptoms, to minimize left ventricular outflow tract obstruction, and to reduce risk of sudden death.

General management: General management includes adequate hydration, advise against competitive sports, avoidance of systemic vasodilators, judicious use of diuretics (all of which would increase left ventricular outflow obstruction), and referral for genetic counselling.

Medical treatment: Medical therapy is indicated in symptomatic patients or in patients with greater than mild degree of left ventricular outflow obstruction (≥25 to 30 mmHg depending on centre).

First line therapy is a selective beta-blocker with no vasodilating properties (atenolol, metoprolol, nadolol). Second line agents include verapamil (a calcium channel blocker but is usually avoided in infants due to concerns of hypotension and cardiac arrest), and disopyramide (a sodium channel blocker, usually less well tolerated in children). If monotherapy fails, combination therapy (commonly a beta-blocker with verapamil) can be given. Diuretics may be given to treat significant pulmonary oedema due to severe left ventricular diastolic dysfunction. Enzyme replacement therapy is indicated in patients with storage diseases amenable to this treatment modality.

Surgical intervention: Surgical myomectomy is considered when symptoms are refractory to medical therapy, the left ventricular outflow gradient is significant (> 60 to 70 mmHg), and/or worsening of mitral regurgitation is evident. Mitral valve repair or replacement may be required for the management of severe mitral regurgitation. Heart transplantation is required in patients with 'burned-out' hypertrophic cardiomyopathy and in those with symptomatic diastolic dysfunction refractory to other treatments.

Device and other interventions: The benefit of dual chamber atrioventricular pacing to reduce the left ventricular outflow gradient has not been substantiated and alcohol septal ablation is not recommended in children. The decision of implantable cardioverter defibrillator implantation for prevention of sudden cardiac death in children is not straightforward. Risk factors for sudden death in adults (HCM SCD risk calculator based on European Society of Cardiology guidelines is valid for patients of 16 years and older) do not apply to young children, and the risk-to-benefit ratio of implantable cardioverter defibrillator implantation may not be obvious. The 2020 American Heart Association guideline recommends consideration of implantable cardioverter defibrillator implantation for primary prevention in paediatric patients with ≥1 of the following major risk factors: family history of hypertrophic cardiomyopathy sudden cardiac death, nonsustained ventricular tachycardia on ambulatory monitor, massive left ventricular hypertrophy, and unexplained syncope.

44.2.2.5 Follow-up

For patients at risk of developing the disease identified by screening (genotype-positive but phenotype-negative at the time of initial assessment), electrocardiogram and echocardiogram performed every 12 months is recommended especially during adolescence.

For diagnosed patients, in particular those on medications, clinical evaluation every 6 to 12 months and electrocardiogram and echocardiogram every 12 months are recommended.

44.2.3 Restrictive Cardiomyopathy

44.2.3.1 Pathology and Pathophysiology

The characteristic pathologic features of restrictive cardiomyopathy are dilation of both atria in the presence of a small or normal sized non-hypertrophic ventricles. Patchy fibrosis may be found in the atria and ventricles. Infiltrative disease (amyloidosis, sarcoidosis, and haemochromatosis) as a cause of restrictive cardiomyopathy is extremely rare in children.

Reduced ventricular compliance is the culprit that leads to increased left and right ventricular filling pressures, reduced impaired cardiac output, pulmonary venous congestion with pulmonary hypertension, and development of pulmonary vascular disease. Enlargement of the two atria predisposes to the occurrence of atrial arrhythmias and thromboembolism. Atrial and ventricular arrhythmias may lead to sudden death.

44.2.3.2 Clinical Presentation and Findings

The clinical manifestations reflect the consequences of increased left and right ventricular filling pressures, arrhythmias, and reduced cardiac output. Hence, younger patients may present with shortness of breath and recurrent episodes of apparent chest infection (probably due to pulmonary venous congestion with or without oedema), while older children may present with palpitations and syncope.

Physical signs are those of respiratory distress and systemic venous congestion (dependent oedema, increased jugular venous pressure, hepatomegaly, and ascites). The pulmonary component of the second heart sound may be accentuated.

44.2.3.3 Investigations

CXR: Biatrial enlargement and pulmonary venous congestion (Fig. 44.3a) are present.

ECG: Electrocardiogram shows the typical features of biatrial enlargement. Other findings include atrial arrhythmias and nonspecific abnormalities of the ST segment and T waves.

Echocardiography: The characteristic echocardiographic features are biatrial enlargement in the presence of normal or small-sized non-hypertrophic ventricles (Fig. 44.3b). Clots may be seen in the atria. Diastolic functional assessment reveals predominant early diastolic filling with short deceleration time and evidence of increased filling pressure. Systolic function of the ventricles is usually preserved until very late stage of the disease. Echocardiographic evaluation provides further clues to differentiate restrictive cardiomyopathy from important differential diagnosis of constructive pericarditis (Fig. 44.3c, d) (Chap. 46).

Cardiac catheterization: Cardiac catheterization provides an assessment of ventricular filling pressures, pulmonary arterial pressure, and pulmonary vascular resistance to monitor disease progression, and to distinguish restrictive cardiomyopathy from constrictive pericarditis (Chap. 46). Endomyocardial biopsy is usually not performed in children given the rarity of paediatric diagnosis of infiltrative disease.

44.2.3.4 Management Strategy

There are no effective medical treatments for diastolic dysfunction. Judicious use of diuretics is important. While diuretics can improve symptoms of pulmonary and systemic venous congestion, over diuresis reduces the preload necessary to maintain cardiac output. Heart rate control to maximize the ventricular filling times may help to reduce symptoms and maintain cardiac output. An antiplatelet agent or anticoagulant is commonly prescribed to reduce the risk of thrombosis. Early heart transplantation offers the only hope for these patients.

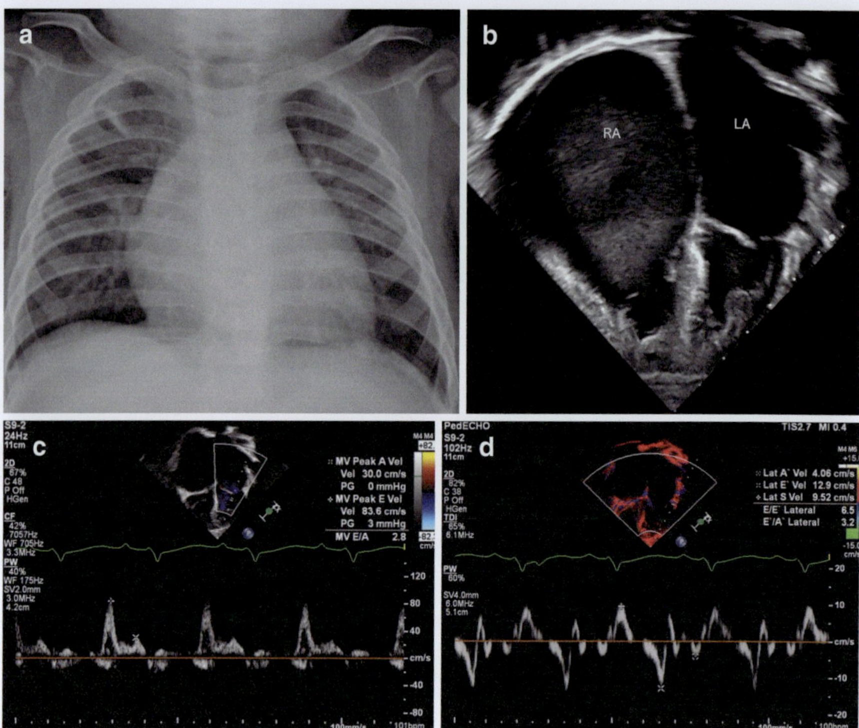

Fig. 44.3 Radiographic and echocardiographic assessment of restrictive cardiomyopathy. (**a**) Chest radiograph showing biatrial enlargement and pulmonary venous congestion (**b**) Characteristic echocardiographic findings of dilation of both right and left atria (**c** and **d**) Transmitral and tissue Doppler imaging provides additional information for diagnosis and differentiation from constrictive pericarditis

44.2.4 Noncompaction Cardiomyopathy

44.2.4.1 Pathology and Pathophysiology

Noncompaction cardiomyopathy is a heterogenous entity. It is believed to be due to an arrest of myocardial development during embryogenesis with failure of compaction of the myocardium. Hence, the myocardium of the ventricle (usually the left ventricle) is seen to consists of two distinct layers, a non-compacted and a compacted layer. Prominent trabeculae and intertrabecular recesses are seen in the non-compacted layer. It may also occur as mixed phenotype with dilated and/or hypertrophic cardiomyopathy.

The pathophysiologic consequences of this developmental myocardial abnormality are systolic and/or diastolic ventricular dysfunction, supraventricular and ventricular arrhythmias, and formation of thrombus within the dilated and poorly contractile left ventricle (originating usually from the intertrabecular recesses).

44.2.4.2 Clinical Presentation and Findings

Patients may present with a cardiac murmur, palpitations due to cardiac arrhythmias, or symptoms of heart failure. The clinical course may appear benign or may be progressive with development of severe heart failure. The course may also be undulating with periods of transient improvement in symptoms and cardiac function. The physical findings may be normal or may be those of dilated or hypertrophic cardiomyopathy.

44.2.4.3 Investigations

CXR: The chest radiograph may appear normal or exhibit features of those of dilated or hypertrophic cardiomyopathy.
ECG: Electrocardiogram is abnormal in most of the patients. There may be features of preexcitation, ST segment abnormalities, T wave inversion, and left ventricular strain pattern.
Echocardiography: A constellation of echocardiographic features has been used to diagnose isolated left ventricular noncompaction (Box 44.3) (Fig. 44.4). Echocardiographic assessment enables the assessment of the mixed phenotype with dilated and/or hypertrophic cardiomyopathy and systolic and diastolic function of the left ventricle.
CMR: Different criteria have been used to establish the diagnosis (Box 44.4).

Box 44.3 Echocardiographic Criteria for Diagnosing Noncompaction Cardiomyopathy
(Jenni et al. Heart 2001;86:666–671)

- thickened myocardium with a two-layered structure consisting of a thin compacted epicardial layer (C) and a much thicker, non-compacted endocardial layer (N) or trabecular meshwork with deep endomyocardial spaces; N/C ratio > 2 (based on the short-axis views with measurement of the N/C ratio at end-systole)
- predominant location of the pathology: mid-lateral, mid-inferior, and apical left ventricular cavity
- Doppler colour flow mapping shows evidence of deep intertrabecular recesses filled with blood from the left ventricular cavity
- absence of coexisting cardiac abnormalities (in isolated noncompaction cardiomyopathy)

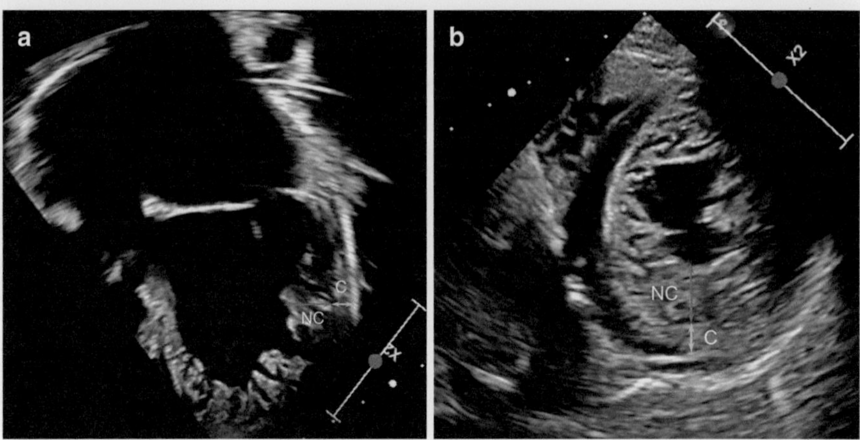

Fig. 44.4 Echocardiographic assessment of noncompaction cardiomyopathy. (**a**) Apical four-chamber and (**b**) parasternal short-axis views illustrating the measurement of the noncompacted and the compacted layers. *C* compacted layer, *NC* noncompacted layer

Box 44.4 Different CMR Criteria Used for Diagnosing Noncompaction Cardiomyopathy

- non-compacted (NC) myocardium: compacted (C) myocardium ratio > 2.3 at end-diastole
- NC myocardium >20% of LV mass
- NC myocardium >25% of LV mass, and NC indexed mass > 15 g/m^2

44.2.4.4 Management Strategy

The lack of consensus on diagnostic criteria potentially leads to under or over diagnosis of noncompaction cardiomyopathy. For isolated left ventricular noncompaction, annual electrocardiogram, echocardiography, and ambulatory Holter monitoring is recommended. For children with concomitant phenotypes of with dilated and/or hypertrophic cardiomyopathy, more frequent evaluation at 6 monthly interval is warranted. The management is based on the phenotype of the concomitant cardiomyopathy. The risk-to-benefit ratio of implantable cardioverter defibrillator implantation to prevent sudden death is unclear. There are little data to support the routine use of an antiplatelet agent or anticoagulant to reduce the risk of thrombosis in noncompaction cardiomyopathy. In the presence of severe left ventricular systolic function, prophylactic aspirin therapy can be considered.

44.3 Clinical Approach to Evaluate the Aetiology of Cardiomyopathies

Apart from arriving at the diagnosis of cardiomyopathy, defining the cardiac phenotype, and assessing the functional severity of heart failure, evaluation of the underlying aetiology is important for counselling, management, and prognostication (Fig. 44.5).

Diagnosis of cardiomyopathy based on clinical and echocardiographic assessment

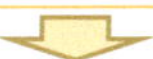

History: growth and development, seizure, decompensation during illnesses, chronic medical conditions (cardiac arrhythmias, childhood cancer requiring to chemotherapy and radiation therapy), maternal condition (gestational diabetes for neonates with hypertrophic cardiomyopathy phenotype), family history (three-generation pedigree)

Physical examination: dysmorphism, syndromic features, growth, neuromuscular assessment

Initial investigations: complete blood count, renal, liver, and thyroid function tests, plasma troponin and creatine phosphokinase, metabolic evaluation (plasma amino acids, urine organic acids, plasma free and total carnitine, acylcarnitine profile, lactate, pyruvate, ammonia), serum selenium level, genetic testing
Investigations to exclude differential diagnosis: Echocardiography, CT, or coronary angiography to exclude ALCAPA in infants with suspected dilated cardiomyopathy (Chapter 41)
Further targeted investigations: e.g. skeletal muscle biopsy, determination of enzyme deficiency in skin fibroblast (Pompe disease)

Fig. 44.5 Approach to the evaluation of the aetiology of cardiomyopathies. *ALCAPA* anomalous origin of the left coronary artery from the pulmonary artery

Cardiac Tumours

45

Cardiac tumours are rare in childhood and may present in utero or postnatally. Majority (90% or more) of primary cardiac tumours in children are benign. About 10% are malignant tumours, which are usually metastatic rather than primary in nature.

45.1 Distribution of Cardiac Tumours in Childhood

Rhabdomyoma is the most common type of cardiac tumour in children, followed by teratoma and fibroma (Table 45.1). It is important to recognize the even benign cardiac tumours can lead to significant haemodynamic compromise and potential life-threatening cardiovascular events.

Table 45.1 Frequency distribution of cardiac tumours in children

Types	Frequency
Benign tumours	
rhabdomyoma	40–60%
teratoma	15–19%
fibroma	12–16%
myxoma	2–4%
haemangioma	5%
others (lymphangioma, haemangiopericytoma, oncocytic tumours)	extremely rare
Malignant tumours	about 10%
rhabdomyosarcomas	
fibrosarcoma	
secondary metastatic tumours (neuroblastoma, leukaemia, lymphoma, melanoma)	

Based on Uzun et al. Orphanet J Rare Dis 2007;2:11

Y.-f. Cheung, *Congenital and Paediatric Acquired Heart Disease in Practice*, https://doi.org/10.1007/978-981-99-2862-0_45

45.2 Pathophysiology

Depending on the nature, location, and size of the cardiac tumours in children, the pathophysiologic consequences and hence the clinical features differ. Small-sized tumours localized within the myocardium may have no pathophysiologic effects. On the other hand, well documented pathophysiologic sequelae of cardiac tumours in children include: (1) obstruction of the inflow and/or outflow of the left or right ventricles by intracavitary tumour ingrowth, (2) cardiac arrhythmias and heart block related respectively to the intramural location or location of tumour in the conduction tissues, (3) heart failure caused by extensive infiltration of myocardium by the tumour tissue, and (4) systemic manifestations due to tumour embolization or an inflammatory response to the tumour tissue.

45.3 Benign Cardiac Tumours

45.3.1 Rhabdomyoma

45.3.1.1 Pathology

Rhabdomyomas are hamartomas with the histologic findings of spider cells, which are swollen myocytes with glycogen-filled vacuoles and striated myofibrils radiating to the cell wall. Rhabdomyomas are usually multiple and located within the ventricular myocardium. Intracavitary extension may obstruct ventricular inflow or outflow. Those located at the atrioventricular junction cause pre-excitation by acting as an accessory pathway. More than 80% of rhabdomyomas regress after birth during early childhood.

Tuberous sclerosis complex is associated with multiple cardiac rhabdomyomas, although its association with a single rhabdomyoma is unclear. Multiple cardiac rhabdomyomas represent the typical neonatal manifestation of this condition. Mutation in the genes *TSC1* and *TSC2* accounts for 75% to 90% of cases of tuberous sclerosis complex. These genes encode respectively the tumour suppressors hamartin and tuberin, which are critical regulators of cell growth and proliferation.

45.3.1.2 Clinical Presentation and Findings

Most of the patients are asymptomatic and the diagnosis is made during fetal echocardiographic screening or postnatal echocardiographic assessment for cardiac murmur or unrelated reasons. Occasionally, patients may present with symptoms of heart failure due to intracardiac obstruction or cardiac arrhythmias. The types of cardiac arrhythmias include atrial or ventricular ectopic beats, Wolff-Parkinson-White syndrome with supraventricular tachycardia, and ventricular tachycardia.

Cardiovascular examination may be normal or may reveal cardiac murmurs and/or signs of heart failure due to ventricular inflow or outflow obstruction. Characteristic skin lesions of tuberous sclerosis including hypomelanotic macules, facial angiofibroma, cephalic plaque over the forehead, shagreen patch usually over the back may be found in older children. However, except for hypomelanotic macules, these lesions are often absent at birth.

45.3.1.3 Management Strategy

Rhabdomyomas characteristically regress spontaneously within usually the first year of life. Hence, most of the patients are managed conservatively with serial electrocardiographic and echocardiographic monitoring. Rarely, surgical resection of the tumour(s) is required in the presence of severe intracardiac obstruction, heart failure, or intractable cardiac arrhythmias. Mammalian target of rapamycin (mTOR) inhibitors (everolimus, sirolimus) may have a role in the management of haemodynamically significant cardiac rhabdomyomas that are difficult to be removed surgically.

45.3.2 Fibroma

45.3.2.1 Pathology

Fibromas are the second most common paediatric cardiac tumour. These are usually solitary tumours derived from the fibroblast and located usually in the ventricular septum or left ventricular free wall. It may become quite large to cause heart failure and ventricular arrhythmias. Central calcification is common and is characteristic of cardiac fibromas.

45.3.2.2 Clinical Presentation and Findings

Symptoms of heart failure and cardiac arrhythmias (usually ventricular arrhythmias) are common modes of presentation.

45.3.2.3 Management Strategy

Fibromas rarely regress and surgical resection of large tumours is usually indicated. Cardiac arrhythmias usually resolve after tumour removal. In children with huge fibromas and little functional myocardium, heart transplantation may be indicated.

45.3.3 Teratoma

45.3.3.1 Pathology

Teratomas are formed by embryonic elements derived from all three germ layers. Nearly all cardiac teratomas are extracardiac but within the pericardial cavity. Teratomas are usually located at the base of the heart at the junction of the ascending aorta and right atrial appendage. They are typically heterogeneous in appearance with solid and multicystic areas. Pericardial effusion is usually present.

45.3.3.2 Clinical Presentation and Findings

Most of the cardiac teratomas present in the fetal or neonatal period. Rapid growth of the tumour in utero may cause cardiac tamponade, fetal hydrops, and death in-utero. Newborn babies and infants may present with symptoms and signs of heart failure, respiratory distress and cyanosis, and cardiovascular collapse due to tamponade. Older children with smaller teratomas may be relatively asymptomatic.

45.3.3.3 Management Strategy

Surgical removal of the tumour and drainage of pericardial effusion prenatally or early postnatally are indicated in the presence of haemodynamic compromise. As malignant transformation of teratomas may occur, tumour resection is also recommended in asymptomatic older children.

45.3.4 Myxoma

45.3.4.1 Pathology

Myxoma is the most common primary cardiac tumour in adults (commonly females) but is rare in children. Derived from multipotent mesenchyme, the tumour consists of cells embedded in a mucoid substance rich in glycosaminoglycans. It is usually solitary, pedunculated, and gelatinous in appearance, and attached to the atrial wall. Most of the myxomas are located in the left atrium (about 80% to 90%), some are in the right atrium, while very few are found in the right or left ventricular endocardium. Myxomas may have a smooth surface or may be villous and friable with the risk of embolization.

45.3.4.2 Clinical Presentation and Findings

Patients may present with constitutional, embolic, and/or cardiovascular symptoms. As the initial presentation may be relatively non-specific, the diagnosis of myxomas may only be made when the cardiac symptoms and signs become obvious.

The classic triad of clinical presentation comprises (1) constitutional symptoms of fever and weight loss, which together with laboratory findings of anaemia and elevated inflammatory markers may suggest connective tissue disease as an initial diagnosis (the cause of these findings is unclear but may be related to production of cytokines and other factors), (2) systemic embolization with stroke or pulmonary embolization depending on the location of the myxoma, (3) cardiac presentations of mitral valvar obstruction including cardiac murmur and symptoms and signs of heart failure. Occasionally, the left atrial myxoma may prolapse through the mitral valve during diastole to cause a ‘diastolic plop’ on auscultation.

Familial occurrence of multiple myxomas suggests the possibility of Carney complex. This is a hereditary disorder (autosomal dominant but may also occur sporadically) most commonly due to mutations in *PRKAR1A*, which encode a subunit of protein kinase A. Clinically, Carney complex is characterized by multiple atrial and extracardiac myxomas, schwannomas, various endocrine tumours, and cutaneous pigmentation abnormalities (lentigines and blue naevi).

45.3.4.3 Management Strategy

Complete surgical excision of the myxoma is the treatment of choice. A recurrence rate of up to 5% has been reported, but the risk is much higher in the presence of family history of myxoma.

45.3.5 Haemangiomas

45.3.5.1 Pathology

Haemangiomas are rare tumours with a heterogeneous nature. It can occur in any of the cardiac cavities and involve any of the myocardial layers.

45.3.5.2 Clinical Presentation and Findings

The presence of multiple haemangiomas in the skin suggests the possibility that the cardiac tumour may be vascular in nature. Depending on location and the extend of the haemangiomas, the infants may be asymptomatic or may develop pericardial effusion, high-output failure, or Kasabach–Merritt syndrome.

45.3.5.3 Management Strategy

Most of the haemangiomas regress during infancy. Surgical resection of large cardiac haemangiomas is difficult due to the vascularity, while medical treatment with propranolol, interferon-α, or steroid can promote the regression of haemangiomas.

45.4 Evaluation of the Nature of Cardiac Tumours

Initial echocardiographic assessment should enable the determination of the location, size, and number of tumour(s) and the haemodynamic consequence. Further definition of the possible nature of the cardiac tumour(s) is important for management, counselling, and prognostication. Clues to the possible nature of the cardiac tumours(s) may be obtained from the history and clinical findings and echocardiographic features (Box 45.1) (Fig. 45.1). Increasingly, computed tomography and cardiac magnetic resonance are used to assess the nature of the cardiac tumours. Positron emission tomography may be necessary if a diagnosis of malignant cardiac tumour is suspected. Myocardial biopsy is usually not performed.

Box 45.1 Clues for Evaluation of the Nature of Cardiac Tumours

Rhabdomyomas

- family history of tuberous sclerosis
- hypomelanotic macules present at birth
- other skin lesions of tuberous sclerosis are found in older children
- echocardiographic features: usually multiple, located at left ventricular free wall or septum, well circumscribed or pedunculated

Fibroma

- echocardiographic features: solitary, well demarcated, and a homogeneous echogenic mass, central calcifications may be evident

Teratoma

- fetal presentation with pericardial effusion, cardiac failure, and hydrops
- echocardiographic features: heterogeneous mass with solid and cystic areas, calcifications may be present, intrapericardial location with accompanying pericardial effusion

Myxoma

- family history of multiple myxomas (Carney complex)
- skin lesions including lentigines and blue naevi (Carney complex)
- constitutional symptoms
- embolic phenomenon
- echocardiographic features: usually a pedunculated solitary mass attached to the endocardial surface of the atrium (most commonly the left atrium), may be smooth or irregular multiple villi, may appear heterogeneous with cystic areas and calcifications, mobile and may prolapse through the mitral valve during diastole

Haemangiomas

- cutaneous haemangiomas and haemangiomas involving other organs
- evidence of Kasabach-Merritt syndrome
- echocardiographic features: an echogenic mass with echolucencies, Doppler colour flow mapping reveals increased vascularity

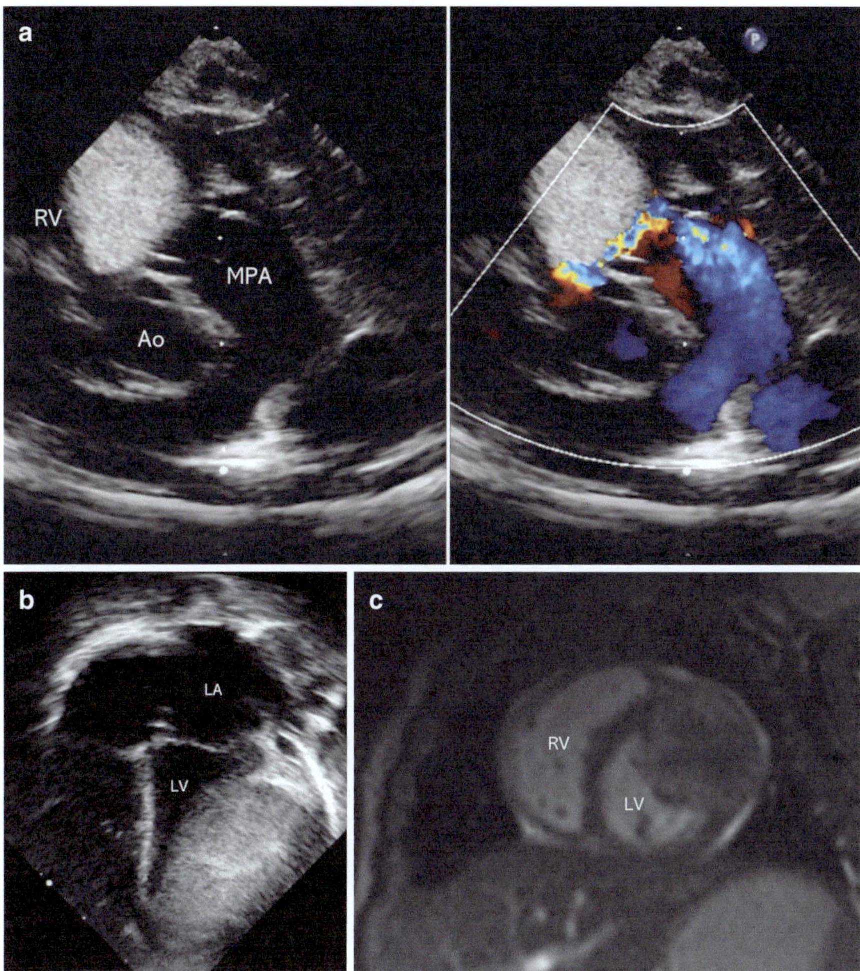

Fig. 45.1 Echocardiographic imaging of cardiac tumours. (**a**) 2D (left panel) and colour flow mapping (right panel) echocardiography showing a large solitary cardiac rhabdomyoma (confirmed by histology) obstructing the right ventricular outflow (**b**) Echocardiographic demonstration of a large solitary fibroma in the left ventricle in an infant (**c**) Cardiac magnetic resonance imaging of this solitary cardiac fibroma. *Ao* aorta, *MPA* main pulmonary artery, *LA* left atrium, *LV* left ventricle, *RV* right ventricle

Pericardial Diseases

46

The pericardium has two layers, a serous visceral layer and a fibrous parietal layer, which enclose the pericardial space with a small amount of serous fluid. Diseases of the pericardium in children include pericarditis with or without pericardial effusion and constrictive pericarditis. Pericarditis can also occur in the presence of myocarditis and is referred to as myopericarditis (when pericarditis is the predominant involvement) or perimyocarditis (when myocarditis is the predominant involvement).

46.1 Pericarditis

Inflammation of the pericardium is the most common pericardial disease. It can be acute, chronic (lasting for >3 months), or recurrent (after a symptom-free period of 4 to 6 weeks or longer from an episode of acute pericarditis) in nature.

46.1.1 Acute Pericarditis

46.1.1.1 Aetiologies

Acute inflammation of pericardium in children can be idiopathic or related to an underlying condition ((Table 46.1). Pericarditis and other cardiovascular sequelae related to COVID-19 infection and mRNA COVID-19 vaccination are discussed in Chap. 61.

Y.-f. Cheung, *Congenital and Paediatric Acquired Heart Disease in Practice*,
https://doi.org/10.1007/978-981-99-2862-0_46

Table 46.1 Causes of acute pericarditis

Category	Condition
Idiopathic	
Infections	Viral (including COVID-19) Bacterial Mycobacterial Fungal
Inflammatory conditions	Autoimmune disorders of connective tissue post pericardiotomy syndrome
Malignancy and its treatment	Primary or secondary malignancies radiation-induced
Others	Uraemia Hypothyroidism Post mRNA COVID-19 vaccination

46.1.1.2 Clinical Presentations and Findings

In infants and young children, the presentation is nonspecific and may include irritability, decreased feeding, and unexplained tachycardia. In older children and adolescents, the characteristic symptom is acute onset of sharp retrosternal pain that worsens with inspiration and improves with leaning forward. The typical finding on examination is a pericardial rub, best heard during inspiration but may disappears with accumulation of significant amount of pericardial fluid. Other symptoms, in particular fever, and signs of underlying conditions may be present.

46.1.1.3 Diagnosis

Initial investigations should include blood workup (white cell count and inflammatory markers), electrocardiographic assessment of PR and ST segment changes, and echocardiographic evaluation of pericardial effusion. Routine viral studies may not be warranted as the yield is low. Additional investigations to identify the underlying aetiology depend on the clinical presentation and suspicion.

The diagnostic criteria based on the 2015 European Society of Cardiology guidelines are shown in Box 46.1.

Box 46.1 Diagnostic Criteria of Acute Pericarditis

Inflammatory pericardial syndrome to be diagnosed with at least 2 of the 4 following criteria

- pericardial chest pain
- pericardial rub
- new widespread ST-elevation or PR depression on ECG
- pericardial effusion

Additional supporting findings

- elevation of markers of inflammation (CRP, ESR, white cell count)
- evidence of pericardial inflammation by imaging (CT, MRI)

46.1.1.4 Management Strategy

The management strategy includes (1) identification and treatment of underlying conditions, (2) monitoring the development and treatment of pericardial effusion, and (3) symptomatic relief of pain.

For symptomatic treatment, non-steroidal anti-inflammatory drugs (NSAIDs) (ibuprofen, naproxen, indomethacin, aspirin) are commonly prescribed until complete resolution of symptoms. Aspirin should be prescribed with caution due to the associated risk of Reye syndrome. Steroid is indicated in patients with underlying autoimmune disorders of connective tissue disease. In other children, steroid has been used conventionally when the response to NSAIDs is unsatisfactory. Recently, colchicine has been incorporated in the management algorithm as an adjunct second line therapy in children with acute pericarditis.

The recognition and management of severe pericardial effusion is described in the section on postoperative pericardial effusion (Chap. 60).

46.1.2 Recurrent Pericarditis

46.1.2.1 Diagnosis

Recurrent pericarditis is diagnosed when symptoms and signs of pericarditis recur after a symptom-free period of 4 to 6 weeks or longer from the first episode of acute pericarditis. While a recurrence rate of 15% to 30% has been reported in adults, recurrence in children is much less frequent. Furthermore, the symptoms and signs may be less florid than those during the initial episode of acute pericarditis.

46.1.2.2 Management Strategy

Treatment of identifiable underlying aetiology as listed in Table 46.1. Non-steroidal anti-inflammatory drugs remain the mainstay of treatment. The addition of colchicine is recommended to improve the treatment response. Further addition of steroid may be considered if the response is incomplete. For patients who are refractory to these agents, discussion with immunologists on the use of immunomodulatory medications including azathioprine, cyclophosphamide, methotrexate, intravenous immunoglobulin, or anakinra (interleukin-1 receptor antagonist) is warranted. In difficult cases, pericardiectomy may be required.

46.2 Constrictive Pericarditis

Constrictive pericarditis occurs when the pericardium thickens with loss of elasticity, which limits the filling of the ventricle during diastole. The term 'constrictive pericarditis' may not be the most accurate description of the condition as inflammation of the pericardium is typically not evident at the time of diagnosis.

46.2.1 Aetiologies

Constrictive pericarditis can be idiopathic or related to previous disease processes that damage the pericardium (Table 46.2).

Table 46.2 Causes of constrictive pericarditis

Category	Condition
Idiopathic	
Infections	Tuberculous Bacterial Viral
Autoimmune disease	Connective tissue disease
Post interventions	Cardiac surgery Radiation-induced

46.2.2 Pathophysiology

The thickened and inelastic pericardium limits volume expansion of the ventricles during diastole and prevents transmission of the normal inspiratory decrease in intrathoracic pressure to the cardiac chambers.

The haemodynamic consequences of constrictive pericarditis are (1) increased filling pressures of all cardiac chambers, (2) increased systemic venous and pulmonary venous pressures, (3) preferential early diastolic filling of the ventricles with little or no late diastolic filling, (4) shifting of ventricular septum to the left during diastole when the right ventricle fills, and (5) failure of the left ventricular diastolic pressure to fall concurrently with the pressure in the pulmonary veins (the latter not enclosed in the pericardial cavity) during diastole, which reduces pulmonary vein-to-left ventricular pressure gradient and left ventricular filling. These contribute to the clinical picture of systemic venous congestion and reduced cardiac output.

46.2.3 Clinical Presentation and Findings

History and examination may reveal an underlying aetiology. The clinical manifestations of constrictive pericarditis reflect the consequences of systemic venous congestion, increased right ventricular filling pressures, and reduced cardiac output. Symptoms include poor growth, easy fatigue, shortness of breath on exertion, and facial and ankle swelling. Signs of systemic venous congestion and fluid retention include ankle oedema, pleural effusion, ascites, and hepatomegaly. Arterial and venous pulse examination reveals pulsus paradoxus and elevated jugular venous pressure without showing decrease during inspiration (Kussmaul sign), respectively.

46.2.4 Investigations

The investigations aim to diagnose the condition and to differentiate it from restrictive cardiomyopathy.

CXR: The cardiac silhouette is usually normal. Pericardial calcification may be present but is uncommon. Pleural effusion may be evident.

ECG: Nonspecific ST and T wave abnormalities and low voltages may be present. Atrial fibrillation occurs in severe constrictive pericarditis.
Echocardiography: Echocardiography is essential in the initial assessment of patients with suspected constrictive pericarditis (Box 46.2).

Box 46.2 Echocardiographic Assessment of Constrictive Pericarditis

Two-dimensional echocardiography
- thickening of pericardium (may be difficult to identify)
- mild to moderate enlargement of both atria
- dilated inferior caval vein and hepatic veins
- septal bouncing during early diastole (initially towards and then away from the left ventricle)
- leftward shifting of ventricular septum during inspiration

Doppler and tissue Doppler echocardiography
- predominance of early diastolic filling (E velocity) and short deceleration time
- significant respiratory variation: >40% increase in tricuspid E velocity during inspiration, ≥25% increase in transmitral E velocity during expiration
- reversed mitral lateral to medial mitral annular early diastolic tissue velocity (e') ratio (normally lateral e' > septal e')
- increased hepatic venous flow reversal with expiration

Strain imaging
- normal left ventricular global longitudinal strain (reduced in restrictive cardiomyopathy)

CT and CMR: These provide information on pericardial thickening and calcification and other features of constrictive pericarditis (dilation of inferior caval vein and hepatic veins, ventricular interdependence). The presence of pericardial thickening is, however, not a prerequisite for diagnosis of constrictive pericarditis.
Cardiac catheterization: Cardiac catheterization provides the gold standard assessment of the characteristic haemodynamics in constrictive pericarditis (Box 46.3).

Box 46.3 Cardiac Catheterization Findings in Constrictive Pericarditis

- increased right and left atrial and ventricular end-diastolic pressures
- increased systemic and pulmonary venous pressures
- prominent y descent of venous and atrial pressure tracings
- square root sign in the left and right ventricular diastolic pressure tracings: early diastolic dip (corresponds to increased early diastolic filling) followed by a plateau (lack of additional filling during the mid and late diastole)
- ventricular pressure discordance during respiration: during inspiration, right ventricular pressure increases while left ventricular pressure decreases
- a bolus of volume expansion may be required in dehydrated patients to unmask the abnormalities highlighted above

46.2.4.1 Differentiation Between Constrictive Pericarditis and Restrictive Cardiomyopathy

Children with constrictive pericarditis present in a similar fashion as restrictive cardiomyopathy clinically with symptoms and signs of systemic venous congestion and heart failure. Features that help to differentiate between the two conditions are shown in Table 46.3.

46.2.5 Management Strategy

Diuretics provide symptomatic relief of the congestive symptoms. In patients with mild pericardial constriction, diuretics and a trial of anti-inflammatory medications may be considered. Pericardiectomy is the definitive treatment for symptomatic patients. It may, however, be challenging in the presence of extensive adhesion and is relatively contraindicated in patients with severe radiation-induced constrictive pericarditis due to extensive pericardial adhesion and concomitant myocardial damage.

Table 46.3 Constrictive pericarditis versus restrictive cardiomyopathy

Parameter	Constrictive pericarditis	Restrictive cardiomyopathy
Clinical signs		
Pulsus paradoxus	Present	Absent
Kussmaul sign	Present	Present
JVP waveform	Prominent x and y descent	Prominent y descent with blunted x descent
Echocardiographic parameters		
Pericardial thickness	Increased in some	Normal
Septal bouncing	Present	Absent
Significant respiratory variation in transmitral and transtricuspid (opposite direction) E velocity	Present	Minimal
Colour M-mode flow propagation	Normal	Decreased
Early diastolic Doppler tissue velocity e' at mitral annulus	Normal or increased	Normal or decreased
Reversed mitral lateral to medial mitral annular e' ratio	Present	Absent
Left ventricular global longitudinal strain	Normal	Reduced
Hepatic venous flow	Reversal of forward flow during expiration	Reversal of forward flow during inspiration
CT/CMR findings		
Thickened pericardium	Present in some	Absent
Late gadolinium enhancement (CMR)	May be pericardial enhancement	Myocardial enhancement in some
Cardiac catheterization findings		
Ventricular pressure discordance during respiration	Present	Absent
RV versus LV end-diastolic pressure (EDP)	Equal	LVEDP usually higher RVEDP
Square root sign	Present	Present

Part X

Acquired Heart Disease

47 Kawasaki Disease

Kawasaki disease (KD) is the commonest acquired heart disease in children in developed countries. It is an acute vasculitis involving medium-sized arteries with systemic inflammation of multiple organs and tissues. This condition, primarily affecting infants and young children, was first described in Japan by Dr. Tomisaku Kawasaki in 1967. Termed initially as mucocutaneous lymph node syndrome due to features of prolonged fever with skin rash and lymphadenopathy, this condition subsequently become known as Kawasaki disease.

47.1 Epidemiology

Kawasaki disease occurs most commonly in young children aged 1 to 2 years, and 80% of patients are younger than 4 years of age. The male to female ratio is about 1.5:1. Although KD occurs worldwide, it is most prevalent in Asian countries, especially in Japan (Table 47.1). The recurrence rate of KD is about 3% to 4% in Japan, and 1% to 2% in North America.

Table 47.1 Reported incidence of Kawasaki disease (per 100,000 < 5 years old)

East		West	
Japan	308	US	25
South Korea	190–220	Canada	20
China	70–120	Australia	9
Taiwan	83	Europe	6–18

Y.-f. Cheung, *Congenital and Paediatric Acquired Heart Disease in Practice*, https://doi.org/10.1007/978-981-99-2862-0_47

Table 47.2 Genes implicated in susceptibility to KD

Gene	Chromosomal location	Function
FCGR2A	1q23	Receptor for IgG Fc fragment, alleles stratify individuals into either strong or weak responders to IgG subclasses and influence clinical phenotypes of infection and inflammation
CASP3	4q34–35	Protease involved in cellular (immune cells and cardiomyocytes) apoptosis
HLA class II	6p21.3	Antigen presentation to T helper cells
BLK	8p23–22	Encodes B-lymphoid tissue kinase that transduces signals downstream of B-cell receptor
ITPKC	19q13.2	Kinase for inositol trisphosphate, acts as a negative regulator of calcineurin/NFAT pathway in T cells
CD40	20q12–13.2	Receptor for CD30 ligand, expressed in antigen-presenting cells, risk alleles associated with increased CD40 ligand cell surface expression and increased serum levels of soluble CD40L in acute phase of KD

47.2 Aetiology and Genetics

Despite intensive research works, the cause of KD remains unknown. Current evidence suggests an immune response, which involves both the innate and adaptive immunity, to a classic yet unidentified antigen.

Several observations suggest genetic influence on predisposition to development of KD: (1) higher incidence of KD in Japanese children and in children of Japanese descent living outside of Japan, (2) an increased likelihood (two-fold increase) of history of KD among parents of a KD patient, and (3) increased incidence among siblings of KD patients (ten-fold increase in relative risk). Genes implicated in susceptibility to KD are shown in Table 47.2.

47.3 Vasculitis and Systemic Inflammatory Processes

Inflammatory damage to the coronary arteries during the acute phase of KD has the most significant impact on long-term outcomes. Coronary arteritis begins about 1 week after disease onset with infiltration of neutrophils, lymphocytes, and macrophages. Severe necrotizing arteritis may damage all three arterial layers and lead to aneurysm formation in the second week of the illness. Rapidly enlarging aneurysms are at risk of rupture and thrombosis. Subacute vasculitis with cellular infiltration may end by the fourth week but may also persist as chronic vasculitis for years. A recently proposed KD arteriopathy model further suggests a luminal myofibroblastic proliferative process that leads to progressive arterial stenosis in the long term.

Structural damage of coronary artery can lead to flow disturbance and endothelial dysfunction. Turbulent flow with energy loss, decreased shear stress, and endothelial dysfunction predispose to thrombus formation within the coronary artery aneurysms.

The inflammatory process also involves other organs and tissues (Box 47.1).

Box 47.1 Systemic Involvement in KD

- lymph nodes: lymphadenopathy
- heart: myocarditis, pericarditis, valvulitis
- lung: interstitial pneumonitis
- gastrointestinal tract: abdominal pain, vomiting, diarrhoea
- liver: hepatitis, hydrops of gallbladder
- pancreas: pancreatitis
- urinary tract: pyuria
- meninges: irritability, aseptic meningitis

47.4 Diagnosis

47.4.1 Classic KD

Classic KD is diagnosed based on clinical criteria (2017 American Heart Association Scientific Statement): (1) fever for at least 5 days (although diagnosed sometimes with only 3 to 4 days of fever) with (2) at least 4 of the 5 of the principal clinical features (Box 47.2).

Box 47.2 Principal Clinical Features of KD

- erythema and cracking of lips, strawberry tongue, and/or erythema of oral and pharyngeal mucosa
- bilateral bulbar conjunctival injection without exudate
- rash: maculopapular, diffuse erythroderma, or erythema multiforme-like
- erythema and oedema of the hands and feet in acute phase and/or periungual desquamation in subacute phase
- cervical lymphadenopathy (≥1.5 cm diameter), usually unilateral

Based on the revised Japanese Circulation Society/Japanese Society for Cardiovascular Surgery 2020 guideline, diagnosis is made clinically when 5 of the 6 criteria are met. The guideline stated that the absolute number of days of fever is not essential and incorporated redness at the BCG (Bacille Calmette-Guérin) inoculation site under the feature of skin rash.

Important differential diagnosis with features of fever, skin rash, and systemic inflammation should be considered and excluded (Box 47.3). Multisystem inflammatory syndrome in children (MIS-C), a new entity recognized during the COVID-19 pandemic with features similar to KD or KD shock syndrome, is discussed in Chap. 61.

Box 47.3 Differential Diagnosis of KD

- viral infections: adenovirus, enterovirus, Ebstein-Barr virus, measles, COVID-19
- bacterial infections: scarlet fever, toxic shock syndrome
- rheumatic conditions: systemic onset juvenile idiopathic arthritis, polyarteritis nodosa
- drug hypersensitivity reactions including Stevens-Johnson syndrome
- other conditions in endemic areas: Rocky mountain spotted fever, leptospirosis

47.4.2 Incomplete KD

Incomplete KD should be considered in infants and children having prolonged fever without explanation, <4 of the principal clinical features, clinical features consistent with KD (Box 47.2), and supportive laboratory and/or echocardiographic findings. The algorithm based on the 2017 American Heart Association Scientific Statement is shown in Fig. 47.1.

47.4.3 Kawasaki Disease Shock Syndrome

Kawasaki disease shock syndrome is defined by the presence of hypotension or clinical signs of poor perfusion. Its incidence is estimated to be about 7%. Clues that suggest KD shock syndrome as the diagnosis rather than other causes of shock (e.g. toxic shock syndrome, septic shock) include the presence of thrombocytosis, a younger age, and echocardiographic findings of coronary arterial abnormalities.

The pathogenesis of KD shock syndrome may be related to myocardial dysfunction and release of inflammatory cytokines that decreases peripheral vascular resistance and increases capillary leak. This mode of KD presentation is associated with more severe systemic inflammation, resistance to intravenous immunoglobulin therapy, and greater risk of coronary arterial complications.

47.4.4 Diagnostic Red Herring

The constellation of certain clinical and laboratory features of KD patients at presentation constitutes diagnostic red herring (Table 47.3). As other features of KD unveil with time together with the lack of response to conventional antibiotic treatment, the correct diagnosis of KD may become apparent. Features that help to distinguish KD from MIS-C are discussed in Chap. 61.

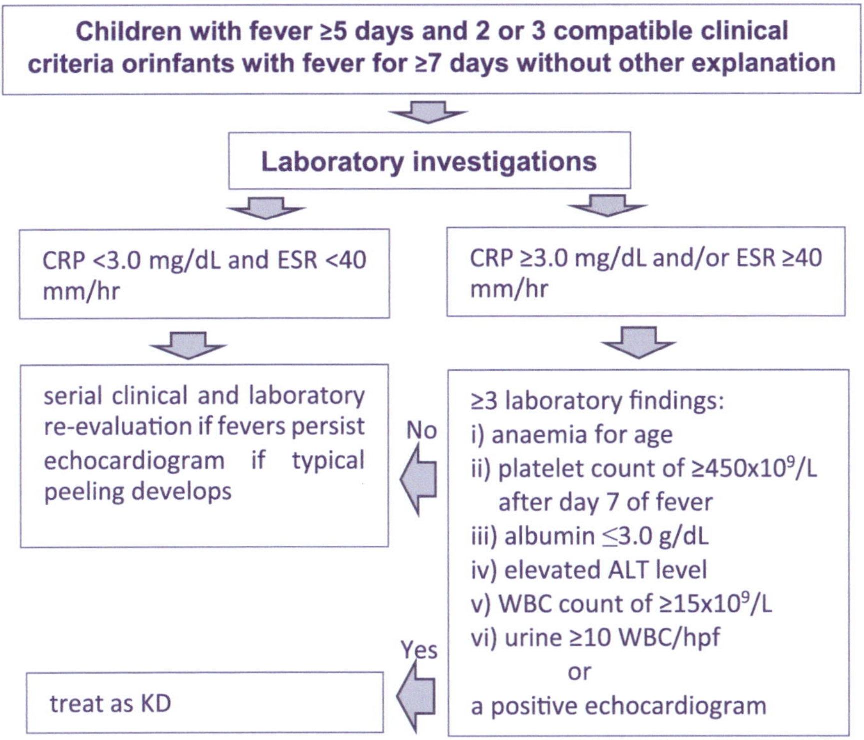

Children with fever ≥5 days and 2 or 3 compatible clinical criteria orinfants with fever for ≥7 days without other explanation

↓

Laboratory investigations

↓ (left branch)

CRP <3.0 mg/dL and ESR <40 mm/hr

↓

serial clinical and laboratory re-evaluation if fevers persist echocardiogram if typical peeling develops

↓ (right branch)

CRP ≥3.0 mg/dL and/or ESR ≥40 mm/hr

↓

≥3 laboratory findings:
i) anaemia for age
ii) platelet count of ≥450x10^9/L after day 7 of fever
iii) albumin ≤3.0 g/dL
iv) elevated ALT level
v) WBC count of ≥15x10^9/L
vi) urine ≥10 WBC/hpf
or
a positive echocardiogram

No → serial clinical and laboratory re-evaluation if fevers persist echocardiogram if typical peeling develops

Yes → treat as KD

Fig. 47.1 Evaluation of suspected incomplete Kawasaki Disease. (Adopted from McCrindle et al. Circulation. 2017;135:e927–e999). *CRP* C reactive protein, *ESR* erythrocyte sedimentation rate, *hpf* high power field, *WBC* white blood cell

Table 47.3 Diagnostic red herring

Presentation	Initial presumptive diagnosis
Fever and pyuria in infants and young children	Urinary tract infection
Fever and irritability in infants with pleocytosis of cerebrospinal fluid	Aseptic meningitis or partially treated meningitis
Fever with enlarged cervical lymph mode	Lymphadenitis (rarely suspicion of Ludwig angina)
Development of skin rash and red eyes after empirical antibiotic treatment	Drug allergy
Shock-like picture with fever and skin rash	Staphylococcal or streptococcal toxic shock syndrome Bacterial sepsis

Given the paucity of signs of KD in infants, especially in those age < 6 months, echocardiography for assessment of coronary arterial abnormalities should be performed in infants with prolonged unexplained fever and laboratory evidence of systemic inflammation.

47.5 Initial Investigations

Markers of inflammation: Erythrocyte sedimentation rate, C reactive protein, and platelet count are characteristically elevated.
Sepsis workup: Pyuria and increased mononuclear cells in the cerebrospinal fluid (with normal glucose and protein levels) may be found.
Liver function test: Increased serum transaminases, hyperbilirubinaemia, and hypoalbuminaemia may be present.
Electrocardiogram: The changes are non-specific. In patients with myocarditis or pericarditis, ST segment changes and T wave abnormalities may be present.
Echocardiography: Echocardiographic assessment should focus on the imaging of coronary arteries for ectasia or aneurysmal dilation and thrombus formation within giant coronary artery aneurysms (Fig. 47.2a, b). Other echocardiographic evaluation should include the assessment of ventricular function, valvar regurgitation, and pericardial effusion. Mild degree of coronary artery dilation can occur in other childhood febrile conditions (Box 47.4).

Box 47.4 Childhood Febrile Illnesses Associated with Mild Coronary Artery Dilation (z score usually <2.5)

- systemic onset juvenile idiopathic arthritis
- vasculitis: polyarteritis nodosa, Takayasu arteritis
- infection: Epstein Barr virus, Rickettsia typhi, COVID-19

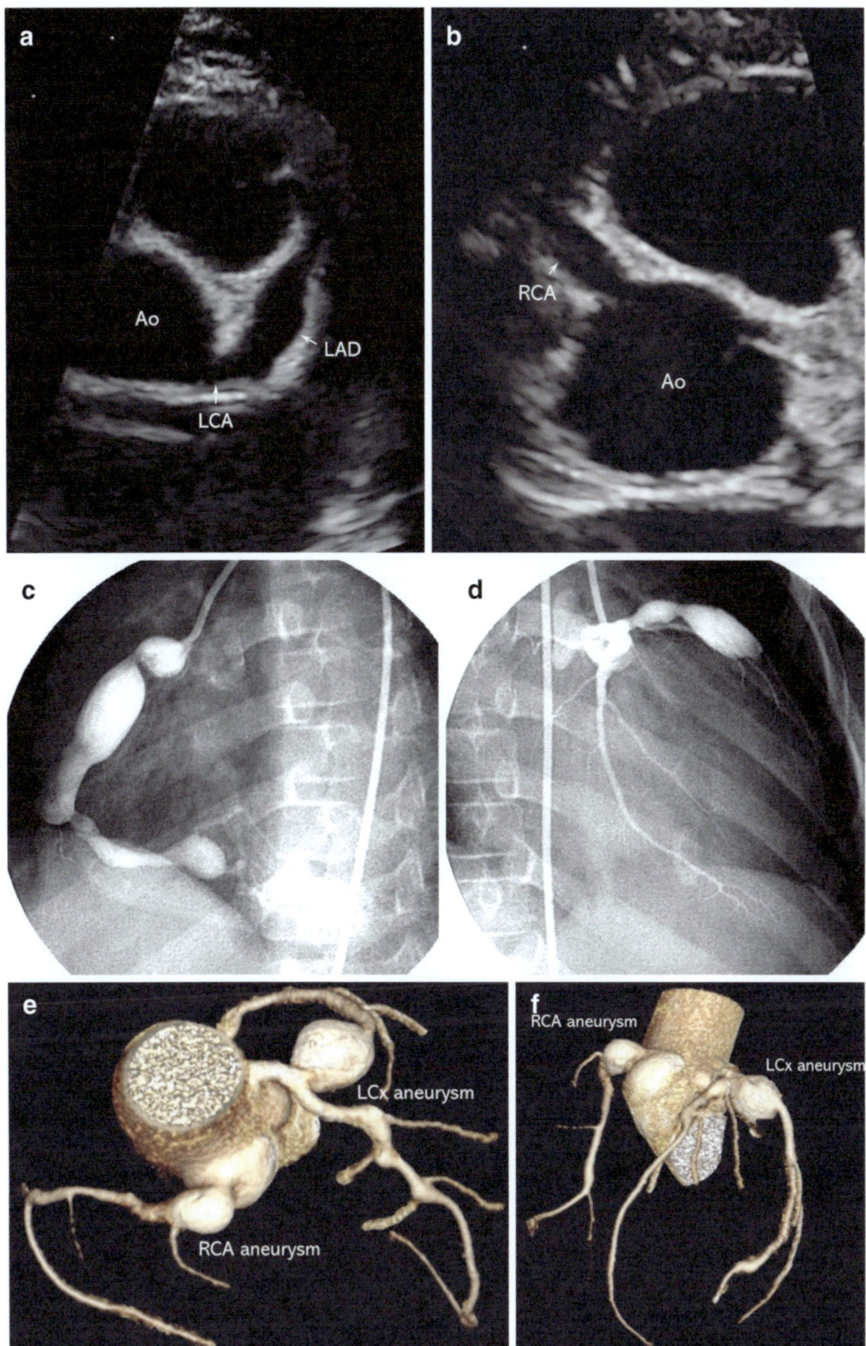

Fig. 47.2 Imaging of coronary artery aneurysms. (**a** and **b**) Echocardiographic (**c** and **d**) angiographic and (**e** and **f**) CT imaging of the right and left coronary artery aneurysms in different patients. *Ao* aorta, *LAD* left anterior descending artery, *LCA* left main coronary artery, *LCx* left circumflex artery, *RCA* right coronary artery

47.6 Acute Management

47.6.1 Initial Treatment

The primary treatment regimen of classic and incomplete KD comprises (1) a single dose of intravenous infusion of immunoglobulin at 2 g/kg given over 10 to 12 h and (2) high dose oral aspirin therapy (Box 47.5).

Box 47.5 Initial Treatment of KD

Intravenous immunoglobulin therapy
- 2 g/kg as a single dose
- given within the first 10 days of illness
- also indicated in patient with delayed diagnosis (later than day 10 of fever) if there is persistent fever, ongoing inflammation (increased ESR or CRP), or documented coronary artery aneurysm(s)

Oral aspirin therapy
- dose varies among centres: 30–50 mg/kg/day or 80–100 mg/kg/day
- duration of high-dose aspirin varies: till afebrile for 48 to 72 h or till day 14 of illness (and afebrile for 48 to 72 h)
- followed by antiplatelet dose of aspirin 3–5 mg/kg/day: to stop if no coronary arterial complications at 6 to 8 weeks of assessment or to continue if coronary arterial abnormalities are present

47.6.2 Management of KD Shock Syndrome

Acute management includes volume expansion, inotropic support, and vasopressors. Differentiation from other causes of shock and correct diagnosis of KD with timely institution of intravenous immunoglobulin is required for the control of inflammation.

47.6.3 Intravenous Immunoglobulin Resistance and Its Management

Resistance to intravenous immunoglobulin treatment, defined as recrudescence or persistence of fever at least 36 h after the end of the intravenous immunoglobulin infusion, occurs about 10% to 20% of patients. Scoring systems to predict resistance to intravenous immunoglobulin treatment and development of coronary arterial complications have been developed by Japanese investigators, but these scores may not apply outside Japan.

Different therapeutic regimens have been used for the management of patients resistant to the initial dose of intravenous immunoglobulin (Box 47.6).

Box 47.6 Regimens Used for Patients with IVIg Resistance

- second dose of 2 g/kg intravenous immunoglobulin
- second dose of intravenous immunoglobulin with prednisolone
- infliximab
- less commonly used regimens: cyclosporin, cyclophosphamide, anakinra, plasma exchange

47.6.4 Risk Stratification Based on Coronary Artery Dimensions

Dimensions of the coronary arteries are normalized for body surface area as z scores (Box 47.7) for risk stratification (Table 47.4).

Box 47.7 Calculation of *z* score of Coronary Arteries

z score = (measured dimension – reference mean)/reference SD

Different formulas are available for calculating z scores (online and app-based z score calculators are available)

These formulas are based on different number of subjects, age range, ethnic groups, methods of calculating body surface area, and regression analysis methods.

Main caveats with implications on management include:

1. same measurement can yield different z scores depending on formula
2. small measurement error may translate into a large difference in z score

Long-term follow-up assessments and management of patients after KD based on the framework proposed in the 2017 American Heart Association Scientific Statement are shown in Fig. 47.3.

Table 47.4 Risk stratification based on coronary artery *z* scores and dimensions based on 2017 American Heart Association Scientific Statement

Coronary arterial abnormality	z score and/or dimension
No involvement	Always <2
Dilation only	2 to <2.5
Small aneurysm	≥2.5 to <5
Medium aneurysm	≥5 to <10 and absolute dimension <8 mm
Large or giant aneurysm	≥10 or absolute dimension ≥8 mm

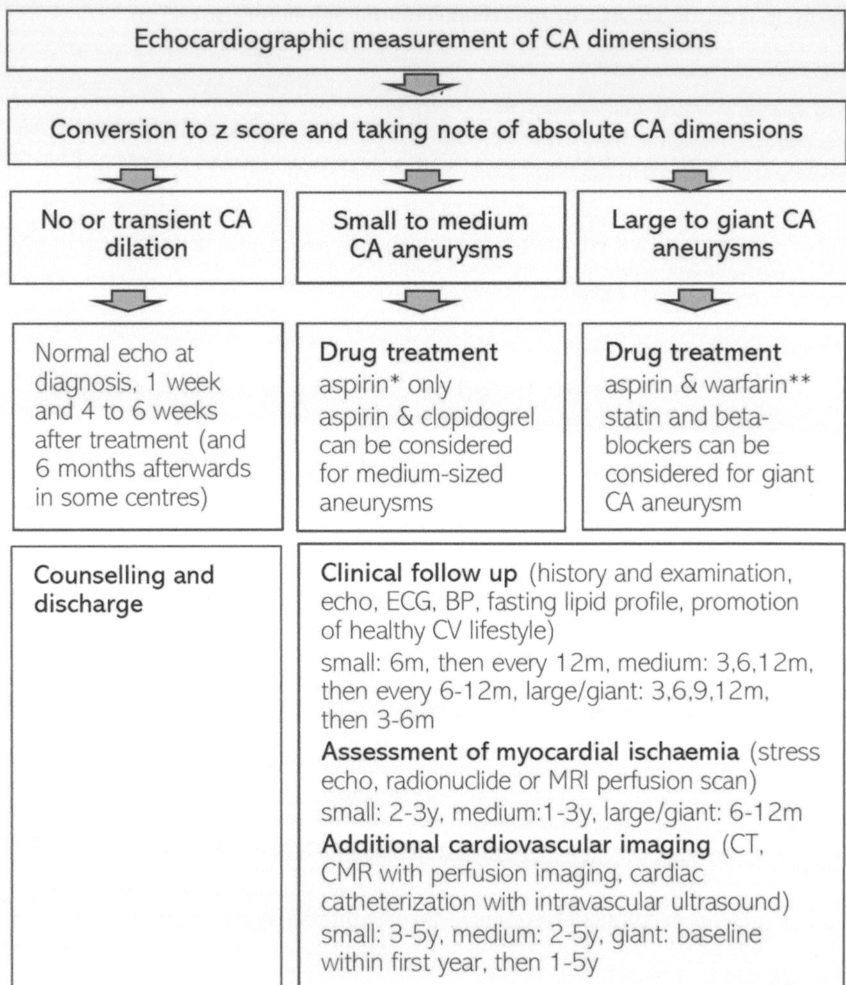

Fig. 47.3 Risk-stratified management of Kawasaki disease based on coronary arterial abnormalities. *dipyridamole if aspirin is to be avoided (e.g. G6PD deficiency). ** warfarin adjustment is difficult in infants and subcutaneous enoxaparin is an alternative. *BP* blood pressure, *CA* coronary artery, *CV* cardiovascular

The focus of long-term monitoring is on coronary arterial complications (Fig. 47.2). Coronary artery aneurysm has been reported to occur in about 25% after KD in the era before the introduction of intravenous immunoglobulin therapy. About 50% to 60% of these patients showed regression of the coronary artery aneurysms. Among patients who have persistent coronary artery aneurysms, a small proportion (about 5%) of patients, especially those with giant coronary artery aneurysms, may develop progressive arterial stenosis and occlusion.

With the introduction of the standard initial treatment with intravenous immunoglobulin and high dose oral aspirin therapy, the rate of coronary artery aneurysm formation has been reduced to less than 5%. Furthermore, the rate of coronary artery aneurysm regression has increased to 75% in the current era.

47.7 Long-Term Management

47.7.1 Medical Thromboprophylaxis

Antiplatelet medications: Aspirin is indicated lifelong in patients with persistent coronary artery aneurysms and should also be considered in those with regressed aneurysms (as endothelial dysfunction may be present). Dual antiplatelet agents (aspirin with clopidogrel) may be considered in patients with medium-sized aneurysms.

Anticoagulation: Warfarin in addition to aspirin is indicated in patients with large or giant aneurysms. Warfarin with dual antiplatelet medications may be considered in patients with large or giant aneurysms together with extensive or distal coronary artery aneurysms. In infants, subcutaneous low molecular weight heparin (enoxaparin) is an alternative as titration of warfarin dose is often difficult.

Statin: Patients with coronary artery aneurysms have dyslipidaemia (lower HDL cholesterol levels) and evidence of low-grade inflammation, increased oxidative stress, and endothelial dysfunction. Statins have the potential beneficial effects of increasing HDL cholesterol, lowering LDL cholesterol, and reducing inflammation, endothelial dysfunction, and oxidative stress and should be considered in patients with coronary artery aneurysms of different sizes.

Beta-blocker: Beta-blockade decreases myocardial oxygen demand. Beta-blockers (e.g. carvedilol, metoprolol) may be considered for KD patients at high risk of myocardial ischaemia due to the presence of large or giant coronary artery aneurysms.

47.7.2 Revascularization

Acute thrombotic occlusion of a coronary artery aneurysm may occur during the acute phase or late after the acute illness in KD patients with coronary artery aneurysms and lead to myocardial infarction and sudden death. In young children, symptoms of myocardial infarction are nonspecific and include irritability, pale looking, vomiting, and shock. Management includes institution of thrombolytic therapy (tissue plasminogen activator) and, in older patients, percutaneous coronary intervention.

Patients with anginal symptoms and documented myocardial ischaemia due to left main coronary artery stenosis or equivalent (with involvement of both the left anterior descending and circumflex arteries) require revascularization. Asymptomatic patients with documented myocardial ischaemia and left main coronary artery involvement (or equivalent) should also be considered for revascularization. Coronary artery bypass graft surgery is usually the intervention of choice for left main coronary artery disease or multivessel coronary artery involvement. Percutaneous coronary intervention may be considered in selected patients with single-vessel disease.

47.8 Counselling

47.8.1 After Treatment of the Acute Illness

General and cardiac aspects: Parents should understand the need of their children to have monitoring for recurrence of fever, further echocardiographic evaluation, and aspirin continued until echocardiographic reassessment at 6 to 8 weeks of illness.
Vaccination: Live attenuated vaccines (including measles and varicella) should be postponed for at least 11 months in patients treated with intravenous immunoglobulin.
Precautions against Reye syndrome: Influenza immunization should be recommended in patients over 6 months of age, especially in those requiring long-term aspirin for coronary aneurysms. Varicella vaccine should also be considered in these patients.

47.8.2 Education of Adolescent Patients

Patients with coronary artery aneurysms require long-term follow up. Education of these patients during their adolescence on their heart condition, the use of cardiac medications, importance of heart-healthy lifestyle, and other issues related to transition to adult care are important (Box 47.8).

Box 47.8 Education of Adolescent KD Patients with Coronary Artery Aneurysms

Cardiac condition

- history of KD and coronary arterial complications
- cardiac events and interventions
- cardiac investigations and results
- recognition of symptoms of myocardial ischaemia or infarction that require urgent medical attention
- cardiac prognosis
- need for lifelong cardiac follow up

Medications

- name and dosages of medications
- reasons for the medications
- the need to monitor anticoagulation (for those taking warfarin)
- drug interactions

Heart-healthy lifestyle

- dietary habits, exercise, alcohol, smoking, obesity, illicit drug use

Transitional issues

- marriage and pregnancy
- predisposition to KD in offspring

Rheumatic Heart Disease

48

Rheumatic heart disease is the leading cause of acquired heart disease causing heart failure in children worldwide but with a skewed distribution. While this condition has almost disappeared in developed countries, as a disease related to poor hygiene and poverty, it poses a major health burden in developing countries.

48.1 Pathogenesis

Acute rheumatic fever follows *Streptococcus pyogenes* (group A *Streptococcus*) infection of the throat and, much less commonly, the skin. The infection precedes onset of acute rheumatic fever by 1 to 5 weeks. This condition is thought to be related to an autoimmune response to *Streptococcus pyogenes* (antigenic or molecular mimicry) in genetically susceptible hosts. Multiple organ systems including the heart, joints, and central nervous system are involved. Recurrent episodes of acute rheumatic fever damage the heart valves and lead to rheumatic heart disease.

48.2 Acute Rheumatic Fever

48.2.1 Clinical Presentation and Findings

Acute rheumatic fever has a peak incidence in children between 5 and 15 years. Symptoms usually appear at about 3 weeks after an episode of group A streptococcal pharyngitis. The streptococcal infection can also be relatively asymptomatic. The clinical presentation is characterized by fever and involvement of multiple organ systems with the heart and the joints being most commonly involved.
Carditis: Carditis occurs in 50% to 70% of patients and is typically a pancarditis. The clinical manifestations are those of pericarditis (chest pain, pericardial rub, pericardial effusion), myocarditis (tachycardia, cardiomegaly, heart failure), and

Y.-f. Cheung, *Congenital and Paediatric Acquired Heart Disease in Practice*, https://doi.org/10.1007/978-981-99-2862-0_48

valvulitis (cardiac murmurs or echocardiographic findings of mitral and aortic regurgitation). Electrocardiogram shows prolongation of PR interval.

Arthritis: Polyarthritis occurs in 60% to 80% of patients. This is characteristically migratory in nature and involves medium and large joints (elbows, wrists, knees, and ankles).

Skin: There are two major skin manifestations: (1) firm and non-tender subcutaneous nodules over the joint extensor surfaces (more commonly observed in patients with carditis), and (2) erythema marginatum, which is a pink, non-pruritic and non-painful rash with pale centre and rounded or serpiginous margins over the trunk and proximal extremities.

Central nervous system: Chorea (Sydenham's chorea or St. Vitus dance) is characterized by abrupt, purposeless, and involuntary movements and is often associated with muscle weakness and emotional lability. It is an uncommon manifestation of acute rheumatic fever and may present late at a few months after streptococcal pharyngitis.

48.2.2 Diagnosis

A definitive diagnostic test for acute rheumatic fever is not available. Diagnosis of acute rheumatic fever is based on the revised Jones criteria. The major revision made in the 2015 AHA Scientific Statement (Gewitz et al. Revision of the Jones criteria for the diagnosis of acute rheumatic fever in the era of Doppler echocardiography. Circulation 2015;131:1806–1818) (1) defined high-risk populations (incidence of acute rheumatic fever >2 per 100,000 school-aged children or all-age rheumatic heart disease prevalence >1 per 1000 population per year), (2) recognized the variability in clinical presentation in these high-risk populations (e.g. lower thresholds for fever and joint manifestations), and (3) included echocardiography for the diagnosis of cardiac involvements.

Diagnosis is made in patients with evidence of preceding group A streptococcal infection (positive throat culture, rapid streptococcal antigen test, or elevated or rising titre of streptococcal antibody) and a combination of major (Table 48.1) and/or minor (Table 48.2) manifestations:

1. initial acute rheumatic fever: 2 major or 1 major plus 2 minor criteria.
2. recurrent acute rheumatic fever: 2 major or 1 major plus 2 minor or 3 minor criteria.

Subclinical carditis refers to echocardiographic evidence of mitral with or without aortic valvar abnormalities. The mitral valve is more commonly involved than the aortic valve. Doppler colour flow echocardiography shows evidence of mitral with or without aortic regurgitation. Morphologic mitral valvar abnormalities include prolapsed or flail leaflets due to chordal rupture, nodularity of leaflet tips and/or mitral annular dilation, while morphologic aortic valvar abnormalities include prolapsed and thickened leaflets and defective coaptation.

Table 48.1 Major manifestations for diagnosis of acute rheumatic fever

Major criteria	
Low-risk populations	Moderate- and high-risk populations
Carditis: clinical and/or subclinical Arthritis: polyarthritis only Chorea Erythema marginatum Subcutaneous nodules	Carditis: clinical and/or subclinical Arthritis: monoarthritis or polyarthritis, polyarthralgia, Chorea Erythema marginatum Subcutaneous nodules

Table 48.2 Minor manifestations for diagnosis of acute rheumatic fever

Minor criteria	
Low-risk populations	Moderate- and high-risk populations
Polyarthralgia Fever (≥38.5 °C) ESR ≥60 mm/h and/or CRP ≥3.0 mg/dL Prolonged PR interval, after accounting for age variability (unless carditis is a major criterion)	Monoarthralgia Fever (≥38 °C) ESR ≥30 mm/h and/or CRP ≥3.0 mg/dL Prolonged PR interval, after accounting for age variability (unless carditis is a major criterion)

48.2.3 Management

Patients with acute rheumatic fever should be managed by (1) treatment of group A streptococcal pharyngitis with penicillin group of antibiotics (see below), regardless of whether or not pharyngitis is still present and even in the absence of a positive throat culture, to eradicate of residual streptococcal carriage of streptococci in the upper respiratory tract, (2) symptomatic treatment of arthritis with aspirin or other nonsteroidal anti-inflammatory drugs for 1 to 2 weeks or longer, (3) medical treatment of heart failure with or without steroid when severe carditis is present, (4) rarely surgical repair of mitral valve when chordal rupture causes severe mitral regurgitation, and (5) if chorea is present, referral to neurologist for consideration of medical treatment (e.g. anticonvulsants).

48.2.4 Prevention

Primary prevention is achieved through diagnosis of group A streptococcal pharyngitis and prompt treatment with penicillin group of antibiotics (phenoxymethylpenicillin or amoxicillin) orally for 10 days or a dose of intramuscular benzathine benzylpenicillin. However, diagnosis and treatment may be not possible in some as about one-thirds of the patients have subclinical infection.

Table 48.3 Guidelines on secondary prophylaxis after acute rheumatic fever (ARF)

Guideline	Recommendations
WHO Expert Consultation Geneva 2004	**Severe valvar disease or after valve surgery**: lifelong prophylaxis **With carditis**: until age 25 years or for 10 years after the last ARF (whichever is longer) **Without carditis**: until age 18 years or for 5 years after the last ARF (whichever is longer)
American Heart Association 2009	**With carditis and residual heart disease**: until age 40 years or for 10 years after last ARF (whichever is longer); lifetime prophylaxis may be needed **With carditis but no residual heart disease**: until age 21 years or for 10 years after last ARF (whichever is longer) **Without carditis**: until age 21 years or for 5 years after last ARF (whichever is longer)
Indian Academy of Paediatrics 2008	**Severe disease or post-intervention patients**: lifelong prophylaxis (may opt to continue until age 40 years) **Healed, mild, or moderate carditis**: until age 25 years or for 10 years after last ARF (whichever is longer) 3.2.: until age 18 years or for 5 years after last ARF (whichever is longer)

Adapted with modifications from Kumar et al. Circulation. 2020:142:e337-e357

Secondary prevention of rheumatic fever with antibiotic prophylaxis is required as acute rheumatic fever frequently recurs with subsequent group A streptococcal pharyngitis and cause rheumatic heart disease. Antibiotic prophylaxis may either be in the form of intramuscular injection of benzathine penicillin G every 4 weeks or oral penicillin V twice daily, although compliance with the latter regimen may be a problem. In patients allergic to penicillin group of antibiotics, sulfadiazine or oral macrolides can be given. Guidelines vary in terms of the duration of secondary prophylaxis, which depends on the severity of carditis and the valvar sequelae (Table 48.3).

48.3 Rheumatic Heart disease

Long-term morbidity and mortality in acute rheumatic fever is related to persistent damage of the valve(s) due to episodes of carditis.

48.3.1 Diagnosis

Rheumatic heart disease is characterized by the persistence of valvar dysfunction following an episode or recurrent episodes of acute rheumatic fever. The valvar lesions include mitral regurgitation (most common), mitral stenosis, mitral regurgitation with stenosis, and mixed mitral and aortic valve disease. Tricuspid and pulmonary valves are rarely involved in the disease process, although functional regurgitation may occur secondary to left-sided valvar disease and pulmonary hypertension. The pathophysiology and clinical findings of these valvar lesions are discussed in Chaps. 14 and 15.

While some of the patients may be diagnosed after an episode of acute rheumatic fever attack, many patients are relatively asymptomatic before the diagnosis of rheumatic heart disease and do not recall history suggestive of acute rheumatic fever. Commonly, patients present in adulthood with shortness of breath on exertion or with complications including atrial arrhythmias, thromboembolism, heart failure, or infective endocarditis.

Echocardiographic features of rheumatic mitral valve abnormalities include thickening and restrictive motion of leaflets, thickening and fusion of chordae, and calcification (Fig. 48.1). Rheumatic aortic valve abnormalities include prolapsed and thickened leaflets and defective coaptation.

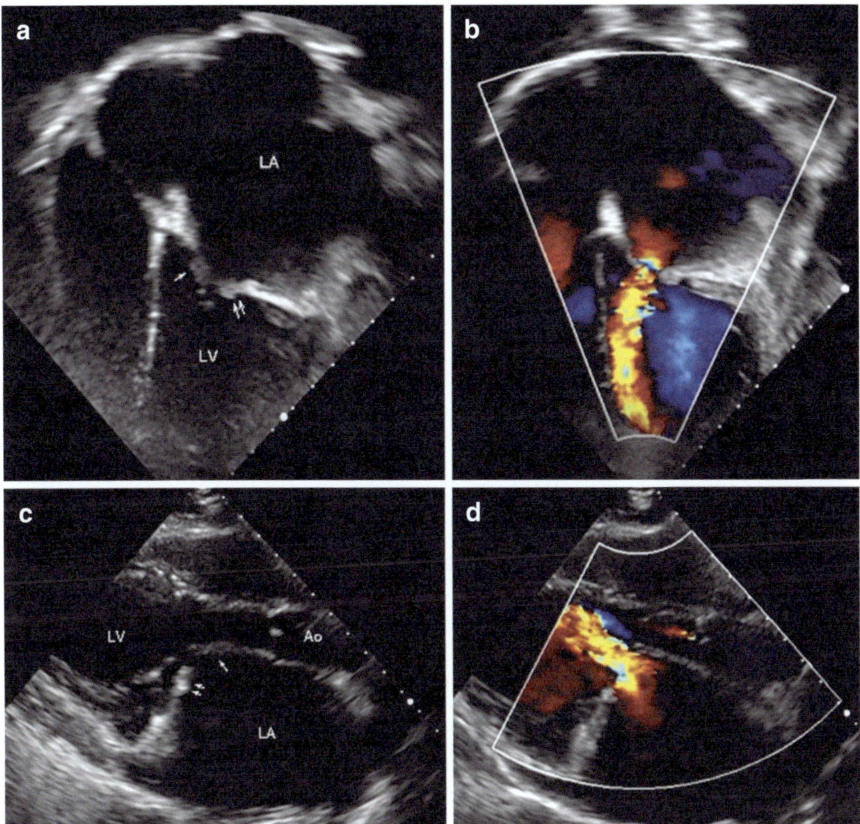

Fig. 48.1 Echocardiographic features of rheumatic valve abnormalities. (**a**) 2D and (**b**) colour Doppler echocardiographic findings from the four-chamber view showing left atrial dilation and severe mitral stenosis due to thickening and restrictive motion of the anterior (single arrow) and posterior (double arrows) mitral valve leaflets (**c**) 2D and (**d**) colour Doppler echocardiographic findings from the parasternal long-axis view showing severe mitral stenosis and mild aortic regurgitation. *Ao* aorta, *LA* left atrium, *LV* left ventricle

48.3.2 Management

Drug treatment has not shown to alter the clinical course of rheumatic heart disease. Medical therapies aim to manage its complications including atrial arrhythmias, thromboembolism, heart failure, or infective endocarditis. Although the current guidelines in developed countries do not recommend antibiotic prophylaxis for patients with rheumatic heart disease, it remains debatable whether these guidelines can be applied similarly to developing countries.

Surgical and transcatheter interventions are indicated in symptomatic patients with severe valve lesions. These include mitral valve repair whenever possible or replacement if necessary for severe mitral regurgitation, mitral balloon valvoplasty for mitral stenosis, and aortic valve repair or replacement or Ross procedure for severe aortic regurgitation. The health care resources, patient education, and issues related to adherence to drug regimen and long-term monitoring in developing countries need to be taken into consideration when deciding on the choice of management.

Infective Endocarditis 49

Infective endocarditis is inflammation of the endocardial lining of the heart, valves, and great arteries caused by infection. Congenital heart defects in children in developed countries and rheumatic heart disease in those in developing countries are the predominant underlying causes of infective endocarditis. Infective endocarditis occurs also in association with indwelling central venous catheters. However, in about 8% to 10% of infective endocarditis in children, no underlying structural heart disease or other risk factors can be identified. Despite improvement in medical care, the mortality rate of infective endocarditis remains high at 5% to 10%.

49.1 Infective Endocarditis

49.1.1 Pathogenesis

The pathogenesis of infective endocarditis is believed to involve (1) damage or denudation of the endothelium, (2) deposition of platelet and fibrin to form nonbacterial thrombotic endocarditis as a nidus, and (3) adherence of bacteria (via adhesins expressed on Gram positive cocci) or fungus in the blood stream to this nidus and followed by proliferation of the bacteria or fungus.

Cardiac endothelium can be damaged or denuded by turbulent blood flow or foreign bodies (e.g. catheters, pacing wire). Cardiac lesions with the highest risk are those that generate high-velocity jets of blood flow (e.g. flow through a ventricular septal defect or across a stenotic valve) and those after repair with foreign materials in close proximity to the highly turbulent flow due to residual lesions. Central venous catheters or pacing wires may rub against the endothelium and damage or interfere with tricuspid valve function to generate turbulent tricuspid regurgitant flow.

Y.-f. Cheung, *Congenital and Paediatric Acquired Heart Disease in Practice*, https://doi.org/10.1007/978-981-99-2862-0_49

Seeding of bacteria into the bloodstream may occur in the following situations: (1) daily activities including chewing of food, toothbrushing, and dental flossing are believed to account for most of the bloodstream seeding, (2) dental procedures that involve manipulation of the gingival or periapical region of teeth or perforation of the oral mucosa cause transient viridans group streptococcal bacteraemia, and (3) in patients with venous catheters or pacing device, entry of bacteria at the skin site or direct infection of the device.

49.1.2 Aetiologic Organisms

The principal pathogenic agents are bacteria, most of which are Gram-positive cocci. The main pathogenic agents are viridans group streptococci, *Staphylococcus aureus*, and *Enterococcus* species. Less common agents are the HACEK group of fastidious Gram-negative bacteria (*Haemophilus parainfluenzae, Haemophilus aphrophilus, Haemophilus paraphrophilus, Actinobacillus actinomycetemcomitans, Cardiobacterium hominis, Eikenella* species, and *Kingella kingae*), other streptococci, and fungus. Rarely, *Coxiella burnetii*, *Brucella*, *Legionella, Bartonella*, and *Chlamydia* are causes of culture-negative endocarditis.

49.1.3 Clinical Presentation and Findings

Children with infective endocarditis present usually with low grade prolonged fever and general complaints of malaise and easy fatigue. The presence of risk factors (underlying congenital or rheumatic heart disease, presence of indwelling catheters and devices) should prompt the consideration of infective endocarditis as a possible diagnosis. Occasionally, patients may present acutely with swinging fever and a septic picture, and in those with valve damage, with symptoms and signs of heart failure.

Clinical findings include extracardiac and cardiac signs. Extracardiac findings are related to bacteraemia or fungaemia, immune-complex related phenomena, and embolic phenomena and complications, while cardiac manifestations depend on the site of infective endocarditis and the valve damage (Table 49.1).

Table 49.1 Extracardiac and cardiac manifestations of infective endocarditis

Phenomenon	Manifestations
Sepsis	Fever with or without shock, splenomegaly
Immune-complex related and embolic phenomena	Splinter haemorrhage, Osler nodes, Janeway lesions, Roth spots, glomerulonephritis with microscopic haematuria and proteinuria
Valve damage	Murmurs of valvar regurgitation, acute heart failure
Embolic complications	Stroke (ischaemic or haemorrhagic), lung abscess, septic emboli to abdominal viscera (gut, liver, kidney) resulting in abscess and infarct

49.1.4 Diagnosis

Infective endocarditis is diagnosed by the modified Duke criteria based either on pathological or clinical findings (Table 49.2). The major and minor clinical criteria are shown in Tables 49.3 and 49.4, respectively. Molecular diagnostics (e.g. PCR) on surgical specimens may help to identify the organism in culture-negative infective endocarditis.

Table 49.2 Modified Duke criteria

Criteria	Definition
Pathological	Microorganisms: demonstrated by culture or histology in a vegetation, a vegetation that has embolized, or an intracardiac abscess, or Pathological lesions: vegetation or intracardiac abscess present, confirmed by histology showing active endocarditis
Clinical	2 major criteria or 1 major plus 3 minor criteria or 5 minor criteria

Table 49.3 Major clinical criteria for diagnosing infective endocarditis (IE)

Major criteria	Definition
Positive blood culture	1. Typical microorganism from 2 separate blood cultures: (a) Viridans streptococci, *Streptococcus bovis*, HACEK group, *Staphylococcus aureus* or (b) Community-acquired enterococci, in the absence of a primary focus OR 2. Microorganisms consistent with IE from: (a) ≥2 positive blood cultures drawn >12 h apart or (b) all of 3 or a majority of ≥4 separate blood cultures (with first and last sample drawn at least 1 h apart) (c) 1 positive blood culture for *Coxiella burnetii* or antiphase-1 immunoglobulin G antibody titre >1:800
Evidence of endocardial involvement	1. Echocardiographic finding of (a) oscillating intracardiac mass on valve or supporting structures (in the path of regurgitant jets or on implanted material in the absence of an alternative anatomic explanation) or (b) abscess or (c) new partial dehiscence of prosthetic valve OR 2. New onset of valvar regurgitation

Adapted with modifications from Li et al. Clin Infect Dis. 2000;30:633-638

Table 49.4 Minor clinical criteria for diagnosing infective endocarditis (IE)

Minor criteria
1. Predisposing heart condition or intravenous drug use
2. Temperature > 38.0 °C
3. Vascular phenomena including major arterial emboli, septic pulmonary infarcts, mycotic aneurysm, intracranial haemorrhage, conjunctival haemorrhages, and Janeway lesions
4. Immunologic phenomena including glomerulonephritis, Osler nodes, Roth spots, and seropositive for rheumatoid factor
5. Positive blood culture (but does not meet a major criterion) or serological evidence of active infection with organism consistent with IE

Adapted with modifications from Li et al. Clin Infect Dis. 2000;30:633-638

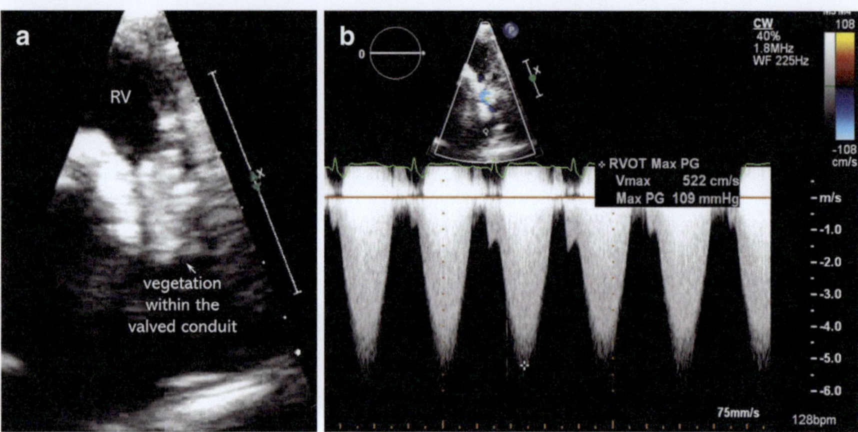

Fig. 49.1 Infective endocarditis involving a right-sided valved conduit. (**a**) Parasternal short-axis view showing a large vegetation in the valved conduit obstructing the right ventricular outflow (**b**) Continuous wave Doppler echocardiography provides an estimation of the pressure gradient across the obstructed conduit

49.1.5 Investigations

Blood culture: Three sets of blood culture are collected within 24 h. An additional 2 to 3 sets of blood culture should be obtained if there is no growth from the initial cultures.

Other blood investigations: Blood tests may show anaemia (due to anaemic of chronic disease or haemolysis), leucocytosis, thrombocytopenia, increased erythrocyte sedimentation rate and C reactive protein, decreased complements, presence of rheumatoid factor, and impaired renal function.

Urine testing: Microscopic haematuria with red cell casts and proteinuria suggest the complication of glomerulonephritis.

Echocardiography: Echocardiogram shows the presence of vegetation (usually in the path of the turbulent jet and adhering to valve or prosthetic materials) and abscess (e.g. aortic root abscess), demonstrates the presence of valvar regurgitation, and enables the assessment of ventricular function (Figs. 49.1 and 49.2). Serial

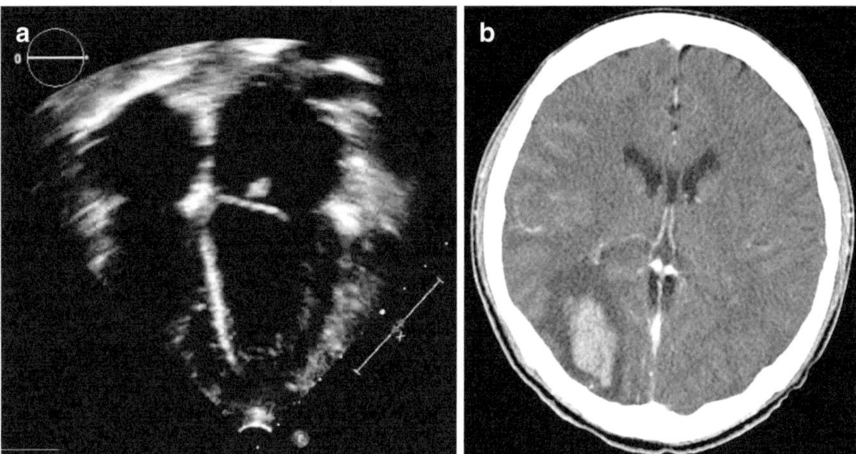

Fig. 49.2 Infective endocarditis involving the mitral valve. (**a**) Apical four-chamber view showing the attachment of a vegetation to the mitral valve leaflet (**b**) Thromboembolism of the left-sided vegetation with development of right cerebral oedema and haematoma in the right parietal-occipital lobe

echocardiographic assessment is indicated to monitor the size of the vegetation, valvar regurgitation, and cardiac function. Transesophageal echocardiography is indicated when transthoracic echocardiographic imaging is unsatisfactory.
ECG: Cardiac arrhythmias including premature beats and complete heart block may occasionally complicate infective endocarditis.

49.1.6 Management Strategy

Antibiotic treatment: Intravenous antibiotic therapy is required for at least 4 weeks and often up to 6 to 8 weeks (Table 49.5). For enteric Gram-negative endocarditis, a duration of at least 6 weeks or more is recommended. Patients with complications may require even longer duration of treatment.
Surgical interventions: Common indications for surgery are persistence of vegetation (especially large vegetation adhered to the mitral valve leaflet) with systemic embolic event, severe mitral or aortic regurgitation leading to acute heart failure, and persistence of bacteraemia despite appropriate antibiotic treatment. Other indications include perivalvar extension causing abscess formation or heart block and fungal endocarditis. The indications for prophylactic surgery to prevent embolic events in children are, however, unclear.

Table 49.5 Antibiotic regimens for infective endocarditis in children

Organism or condition	Recommended antibiotics	Alternative choice of antibiotics
Native valve infection (initial empirical therapy or culture-negative)	Ampicillin/sulbactam plus gentamicin ± vancomycin	Vancomycin plus gentamicin
Endocarditis with vascular cannulae (initial empirical therapy or culture-negative)	Vancomycin plus gentamicin plus cefepime or ceftazidime	
Streptococci (highly sensitive to penicillin)	Penicillin G or ceftriaxone	Vancomycin or ceftriaxone or a first-generation cephalosporin
Streptococci (relatively resistant to penicillin)	Penicillin G plus gentamicin (for first 2 weeks, or whole course for enterococci)	Vancomycin plus gentamicin for enterococci Ampicillin plus ceftriaxone (for aminoglycoside-resistant enterococci) Ceftriaxone plus gentamicin (not for enterococcal endocarditis)
Staphylococci (usually resistant to penicillin G)	Oxacillin or nafcillin ± gentamicin (for 3–5 days)	Vancomycin or a first-generation cephalosporin
Methicillin-resistant *Staphylococcus aureus*	Vancomycin	Daptomycin
Staphylococci with vancomycin resistance or vancomycin intolerance	Daptomycin	
(For staphylococci infection with prosthetic materials)	(Plus rifampicin plus gentamicin for first 2 weeks)	
Gram-negative enteric bacilli	Ceftazidime, cefepime, cefotaxime, or ceftriaxone plus gentamicin (or tobramycin or amikacin)	A broad-spectrum penicillin plus gentamicin (or tobramycin or amikacin)
HACEK group	Ceftriaxone or cefotaxime or ampicillin-sulbactam	Ampicillin plus aminoglycoside
Fungi (*Candida* or *Aspergillus* species)	Surgical resection plus amphotericin B ± flucytosine	If surgery cannot be performed, amphotericin B followed by possibly lifelong imidazole suppression

Adapted with modifications from Baltimore et al. Circulation. 2015;132:1487-1515

49.2 Prevention of Infective Endocarditis

Antibiotic prophylaxis for the prevention of infective endocarditis used to be recommended in a wide spectrum of congenital heart patients undergoing dental and other medical procedures. Nonetheless, the following factors have led to current recommendations that limit the use of prophylactic antibiotics: (1) bacteraemia occurs in daily activities including chewing of food, toothbrushing, and dental flossing cause bacteraemia, (2) estimated risk of infective endocarditis after dental procedures is very low, (3) lack of evidence-based data to demonstrate efficacy of antibiotic prophylaxis, and (4) use of antibiotics may be associated with anaphylaxis, albeit the risk is low, and emergence of bacterial resistance.

The current guidelines are the 2007 American Heart Association (AHA) guideline, 2015 European Society of Cardiology (ESC) guideline, and the NICE (National Institute for Health and Care Excellence) guideline from United Kingdom. Whereas the American Heart Association and the European Society of Cardiology guidelines limit the use of prophylactic antibiotics to patients with the highest risk of infective endocarditis, the NICE guideline recommends that prophylactic antibiotics should not routinely be given to cardiac patients undergoing dental and non-dental procedures.

49.2.1 Counselling and General Recommendations

Patients at high risk of infective endocarditis should be counselled on the followings: (1) symptoms of and predisposing risk factors for infective endocarditis, (2) importance of dental hygiene and the need for regular dental assessment, (3) need for good skin care and timely disinfection of wounds, (4) ear piercing and tattooing are discouraged and, if undertaken, should be performed in sterile condition, and (5) need to seek early consultation and antibiotic treatment for possible bacterial infection. Central and peripheral catheters should be removed early if possible and meticulous line care is required.

49.2.2 High Risk Cardiac Conditions

The current AHA (Wilson et al. Prevention of infective endocarditis: guidelines from the American Heart Association. Circulation. 2007;116:1736–1754) and ESC (Habib et al. 2015 ESC Guidelines for the management of infective endocarditis. Eur Heart J 2015;36:3075–3123) guidelines limit the use of prophylactic antibiotics to patients with cardiac conditions at highest risk of infective endocarditis and who are undergoing at risk procedures (Box 49.1).

Box 49.1 Cardiac Conditions for Which Antibiotic Prophylaxis is Indicated for Patients Undergoing at Risk Procedures

2007 AHA guideline

- prosthetic cardiac valve or prosthetic material used for cardiac valve repair
- previous infective endocarditis
- unrepaired cyanotic congenital heart disease, including palliative shunts and conduits

- completely repaired congenital heart defect with prosthetic material or device whether placed by surgery or by catheter intervention, during the first 6 months after the procedure
- repaired congenital heart disease with residual defects at the site or adjacent to the site of a prosthetic patch or prosthetic device (which inhibit endothelialization)
- cardiac transplantation recipients who develop cardiac valvulopathy

2015 ESC guideline

- patients with any prosthetic valve, including a transcatheter valve, or those in whom any prosthetic material was used for cardiac valve repair
- patients with a previous episode of infective endocarditis
- any type of cyanotic congenital heart disease
- any type of congenital heart disease repaired with a prosthetic material, whether placed surgically or by percutaneous techniques, up to 6 months after the procedure or lifelong if residual shunt or valvular regurgitation remains

Table 49.6 2007 AHA guideline on the need for prophylactic antibiotics

Procedure	Recommendation
Dental procedure	Recommended for procedures involving manipulation of gingival tissue or periapical region of teeth or perforation of oral mucosa No need for the following procedures: routine anaesthetic injections through noninfected tissue, taking dental radiographs, placement of removable prosthodontic or orthodontic appliances, adjustment of orthodontic appliances, placement of orthodontic brackets, shedding of deciduous teeth, and bleeding from trauma to the lips or oral mucosa
Respiratory tract procedure	Reasonable for invasive procedure involving incision of biopsy of the respiratory mucosa (e.g. tonsillectomy and adenoidectomy) No need for bronchoscopy unless the procedure involves incision of the respiratory tract mucosa
Gastrointestinal or urogenital procedures	No need for patients undergoing these procedures, including diagnostic esophagogastroduodenoscopy or colonoscopy
Skin and soft tissue procedure	Recommended for involving infected skin, skin structure, or musculoskeletal tissue

49.2.3 At-Risk Procedures

The AHA (Table 49.6) and ESC (Table 49.7) guidelines provide recommendations on the need for prophylactic antibiotics in high-risk cardiac patients (Box 49.1) undergoing at risk procedures.

Table 49.7 2015 ESC guideline on the need for prophylactic antibiotics

Procedure	Recommendation
Dental procedure	Considered for dental procedures requiring manipulation of gingival or periapical region of teeth or perforation of oral mucosa No need for local anaesthetic injections in non-infected tissues, treatment of superficial caries, removal of sutures, dental X-rays, placement or adjustment of removable prosthodontic or orthodontic appliances or braces or following the shedding of deciduous teeth or trauma to the lips and oral mucosa
Respiratory tract procedure	Not recommended for respiratory tract procedures, including bronchoscopy, laryngoscopy, or transnasal or endotracheal intubation
Gastrointestinal or urogenital procedures or transesophageal echocardiography	Not recommended for gastroscopy, colonoscopy, cystoscopy, vaginal or caesarean delivery or transesophageal echocardiography
Skin and soft tissue procedure	Not recommended for these procedures

Table 49.8 AHA guideline on prophylactic antibiotics for high-risk dental procedures

		Regimen: single dose 30 to 60 min before procedure	
Situation	Agent	Adults	Children
Oral	Amoxicillin	2 g	50 mg/kg
Unable to take oral medication	Ampicillin OR Cefazolin or ceftriaxone	2 g IM or IV 1 g IM or IV	50 mg/kg IM or IV 50 mg/kg IM or IV
Allergic to penicillin or ampicillin—oral	Cephalexin[a, b] OR Azithromycin or clarithromycin OR Doxycycline	2 g 500 mg 100 mg	50 mg/kg 15 mg/kg 2.2 mg/kg (<45 kg) 100 mg (>45 kg)
Allergic to penicillin or ampicillin and unable to take oral medication	Cefazolin or ceftriaxone[b]	1 g IM or IV	50 mg/kg IM or IV

Reprinted with permission Circulation. 2021;143:e963-e978©2021 American Heart Association, Inc.

[a]or other first- or second-generation oral cephalosporin in equivalent adult or paediatric dosing

[b]cephalosporins should not be used in an individual with a history of anaphylaxis, angioedema, or urticaria with penicillin or ampicillin

49.2.4 Prophylactic Antibiotics Regimen

The 2021 AHA (Tables 49.8 and 49.9) and 2015 ESC (Tables 49.10 and 49.11) guidelines also provide recommendations on the choice of prophylactic antibiotics.

Table 49.9 AHA guideline on prophylactic antibiotic for other procedures

Procedure	Antibiotic regimen
Invasive respiratory tract procedure	Contain an agent active against viridans group streptococci or *Staphylococcus aureus* (vancomycin for MRSA)for invasive procedures that involve the incision of respiratory mucosa (e.g. tonsillectomy) or the treatment of an established infection
Gastrointestinal or urogenital procedures	Contain an agent active against enterococci for patients with established gastrointestinal or urogenital tract infection or if antibiotic is indicated to prevent wound infection or sepsis
Skin and soft tissue procedure	Contain an agent active against staphylococci and beta-haemolytic streptococci for infected skin, skin structure, or musculoskeletal tissue

Table 49.10 ESC guideline on prophylactic antibiotics for high-risk dental procedures

		Single dose 30 to 60 min before procedure	
Situation	Antibiotic	Adults	Children
No allergy to penicillin or ampicillin	Amoxicillin or ampicillin[a]	2 g orally or IV	50 mg/kg orally or IV
Allergy to penicillin or ampicillin	Clindamycin	600 mg orally or IV	20 mg/kg orally or IV

[a]alternatively, cephalexin 2 g IV for adults or 50 mg/kg IV for children, cefazolin or ceftriaxone 1 g IV for adults or 50 mg/kg IV for children; cephalosporins should not be used in patients with anaphylaxis, angioedema, or urticaria after intake of penicillin or ampicillin due to cross-sensitivity

Table 49.11 ESC guideline on prophylactic antibiotic for other procedures

Procedure	Antibiotic regimen
Invasive respiratory tract procedure	Contain an anti-staphylococcal drug for a procedure to treat an established infection
Gastrointestinal or urogenital procedures	Contain an agent active against enterococci for patients with established gastrointestinal or urogenital tract infection or if antibiotic is indicated to prevent wound infection or sepsis
Skin and soft tissue procedure	Contain an agent active against staphylococci and beta-haemolytic streptococci for infected skin, skin structure, or musculoskeletal tissue

Cardiovascular Involvement in Systemic Disease

50

Structural cardiac malformations can occur as part of the syndromic disorders with systemic involvement (Chap. 62). The heart may also be affected by systemic disease or by the treatment of systemic disorders.

50.1 Autoimmune Connective Tissue Disorders

Involvements of pericardium, myocardium, endocardium, and cardiac conduction tissues are well documented in autoimmune connective tissue disorders (Table 50.1).

Table 50.1 Cardiac involvements in autoimmune connection tissue disorders

Connective tissue disorders	Cardiac involvements
Systemic lupus erythematosus	Pericarditis Myocarditis Libman-Sacks endocarditis (fibrin clumps with mononuclear cells adherent to the mitral and/or aortic valves) causing valvar regurgitation and/or stenosis Coronary arteritis causing aneurysmal dilation Cardiac arrhythmias (premature beats, atrial arrhythmias, and heart block)
Juvenile idiopathic arthritis	Pericarditis Myocarditis and endocarditis (uncommon) Coronary arterial dilation
Juvenile systemic sclerosis (scleroderma)	Myocardial fibrosis causing cardiomyopathy Fibrosis of conduction tissue Pericardial effusion Pulmonary fibrosis causing pulmonary hypertension and right heart failure
Mixed connective tissue disease	Pericarditis Myocarditis Mitral valve prolapse Intimal hyperplasia of coronary arteries Pulmonary hypertension

Y.-f. Cheung, *Congenital and Paediatric Acquired Heart Disease in Practice*,
https://doi.org/10.1007/978-981-99-2862-0_50

50.2 Cardiorenal Syndrome

Acute or chronic dysfunction of the kidney causes cardiac dysfunction and vice versa. Cardiorenal syndrome refers to this bidirectional functional cross talk between the heart and the kidneys. With regard to the cardiac involvement in children with renal dysfunction, chronic renocardiac syndrome is the most commonly recognized cardiorenal syndrome in children. It is characterized by the occurrence of various cardiovascular morbidities in children with primary chronic kidney disease. The cardiovascular abnormalities include left ventricular hypertrophy, left ventricular diastolic dysfunction, and increased arterial stiffness.

While the pathophysiological mechanism of chronic renocardiac syndrome is unclear, several factors predispose to alteration of myocardium and development of cardiac dysfunction; (1) increased cardiac preload due to salt and water retention, (2) increased afterload and profibrotic effects on the heart due to activation of the renin-angiotensin-aldosterone system and increased systemic arterial stiffness, and (3) increased prevalence of cardiovascular risk factors (hypertension, obesity, dyslipidaemia, chronic anaemia, and chronic inflammation).

50.3 Neuromuscular Disorders

Inherited neuromuscular disorders affect not only skeletal muscle but can also cause cardiomyopathy and/or cardiac arrhythmias. Development and progression of cardiac abnormalities can be dissociated from the development of skeletal myopathy.

Cardiomyopathies (usually dilated cardiomyopathy) occur in different types of neuromuscular disorders: (1) X-linked recessive muscular dystrophies (Duchenne and Becker muscular dystrophies), (2) limb-girdle muscular dystrophies, (3) mitochondrial myopathies (Barth syndrome being associated with either dilated, hypertrophic or noncompaction cardiomyopathy, Friedreich ataxia with hypertrophic cardiomyopathy), (4) myotonic dystrophies (especially nemaline myopathy), (5) congenital myopathies, and (6) myofibrillar myopathies (usually in adulthood).

Cardiac arrhythmias are common in certain types of neuromuscular disorders, notably Duchenne and Becker muscular dystrophies, Emery-Dreifuss dystrophy, certain types of limb-girdle muscular dystrophies, myotonic dystrophy, and mitochondrial myopathies.

Early evaluation with regular echocardiographic and electrocardiographic monitoring and, increasingly, cardiac magnetic resonance before the appearance of cardiac symptoms with institution of medical therapies (angiotensin-converting enzyme inhibitors, beta-blockers, diuretics, and aldosterone antagonists) may have positive impact on long-term outcomes. In patients with Duchenne muscular dystrophy, glucocorticoids may slow the progression of cardiac disease.

50.4 Endocrine Disorders

Infants of mothers with poorly controlled diabetes mellitus have increased risk of having congenital cardiac malformations and hypertrophic cardiomyopathy. The hypertrophic myocardium usually regress within the first few weeks after birth. In babies with shortness of breath due to mild degree of left ventricular diastolic dysfunction and evidence of increased fluid in the lungs, short duration of low dose diuretics and rarely beta-blocker therapy may be required.

Hyperthyroidism causes a high cardiac output state through activation of the sympathetic nervous systemic and direct myocardial stimulation by triiodothyronine (T3) to produce effects similar to those of beta-adrenergic stimulation. High output cardiac failure and tachycardia-induced cardiomyopathy are not commonly encountered in children. The cardiovascular effects are usually reversible with adequate treatment of the thyroid disorder. Congenital hypothyroidism in newborns and hypothyroidism in older children may be associated with sinus bradycardia and pericardial effusion, both of which will resolve with thyroxine replacement.

50.5 Childhood Cancers

Cardiovascular involvements in children with cancers are related to (1) chemotherapeutic agents, (2) radiation therapy, and (3) cardiometabolic risk factors rather to the underlying malignancies.

Among the chemotherapeutic agents used for the treatment of childhood malignancies, anthracyclines are the most notorious agents that cause cardiotoxicity both during the acute phase of treatment and in the long term. Mechanisms of anthracycline-induced cardiotoxicity include oxidative stress, alterations of mitochondrial structure and function, damage to the mitochondria genome through interfering with topoisomerase II-β activity, and reduction in cardiac progenitor cells. Cardiotoxicity is manifested as systolic and/or diastolic dysfunction, prolongation of QT interval, and cardiac arrhythmias. Risk factors for anthracycline-induced cardiotoxicity include higher cumulative dose of anthracyclines, younger age, female sex, concomitant radiation and other chemotherapeutic therapy, and genetic variants that affects anthracycline transport and metabolism. Dexrazoxane, an iron-chelating agent, has been shown to protect against anthracycline-induced cardiotoxicity in childhood leukaemias and other cancers, although there are concerns about the possibility of an increased risk of second malignancies.

Nonanthracycline agents including alkylating agents (cyclophosphamide, ifosfamide), cisplatin, and tyrosine kinase inhibitors are also associated with cardiotoxicity.

Radiation therapy may induce inflammation and fibrosis of the pericardium, myocardium, valves, conduction system, and arteries. Hence, radiation-induced cardiovascular disease includes constrictive pericarditis, restrictive cardiomyopathy, fibrosis of mitral and aortic valves, heart block, and fibrosis and thickening of the aorta, carotid arteries, and pulmonary arteries.

Among long-term childhood cancer survivors, cardiometabolic risk factors for premature atherosclerosis and cardiac dysfunction are prevalent. These survivors are at increased risk of obesity, insulin resistance, dyslipidaemia, hypertension, and among those exposed to cranial radiation or surgery, growth hormone deficiency.

50.6 Inborn Errors of Metabolism

50.6.1 Disorders of Fatty Acid Metabolism

The heart utilizes fatty acids for energy production. Fatty acid beta-oxidation, which takes place in the mitochondria, normally provides up to 70% of ATP production for cardiac contraction. While short- and medium-chain fatty acids can enter the mitochondria directly, long-chain fatty acids are transported by way of the carnitine shuttle cycle. Disorders of fatty acid metabolism can hence be due to carnitine transport defects, disruption of the carnitine shuttle cycle, and fatty acid oxidation defects.

50.6.1.1 Carnitine Transport and Cycle Defects

Carnitine is essential for transferring long-chain fatty acids across the mitochondrial membrane for beta-oxidation and subsequent energy production through fatty acid metabolism.

Carnitine deficiency results in recurrent hypoketotic hypoglycaemia and muscle weakness. Cardiac manifestations include dilated cardiomyopathy (which manifests usually during infancy), hypertrophic cardiomyopathy (apparent usually beyond the first year of age), and cardiac arrhythmias. Carnitine deficiency can be (1) primary due to mutations in *SLC22A5,* which encodes the high-affinity carnitine transporter OCTN2 in the plasma membrane, or (2) secondary to other inherited or acquired metabolic defects (e.g. organic acidaemias, defects of fatty acid oxidation). Oral supplementation with L-carnitine rapidly improves muscle weakness and cardiac function.

Disruption of the carnitine cycle with cardiomyopathy as a clinical manifestation can be related to deficiency of carnitine-acylcarnitine translocase (which transports carnitine and carnitine-fatty acid complexes across the mitochondrial membrane) or carnitine palmitoyltransferase type 2 (which removes the carnitine from the long-chain fatty acyl-CoA).

50.6.1.2 Fatty Acid Oxidation Defects

Fatty acid oxidation defects lead to deficiency of energy production. These autosomal recessive disorders include defects in the beta-oxidation of long-chain fatty acids (e.g. very-long-chain acyl-CoA dehydrogenase and long-chain 3-hydroxyacyl-CoA dehydrogenase deficiencies) and medium- and short-chain fatty acids (e.g. medium-chain acyl-coenzyme A dehydrogenase and multiple acyl-coenzyme A dehydrogenase deficiencies). Patients usually present during infancy and early childhood with clinical manifestations ranging from failure to thrive and mild hypotonia to metabolic crisis (metabolic acidosis, nonketotic hypoglycaemia, hyperammonaemia), cardiomyopathy, skeletal myopathy, hepatomegaly with liver failure, and neonatal death.

50.6.2 Glycogen Storage Diseases

Glycogen storage diseases are caused by inborn errors of glucose and glycogen metabolism. Pathogenic variants in genes encoded for proteins involved in glycogen synthesis, degradation, or regulation result in abnormal storage of glycogen. Depending on the type, the liver, skeletal muscle, or myocardium and cardiac conduction tissues can be affected.

Hypertrophic cardiomyopathy is the main cardiac phenotype. It occurs in several types of glycogen storage disease with also skeletal muscle involvement (muscle weakness, hypotonia): (1) lysosomal acid maltase deficiency (Pompe disease), (2) lysosome-associated membrane protein 2 deficiency (Danon disease), and (3) muscle glycogen synthase deficiency. Cardiac arrhythmias with muscle weakness have been reported in glycogenin-1 deficiency.

50.6.3 Mucopolysaccharidosis

Mucopolysaccharidoses are caused by the deficiency of enzymes involved in the degradation of glycosaminoglycans. Accumulation of partially degraded glycosaminoglycans in the lysosomes causes cellular dysfunction. These lysosomal storage disorders are classified into different types based on the clinical features (soft tissue, skeletal, and/or central nervous system manifestations) and the type of enzyme deficiency. All types of mucopolysaccharidoses, except type II (X-linked), are autosomal recessive disorders.

The myocardium, endocardium, valves, and vessels can be affected by the underlying disorder (Box 50.1). Additionally, severe pulmonary disease with hypoxaemia can result in pulmonary hypertension and right heart failure.

Box 50.1 Cardiovascular Involvements in Mucopolysaccharidoses

- cardiomyopathy
- valvar thickening with regurgitation or stenosis (usually involving the mitral and aortic valves) (Fig. 50.1)
- arterial narrowing (coronary and other systemic arteries)
- aortic root dilation and aneurysms
- cor pulmonale

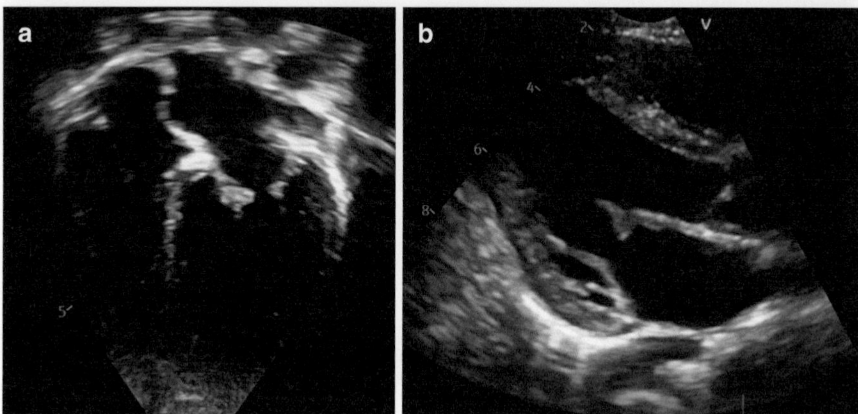

Fig. 50.1 Valve involvement in mucopolysaccharidoses. (**a**) Apical four-chamber and (**b**) parasternal long-axis views showing thickening of the mitral valve leaflets

50.7 Mitochondrial Diseases

Primary mitochondrial diseases are caused by mutations in nuclear and mitochondrial DNA. Multisystem involvement in characteristic in infants and children with primary mitochondrial disease. Clinical manifestations include failure to thrive with feeding problems, neurological abnormalities (hypotonia, seizure, developmental delay or regression, muscle weakness, spasticity, dystonia, and visual and hearing impairment), and cardiac abnormalities (cardiomyopathies, cardiac arrhythmias, and conduction defects). The cardiac involvements in mitochondrial disease encountered during infancy and childhood are shown in Table 50.2.

Table 50.2 Cardiac involvements in mitochondrial disease encountered during infancy and childhood

Mitochondrial disease	Cardiac involvements
Mitochondrial encephalomyopathy, lactic acidosis and stroke-like episodes (MELAS)	Cardiomyopathies (dilated, hypertrophic, restrictive, noncompaction), pre-excitation, first degree heart block
Barth syndrome	Cardiomyopathies (dilated, noncompaction), ventricular arrhythmias coronary arterial dilation
Leigh syndrome	Cardiomyopathies (dilated, hypertrophic), bradycardia, pre-excitation
Myoclonus, epilepsy and ragged red fibres (MERRF)	Cardiomyopathies (dilated, hypertrophic, histiocytic), pre-excitation

Part XI

Critical Care Issues Post Cardiac Surgery

51 Fluid Management

Fluid management of paediatric patients after cardiac surgery is important as fluid overload occurs commonly after cardiac surgery.

51.1 Fluid Overload

Fluid overload occurs after cardiac surgery due to (1) systemic inflammation and capillary leak after cardiopulmonary bypass, (2) acute kidney injury with reduced fluid removal, (3) the need for extra fluid boluses to maintain cardiac output (e.g. in patients with right ventricular dysfunction and those after Fontan operation), and (4) increased release of antidiuretic hormone. Morbidities associated with fluid overload include impaired function of the heart, lungs, and the kidney, prolonged stay in intensive care unit and hospital, and worse overall survival.

51.2 Fluid Management

There are no standard guidelines on the fluid regimens in terms of the type and amount of fluid in the postoperative period for children after cardiac surgery and the practice varies among institutions. Most of the centres adopt different levels of fluid restriction in the first few days after surgery. The calculation of 100% fluid maintenance is shown in Box 51.1.

Y.-f. Cheung, *Congenital and Paediatric Acquired Heart Disease in Practice*, https://doi.org/10.1007/978-981-99-2862-0_51

Box 51.1 Calculation of 100% Fluid Maintenance

Holliday-Segar formula
first 10 kg: 100 mL/kg/day
11–20 kg: 1000 mL + 50 mL/kg (for each kg > 10 kg)/day
>20 kg: 1500 mL + 20 mL/kg (for each kg > 20 kg)/day

Based on body surface area
1500 mL/m^2/day

For cardiac surgery requiring cardiopulmonary bypass, the total fluid intake is usually limited initially to 50% (varies from 25% to 75% among centres) of normal maintenance within the first 24 h of surgery, with gradual increase by 25% per day to 100%. In patients with right ventricular dysfunction and restrictive physiology and in post Fontan patients, the increase per day may be slower and kept at about 75% of maintenance or even less for a longer period of time.

For cardiac surgery not requiring cardiopulmonary bypass, total fluid intake is usually limited initially to 75% (50% in some centres) of normal maintenance within the first 24 h, with gradual increase by 25% per day to 100%.

51.3 Type of Maintenance Fluid

The type of fluid to be used for maintenance infusion also differs among centres. In neonates, dextrose, with addition of electrolytes, is commonly given. In older children, 0.9% or 0.45% NaCl is commonly given. For adolescents, Ringer's lactate or Plasmalyte may be used. Importantly, hypotonic fluids, if used, should be given with caution in children and the potential complication of hyponatraemia should be monitored.

52 Use of Inotropes and Vasoactive Medications

Inotropes increase cardiac contractility, while vasoactive medications induce vasoconstriction (vasopressors) or vasodilation (vasodilators). Many drugs have both inotropic and vasoactive effects. These classes of medications constitute important components in the management of infants and children after cardiac surgery and those with acute cardiovascular decompensation due to underlying cardiac or noncardiac disease. Evidence-based guidelines are, however, lacking. There is hence a strong institutional preference on the choice, dose, and duration of these medications for the management of children after cardiac surgery and those with cardiac decompensation.

52.1 Targets of Inotropes and Vasoactive Medications

Inotropes and vasoactive medications exert their effects on the heart and blood vessels through activation of the specific receptors or other mechanisms (Table 52.1).

Y.-f. Cheung, *Congenital and Paediatric Acquired Heart Disease in Practice*, https://doi.org/10.1007/978-981-99-2862-0_52

Table 52.1 Receptors of inotropes and vasoactive medications

Receptors	Predominant location in cardiovascular system	Cardiovascular effects on stimulation
α1	Arterioles (α1 is the predominant α receptor in vascular smooth muscle)	Vasoconstriction
β1	Heart (β1 is the predominant β receptor in the heart)	Increase in heart rate and contractility
β2	Arterioles (β2 is the predominant β receptor in vascular and non-vascular smooth muscle)	Vasodilation
D1	Dopaminergic postsynaptic receptor mainly in coronary, renal, mesenteric, and cerebral beds	Vasodilation
D2	Dopaminergic presynaptic receptor in vasculature and renal tissues	Vasodilation
Vasopressin V1a receptor	Vascular smooth muscle	Activate protein kinase C, which in turn increases intracellular calcium to produce smooth muscle contraction

52.2 Inotropes and Vasoactive Medications

52.2.1 Catecholamines

Catecholamines exert cardiovascular actions through primarily α1, β1, β2, and dopaminergic receptors. Some of the catecholamines act predominantly through stimulation of α1 receptor, while some act predominantly through stimulation of β receptors. Some may act on more than one receptor to exert multiple actions, while some have dose-dependent activation of different receptors. The pharmacologic effects of these commonly used catecholamines are shown in Table 52.2. The properties of catecholamines and their clinical implications are further discussed.

52.2.1.1 Dopamine

The clinical significance of so-called ‘renal dose’ dopamine remains controversial. At a low dose of 0.5 to 3 μg/kg/min, dopamine has been shown to stimulate dopaminergic D1 postsynaptic receptors (mainly in coronary, renal, mesenteric, and cerebral beds) and D2 presynaptic receptors (in vasculature and renal tissues) to promote vasodilation and to increase blood flow to these tissues. However, dopamine has not been shown clinically to increase glomerular filtration rate or to exert renal protective effects. At intermediate doses (5 to 10 μg/kg/min), dopamine exerts predominant β-adrenergic effects to cause inotropic and chronotropic effects with only a mild increase in systemic vascular resistance. At higher doses (> 10 μg/kg/min), the α1-adrenergic effect becomes dominant and results in significant vasoconstriction.

Table 52.2 Vasoactive medication receptor activity and clinical effects

Drug	α1	β1	β2	D1/D2	Predominant cardiovascular effects
Dopamine (μg/kg/min)					
2 to 4	0	+	0	++	↑ CO
5 to 10	+	++	0	++	↑ CO, ↑ SVR
10 to 20	++	++	0	++	↑↑ SVR
Dobutamine	+	+++	++	0	↑ CO, ↓ SVR
Isoprenaline	0	+++	+++	0	↑ CO, ↓ SVR
Adrenaline	+++ (high dose)	+++	++	0	↑↑ CO ↓ SVR (low dose) ↑ SVR (high dose)
Phenylephrine	+++	0	0	0	↑↑ SVR
Noradrenaline	+++	++	0	0	↑↑ SVR

CO cardiac output, *SVR* systemic vascular resistance

52.2.1.2 Dobutamine

Dobutamine has a strong affinity to β-receptors to exert cardiac inotropic and chronotropic effects and cause mild vasodilation. The net effect is an increase in cardiac output with decrease in systemic vascular resistance. However, dobutamine significantly increases myocardial oxygen consumption and is also proarrhythmic.

52.2.1.3 Adrenaline

At low dose, the β-adrenergic effects of adrenaline are more pronounced, while at high dose, α1-adrenergic effects become obvious. Hence, low dose adrenaline infusion increases cardiac output and decreases systemic vascular resistance, while high dose infusion increases both the cardiac output and systemic vascular resistance.

52.2.1.4 Noradrenaline

Norepinephrine is potent α1-adrenergic receptor agonist that exerts primarily a vasoconstrictive effect. It has modest β-agonistic action with mild inotropic and minimal chronotropic effects. It increases systolic and diastolic blood pressure, left ventricular afterload (which may impair cardiac output), and coronary perfusion.

52.2.1.5 Isoprenaline

Isoprenaline is a potent nonselective β-adrenergic agonist that exerts inotropic, chronotropic effects, and systemic and pulmonary vasodilatory effects. The systemic vasodilatory effect may counteract its effect on stroke volume and limit the increase in cardiac output. The use of isoprenaline is further limited by its significant chronotropic effect and the increase in myocardial oxygen consumption. It is primarily used for the management of infants and children with bradycardia due to complete heart block.

52.2.2 Phosphodiesterase Inhibitor

Milrinone inhibits phosphodiesterase type III and is the most commonly used phosphodiesterase inhibitor for cardiovascular indications in paediatric critical care. Inhibition of phosphodiesterase increases cAMP, in turn increasing intracellular calcium to augment cardiac contractility and enhancing reuptake of calcium during diastole to enhance myocardial relaxation (lusitropic effect). Furthermore, the increased cAMP in vascular smooth muscles leads to vasodilation and reduces afterload. There are data to suggest that milrinone may prevent low cardiac output syndrome in infants and children after cardiac surgery.

52.2.3 Calcium Sensitiser

Levosimendan is the most commonly used calcium sensitiser in the paediatric critical care setting. Calcium sensitizers have two mechanisms of actions: (1) through calcium-dependent binding to troponin C to enhance ventricular contractility, and (2) opening of ATP-dependent potassium channels on vascular smooth muscle to cause arteriolar and venous dilation. The combined effects are augmentation of cardiac contractility with decrease in systemic vascular resistance. There are data to suggest that levosimendan may prevent low cardiac output syndrome in infants and children after cardiac surgery when used as an adjunct therapy to other vasopressors.

52.2.4 Other Vasoactive Medications

52.2.4.1 Vasopressin

Vasopressin (antidiuretic hormone), synthesized in the hypothalamus, stimulates V1a receptors in the vascular smooth muscle to activate protein kinase C, which in turn increases intracellular calcium to produce smooth muscle contraction. It may have a negative impact on cardiac output due to increase in systemic vascular resistance and reflex increase in vagal tone. It is used as a second-line agent in vasodilatory shock and other causes of vasoplegia refractory to other treatments.

52.2.4.2 Vasodilators

Vasodilators are used to reduce systemic vascular resistance and left ventricular afterload in paediatric cardiac patients with reduced cardiac output but with normal or increased systemic arterial pressure.

Sodium Nitroprusside

Sodium nitroprusside, a salt that comprises ferrous iron, nitric oxide and cyanide, dilates both arteries and vein by releasing nitric oxide. The haemodynamic effects are reduction in afterload and preload. Nitroprusside has the advantages having a rapid onset of action (with minutes) and a short duration of effect (about 10 min), hence rendering it highly titratable.

Cyanide and thiocyanate are produced during metabolism of sodium nitroprusside. Hence, there is a possibility of cyanide and thiocyanate toxicity administered at high doses or for a long period. Cyanide toxicity, occurring usually at doses ≥10 μg/kg/min, manifests as lactic acidosis, shortness of breath, confusion, lethargy, seizure, cardiac dysfunction, and death. Increased level of thiocyanate is also mildly neurotoxic. Nonetheless, most paediatric data do not suggest a relationship between elevated cyanide and thiocyanate levels and development of toxicity. Rarely, methaemoglobinaemia may occur. As yet, there is no consensus as to how to monitor for cyanide and thiocyanate toxicity during administration of sodium nitroprusside.

Nitroglycerin

Nitroglycerin is converted by mitochondrial aldehyde dehydrogenase to nitric oxide to cause dilation of the veins (which is the more dominant effect) and arteries. The use of nitroglycerin avoids cyanide and thiocyanate toxicity of nitroprusside, although the vasodilation effect of nitroglycerin is less than that of nitroprusside.

52.3 Complications Related to the Use of Inotropes and Vasoactive Medications

High doses of inotropes and vasopressor can cause significant complications. These include (1) excessive local vasoconstriction, especially in the presence of extravasation, leading to skin necrosis, (2) severe systemic vasoconstriction leading to necrosis and gangrenous changes of the extremities, gastric and intestinal ischaemia, and impaired renal perfusion and renal failure, (3) cardiac arrhythmias, and (4) myocardial ischaemia due to an increase in myocardial oxygen consumption. High doses of vasodilators cause systemic hypotension and, when nitroprusside is used, possible cyanide and thiocyanate-related toxicities.

Central Venous and Left Atrial Parameters

53

53.1 Central Venous Parameters

The central venous catheter in children undergoing cardiac surgery enables the monitoring of central venous pressure, assessment of pressure waveform, and sampling of blood for assessment of central venous oxygen saturation (ScvO2) to facilitate postoperative management.

53.1.1 Central Venous Pressure

Central venous pressure provides an estimation of the right atrial and right ventricular filling pressure and is also used as a surrogate of right ventricular end-diastolic volume. The normal central venous pressure ranges from 2 to 8 mmHg.

Progressive decrease in central venous pressure in the presence of other indices of low cardiac output syndrome (Chap. 55) warrants a trial of fluid bolus to determine the preload responsiveness in children after cardiac surgery. The relationship between central venous pressure and volume status is, however, not linear. Whereas the trend of decrease in central venous pressure probably reflects progressive depletion of intravascular volume depletion, a static measurement of normal or increased central venous pressure may not provide accurate information of the intravascular volume status.

Apart from the volume status, other factors in congenital heart patients after surgery can lead to an increase or a decrease in central venous pressure (Table 53.1). It is important therefore to consider these factors when interpreting and managing an abnormal central venous pressure in postoperative congenital heart patients.

Y.-f. Cheung, *Congenital and Paediatric Acquired Heart Disease in Practice*, https://doi.org/10.1007/978-981-99-2862-0_53

Table 53.1 Factors other than volume status affecting central venous pressure in children after surgery for congenital heart disease

Factors	Effect on central venous pressure
Ventricular dysfunction	
Systemic ventricular dysfunction	Increase
Right ventricular systolic dysfunction	Increase
Restrictive right ventricular physiology	Increase
Single ventricular physiology	
Bidirectional cavopulmonary connection	Increase
Fontan procedure	Increase
Residual valvar lesions and shunt	
Tricuspid regurgitation	Increase
Tricuspid stenosis	Increase
Left ventricular-to-right atrial shunt	Increase
Cardiac arrhythmias	
Atrioventricular dyssynchrony	Increase
Tachyarrhythmias	Increase
Tamponade	
Pericardial effusion	Increase
Tension pneumothorax	Increase
Mechanical ventilation	
High mean airway pressure	Increase
High positive end-expiratory pressure	Increase
Venous capacitance	
Venodilation (e.g. nitrates)	Decrease
Venoconstriction (e.g. adrenaline, noradrenaline)	Increase

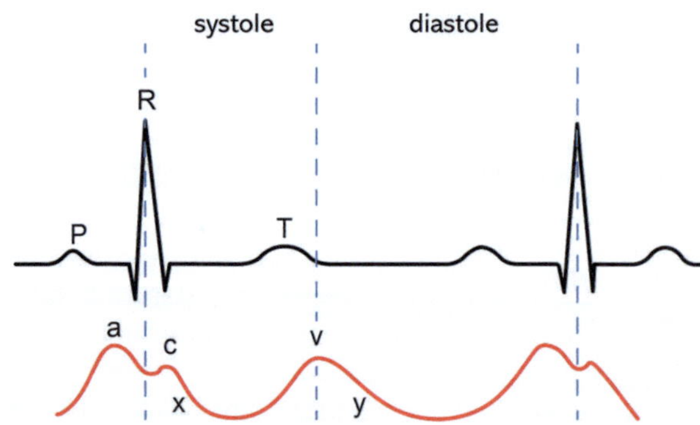

Fig. 53.1 Central venous pressure waveform. Central venous waves in relation to the electrocardiogram and the cardiac cycle

53.1.2 Central Venous Pressure Waveform

The normal central venous pressure waveform consists of 3 peaks (a, c, and v waves) and 2 descents (x and y descents) (Fig. 53.1). The origins of these waves and descents are described in Table 53.2.

Central venous pressure waveform can provide additional clues to the underlying causes of hemodynamic disturbances in children after cardiac surgery. Typical examples are (1) canon a wave occurring in cardiac arrhythmias that result in the

Table 53.2 Origins of the central venous pressure waves and descents

Wave or descent	Origin
a wave	Produced by right atrial contraction and occurs just after P wave
c wave	Due to isovolumic ventricular contraction that forces the tricuspid valve to bulge into the right atrium
x descent	Pulling of tricuspid away from the right atrium during right ventricular ejection
v wave	Filling of the right atrium late ventricular systole
y descent	Opening of the tricuspid valve with rapid emptying of blood into the right ventricle during early diastole

right atrium contracting against a closed tricuspid valve (junctional rhythm, complete heart block, right ventricular pacing), (2) fusion of the c and v waves (cv wave) in tricuspid regurgitation with attenuation of the x descent, (3) large a waves in conditions with restrictive right ventricular filling and tricuspid stenosis (the y descent is also attenuated because of the slow filling of the right ventricle).

53.1.3 Central Venous Oxygen Saturation (ScvO2)

Measurement of ScvO2, with blood sampled from the central venous line, aims to provide a surrogate assessment of mixed venous oxygen saturation (SvO2) in practice.

Assessment of SvO2, which requires pulmonary arterial sampling, provides an assessment of the balance between oxygen delivery and oxygen consumption, early detection of tissue hypoxaemia, and guidance of the response to treatment. The physiological significance of SvO2 in shown in Box 53.1.

Box 53.1 Physiological Significance of SvO2

VO2 = CO × (Ca–Cv) (based on Fick principle)

VO2 is oxygen consumption

CO is cardiac output

Ca (arterial oxygen content) = 1.34 × haemoglobin × SaO2 (×10 to convert mL/dL to mL/L)

Cv (venous oxygen content) = 1.34 × haemoglobin × SvO2 (×10 to convert mL/dL to mL/L)

CO = VO2/(Ca–Cv)

Ca-Cv represents the arteriovenous difference in oxygen content

Rearranging the equation and substituting Ca and Cv

SvO2 = SaO2 – [VO2/(CO × haemoglobin × 1.34 × 10)]

Hence, the SvO2 depends on the balance between oxygen consumption and cardiac output, arterial oxygen saturation, and haemoglobin level. The normal mixed venous oxygen saturation is about 70% to 75%, reflecting that the body tissue is normally extracting about 25% to 30% of oxygen carried in the arterial blood.

A low SvO2 may therefore reflect low cardiac output, reduced arterial oxygenation, anaemia, or increased oxygen consumption (e.g. sepsis) (Table 53.3), and is useful in guiding timely assessment (Fig. 53.2) and interventions (Box 53.2) before cardiovascular deterioration of cardiac patients in the early postoperative period. Nonetheless, a normal or high SvO2 does not exclude such disturbances. A high SvO2 may occasionally be due to poor extraction of oxygen by tissues with extensive cell death. Assessment of SvO2 requires, however, insertion of a pulmonary arterial catheter, which is not routinely performed in children after cardiac surgery.

Compared with the assessment of SvO2, determination of ScvO2 is more convenient given that blood sampling is only required from the central venous line. In healthy subjects, ScvO2 is slightly lower than SvO2, although the ScvO2 value may

Table 53.3 Causes of low SvO2 or ScvO2

Decreased oxygen delivery	Increased oxygen consumption
Low cardiac output syndrome	Sepsis
Hypoxaemia due to pulmonary and ventilatory abnormalities	Increased metabolic demand (e.g. fever, irritability, pain, respiratory distress)
Decreased oxygen carrying capacity (haemorrhage, anaemia)	

Clinical

- assess ventilation and respiratory system
- assess for adequacy of analgesia and sedation
- assess for evidence of low cardiac output syndrome
- assess for haemorrhage and anaemia

Imaging

- CXR for pulmonary causes of hypoxaemia
- echocardiogram to assess cardiac causes of low cardiac output syndrome

Blood investigations

- blood count for anaemia
- arterial blood gas
- blood culture if sepsis is suspected

Fig. 53.2 Assessment of low SvO2 or ScvO2. *CXR* chest X ray

vary with the location of sampling and cardiac and other conditions (e.g. shock) that redistribute flow between the upper and lower parts of the body.

In most situations, ScvO2 has a similar trend as SvO2. Hence, a low ScvO2 in the absence of significant anaemia or hypoxaemia is a good indicator of low cardiac output and should prompt immediate assessment and treatment of the underlying cause. The trend of change in ScvO2 reflects the change in cardiac output, albeit in a non-linear fashion, assuming that haemoglobin and arterial oxygen content remain relatively stable during the period of assessment. Nonetheless, similar to SvO2, a normal or high ScvO2 can also be falsely reassuring. Hence, assessment of the ScvO2 trend is preferred to isolated interpretation of a single ScvO2 reading.

In cyanotic and acyanotic patients, the ScvO2 can also be used to estimate the oxygen extraction ratio (SaO2 – ScvO2)/SaO2 and a value exceeding 25 to 30% should alert an increase oxygen extraction and prompt investigations of the underlying cause.

Box 53.2 Management of Low SvO2 or ScvO2

- optimize ventilation and treat respiratory cause
- increase oxygen supply
- treat fever and sepsis
- optimize analgesia and sedation
- trial of volume bolus
- inotropic support to increase systemic cardiac output
- transfuse blood if indicated

53.2 Left Atrial Pressure

Insertion of a left atrial catheter in children undergoing cardiac surgery enables the monitoring of left atrial pressure, an estimation of left ventricular end-diastolic pressure, and more accurate assessment of the volume status (especially in patients with right ventricular dysfunction and restrictive right ventricular physiology). The normal left atrial pressure is 1 to 2 mmHg higher than the right atrial pressure and ranges from 4 to 10 mmHg.

The left atrial pressure waveform is similar to the central venous pressure waveform. It consists of 3 peaks (a, c, and v waves) and 2 descents (x and y descents) with origins of these waves and descents as described in Table 53.2 but related to changes and motion of left-sided structures.

Apart from the volume status, other factors in congenital heart patients after surgery can also alter the left atrial pressure (Table 53.4). It is important therefore to consider these factors when interpretating and managing an abnormal left atrial pressure in postoperative congenital heart patients.

Table 53.4 Factors other than volume status affecting left atrial pressure in children after surgery for congenital heart disease

Factors	Effect on left atrial pressure
Ventricular dysfunction	
Left ventricular systolic and diastolic dysfunction	Increase
Left ventricular hypertrophy	Increase
Residual valvar lesions and shunt	
Mitral regurgitation	Increase
Mitral stenosis	Increase
Left-to-right shunt	Increase
Cardiac arrhythmias	
Atrioventricular dyssynchrony	Increase
Tachyarrhythmias	Increase
Tamponade	
Pericardial effusion	Increase

Off Target Arterial Oxygen Saturation 54

For patients with a biventricular circulation and the absence of right-to-left cardiac or pulmonary shunt, the arterial oxygen saturation (SaO_2) is 100%. Nonetheless, the targets of SaO_2 differ among different congenital heart conditions after palliative or corrective surgery. Understanding the causes of deviation from the target SaO_2, which may precede significant haemodynamic deterioration in certain cardiac conditions, is important for timely institution of treatment and planning of further management.

54.1 Biventricular Circulation

54.1.1 Post Relief of Severe Right Ventricular Outflow Obstruction

A low SaO_2 (usually between 70 and 85% and with normocarbia) may persist in the first few days after relief of right ventricular obstruction in neonates with critical pulmonary stenosis and pulmonary atresia with an intact ventricular septum. The restrictive filling of hypertrophic, poorly compliant, and, in some patients, hypoplasia of the right ventricle, promotes right-to-left atrial shunting to cause a low SaO_2.

Doppler colour flow mapping and bubble contrast echocardiography, with injection of agitated saline contrast in any of the peripheral veins, help to define the cause of a low SaO_2 and to ascertain the level and severity of intracardiac right-to-left atrial shunt. Maintenance of prostaglandin E may be required initially but can usually be weaned off in less than 2 weeks after intervention. In neonates with persistently low SaO_2, particularly in those hypertrophic and hypoplastic right ventricles, insertion of a systemic-to-pulmonary arterial shunt or ductal stenting (performed sometimes at the same time when the pulmonary valve is perforated in pulmonary atresia with an intact ventricular septum) is required.

Y.-f. Cheung, *Congenital and Paediatric Acquired Heart Disease in Practice*, https://doi.org/10.1007/978-981-99-2862-0_54

54.1.2 Post Repair of Conditions at Risk of Right Ventricular Dysfunction

Patients at risk of postoperative right ventricular dysfunction (significant preoperative right ventricular hypertrophy and/or dysfunction or anticipated postoperative acute rise in right ventricular afterload due to pulmonary hypertensive crisis) may benefit from leaving the oval foramen patent or creation of a small interatrial communication to augment cardiac output by allowing right-to-left atrial shunt flow. Patients undergoing, for example, repair of truncus arteriosus, tetralogy of Fallot, and Ebstein anomaly may benefit from this approach. A low SaO_2 (usually about 80–90%) and normocarbia are characteristic of the intended right-to-left atrial shunt in these patients.

54.1.3 Inadvertent Creation of a Right-to-Left Atrial Shunt

A prominent Eustachian valve can be mistaken as part of the atrial septum. Closure of the valve to the atrial septum during supposedly closure of an atrial septal defect results in inadvertent diversion of blood from the inferior caval vein to the left atrium and significant decrease in SaO_2 (down to 70% or even lower). The prominent Eustachian valve, especially in patients with pulmonary atresia with an intact ventricular septum, may also interfere with device occlusion of an associated atrial septal defect. Bubble contrast echocardiography with injection of agitated saline into a peripheral vein in the lower limb would unveil this inadvertently created right-to-atrial shunt.

54.1.4 Right-to-Left Intrapulmonary Shunt

In the presence of a structurally normal heart with bubble contrast echocardiographic assessment showing the absence of a right-to-left cardiac shunt, a low SaO_2 may be caused by intrapulmonary right-to-left shunting due to pulmonary arteriovenous malformations (Chap. 36).

54.2 Univentricular Circulation

54.2.1 Unexpected Degree of Cyanosis After Fontan Procedure

An SaO_2 of more the 90% is usually expected in patients with satisfactory haemodynamics after the Fontan procedure (Chap. 19). Causes of exaggerated degree of cyanosis include: (1) increased right-to-left shunting through the fenestration due to high pulmonary vascular resistance (lung collapse, pneumonia, pneumothorax, pleural effusion, unfavourable pulmonary vasculature), (2) pulmonary veno-venous collaterals that drain into the pulmonary venous atrium, (3) pre-existing pulmonary arteriovenous fistulas, (4) bilateral hepatic venous drainage with some of the hepatic veins not incorporated into the Fontan circuit and draining separately into the pulmonary venous atrium (usually in the setting of heterotaxy syndrome), and (5) ventricular dysfunction (which increases oxygen extraction and decreases mixed venous oxygen saturation).

54.3 Post Insertion of Systemic-to-Pulmonary Arterial Shunt

54.3.1 Low SaO_2

A low SaO_2 (<70%) after insertion of a systemic-to-pulmonary arterial shunt may be caused by inadequate pulmonary flow or respiratory conditions (Table 54.1). This requires immediate assessment (Fig. 54.1) and appropriate actions to rectify the situation (Box 54.1).

Table 54.1 Causes of low SaO_2 after insertion of a systemic-to-pulmonary arterial shunt

Inadequate pulmonary flow	Respiratory conditions
Shunt stenosis or blockage	Endotracheal tube problems
Small size of the shunt	Pneumothorax
Small branch pulmonary arteries	Pneumonia
Branch pulmonary arterial stenosis	Pleural effusion
Inadequate flow due to systemic hypotension	Lung atelectasis

Clinical

- assess ventilation and respiratory system
- listen for shunt murmur
- assess for evidence of low cardiac output syndrome

Imaging

- CXR for pulmonary oligaemia, differential flow and pulmonary causes
- echocardiogram to assess shunt flow, branch pulmonary arterial stenosis and size
- CT and/or cardiac catheterization (with preparation for intervention)

Blood investigations

- arterial blood gas
- coagulation profile

Fig. 54.1 Assessment of low SaO_2 in a shunted infant. Abbreviations: *CT* computed tomography, *CXR* chest X ray, *SaO_2* arterial oxygen saturation

Box 54.1 Management of Low SaO_2 in a Shunted Infant

- optimize ventilation and treat respiratory cause
- trial of volume bolus
- start systemic vasoconstrictor (e.g. noradrenaline) to promote pulmonary blood flow
- inotropic support to increase systemic cardiac output
- urgent surgical revision or transcatheter recanalization of shunt
- review the regimen of anticoagulation

54.3.2 High SaO_2

A high SaO_2 > 85–90% in neonates and infants after insertion of a systemic-to-pulmonary arterial shunt indicates high pulmonary blood flow (Table 54.2). This finding should alert the possibility of cardiovascular deterioration due to pulmonary steal from systemic and coronary circulation. This requires immediate assessment to diagnose the cause (Fig. 54.2) and actions to manage the situation (Box 54.2). There are patients, despite having a higher-than-expected SaO_2, who are relatively stable with adequate systemic perfusion as their cardiac output remains adequate.

Table 54.2 Causes of a high SaO_2 after insertion of a systemic-to-pulmonary arterial shunt

Excessive pulmonary flow	Ventilatory conditions
Large size of the inserted shunt	Administration of high FiO_2
Persistence of a large arterial duct	
Presence of multiple aortopulmonary collaterals	

Clinical
- assess for evidence of impaired systemic perfusion
- note the wide pulse pressure and low diastolic blood pressure
- feel for bounding pulses
- look for signs of respiratory distress due to increased pulmonary flow
- listen for shunt and ductal murmur

Cardiac investigations
- chest radiograph to assess pulmonary plethora and oedema
- echocardiogram to assess shunt and ductal flow and evidence of aortopulmonary collaterals
- ECG to assess myocardial ischaemia due to coronary steal

Blood investigations
- arterial blood gas and lactate level
- coagulation profile

Fig. 54.2 Assessment of high SaO_2 in a shunted infant. Abbreviations: *ECG* electrocardiogram, *SaO_2* arterial oxygen saturation

Box 54.2 Management of High SaO_2 in a Shunted Infant

In infants with respiratory distress and poor peripheral circulation and rising lactate
- intubate and ventilate if already extubated
- ventilated with FiO_2 0.21 and allow permissive hypercapnia (to increase pulmonary vascular resistance)
- trial of volume bolus
- start systemic vasodilator if systolic and diastolic pressure allows and in the absence of evidence of coronary steal
- give vasoconstrictor (noradrenaline or vasopressin) in the presence of low diastolic pressure (with or without ECG evidence of myocardial ischaemia) (need to watch out for further systemic hypoperfusion)
- inotropic support to increase systemic cardiac output
- urgent ductal ligation if a large arterial duct is present
- downsize the shunt if necessary

In clinically stable infants with mild respiratory distress
- off supplemental oxygen
- maintain fluid restriction
- start diuretics
- monitor for closure of the arterial duct and ligate or occlude if necessary

Low Cardiac Output Syndrome 55

Low cardiac output syndrome refers to the phenomenon of reduced cardiac output after cardiac surgeries that require cardiopulmonary bypass, occurring usually at about 6–18 h post operation.

55.1 Pathophysiology

The myocardial response to cardiopulmonary bypass, alteration of ventricular loading, and haemodynamic consequences of residual anatomic lesions act in concert to cause low cardiac output syndrome.

Several factors related to cardiopulmonary bypass contribute to myocardial dysfunction: (1) activation of systemic inflammatory response, (2) myocardial ischaemia during aortic cross clamping, (3) inadequate myocardial protection, (4) the need for ventriculotomy, and (5) reperfusion injury. Apart from systolic dysfunction, diastolic dysfunction may also occur after paediatric cardiac surgery, a typical example is the restrictive right ventricular physiology after repair of tetralogy of Fallot (Chap. 27).

Loading of the heart may be altered postoperatively and may affect cardiac function: (1) unloading of the preoperative volume and/or pressure overloaded ventricles by the surgical procedure, (2) residual lesions may increase volume and/pressure load and worsen ventricular function as postoperative ventricular contractile reserve is reduced, (3) decreased preload may result from hypovolaemia and capillary leak due to the systemic inflammatory response, and (4) increased afterload to the right ventricle due to pulmonary hypertension, increased airway pressure, pleural effusion and pneumothorax, and to the left ventricle from an increased systemic vascular resistance relating to the systemic inflammatory response after cardiopulmonary bypass.

Y.-f. Cheung, *Congenital and Paediatric Acquired Heart Disease in Practice*, https://doi.org/10.1007/978-981-99-2862-0_55

Preservation or creation of a right-to-left atrial shunt may improve systemic ventricular filling and the cardiac output. Leaving the patent oval foramen unclosed is hence beneficial for maintenance of the systemic cardiac output in children with a restrictive right ventricular physiology after repair of tetralogy of Fallot, while creation of a fenestration during Fontan operation may benefit patients with less favourable pulmonary arterial anatomy and/or slightly elevated pulmonary arterial resistance.

55.2 Diagnosis

Well-defined diagnostic criteria for low cardiac output syndrome are not available. Diagnosis is based on clinical signs of reduced cardiac output, unfavourable physiological monitoring parameters, and worsening of blood parameters that suggest worsening of oxygen delivery to the peripheral tissues (Table 55.1). Additional useful parameters for assessment and monitoring include central venous pressure, left atrial pressure, pulse index contour cardiac output (PiCCO), and near-infrared spectroscopy (NIRS) monitoring.

Assessment of the trend of changes is more important that a single time point evaluation of these signs and parameters. The ability to act early based on subtle unfavourable changes is the key to the management of low cardiac output syndrome after paediatric cardiac surgeries.

Table 55.1 Diagnosis of low cardiac output syndrome

Clinical signs	Physiologic monitoring parameters	Blood parameters
• tachycardia • weak pulse volume • cold extremities • prolonged capillary refill	• tachycardia • increased core-to-peripheral temperature gradient • decreased urine output • reduced pulse pressure from the arterial line • a narrow amplitude pulse oximetry photoplethysmogram • systemic hypotension (a late sign due to an initial compensatory response)	• increasing level of lactate • metabolic acidosis • progressive decrease in central venous oxygen saturation

55.3 Further Investigations

CXR: Chest radiography may reveal pneumothorax or pleural effusion as the cause of low cardiac output syndrome.
ECG: Complete heart block, junctional ectopic tachycardia, and other types of cardiac arrhythmias may cause low cardiac output syndrome.
Echocardiography: Echocardiographic assessment may unveil ventricular dysfunction, residual cardiac lesions, atrioventricular valvar regurgitation, and cardiac tamponade.
Blood investigations: Worsening of metabolic acidosis, rising lactate level, progressive decrease in central venous oxygen saturation, and deterioration of renal and liver function are indicative of worsening tissue oxygenation.

55.4 Management Strategy

Timely institution of therapeutic measures is vital for the prevention of end-organ damage. The management strategy aims to increase systemic oxygen delivery and to restore balance between oxygen delivery and demand through addressing the postoperative cardiac, vascular, pulmonary, and possible endocrine perturbation (Box 55.1).

Box 55.1 Management of Low Cardiac Output Syndrome

Augment cardiac output
- optimize preload
- augment cardiac contractility with inotropes
- maintain sinus rhythm and restore atrioventricular synchrony if possible
- reduce high systemic vascular resistance with milrinone and/or systemic vasodilators to improve systemic ventricular output
- reduce pulmonary vascular resistance with inhaled nitric oxide and other pulmonary vasodilators to increase right ventricular output
- relieve pericardial tamponade and tackle significant residual cardiac lesion(s)
- mechanical circulatory support

Restore systemic vascular function
- reduce high systemic vascular resistance with milrinone and/or systemic vasodilators to improve systemic ventricular output
- start vasopressors to maintain perfusion pressure in the presence of vasoplegia (beware of worsening cardiac output with significant increase in systemic vascular resistance)

Pulmonary support

- institute positive pressure ventilatory support to unload respiratory muscles and increase systemic cardiac output (beware that excessively high intrathoracic pressure would increase pulmonary vascular resistance and impair right ventricular output)
- sedate, provide adequate pain relief, and paralyze, if necessary, for better ventilatory support and to decrease oxygen consumption

Address possible endocrine perturbation

- consider relative adrenal insufficiency especially in infants after cardiac surgery with low cardiac output syndrome refractory to management and give hydrocortisone
- worth replenishing triiodothyronine (T3) in infants and young children with postoperative thyroid dysfunction

56 Pulmonary Hypertensive Crisis

Postoperative pulmonary hypertension is a common problem in children after cardiac surgery. Pulmonary hypertensive crisis is characterized by an acute increase in pulmonary arterial resistance and pressure that result in acute right ventricular failure and is potentially lethal.

56.1 Pathophysiology

The pulmonary vascular reactivity is increased after surgery for congenital heart disease. Mild stimuli (e.g. suctioning of endotracheal tube, irritability of patient) may trigger pulmonary vasospasm and cause an acute increase in pulmonary vascular resistance and pulmonary arterial pressure. This results in acute right ventricular failure, increased tricuspid regurgitation, decrease in right and left ventricular cardiac output, systemic hypotension, myocardial ischaemia, and increased airway resistance.

56.2 Risk Factors

The occurrence of postoperative pulmonary hypertensive crisis represents an interplay between the underlying cardiac condition, patient factors, cardiopulmonary bypass, outcomes of cardiac surgery, and the postoperative critical care milieu.
Underlying cardiac conditions: The pulmonary vasculature is reactive in cardiac conditions with increased pulmonary arterial flow (large ventricular septal defect, atrioventricular defect, truncus arteriosus, transposition of the great arteries with ventricular septal defect), pulmonary venous obstruction (obstructed total anomalous pulmonary venous connection), and left atrial hypertension (Shone complex, mitral stenosis and regurgitation).

Y.-f. Cheung, *Congenital and Paediatric Acquired Heart Disease in Practice*, https://doi.org/10.1007/978-981-99-2862-0_56

Patient factors: The risk is increased in patients with Down syndrome and in infants with delayed repair of large left-to-right shunts (beyond 6 months of age) and truncus arteriosus (beyond 2–3 months of age).
Cardiopulmonary bypass: Cardiopulmonary bypass, hypothermia, and circulatory arrest cause injury (inflammatory response and ischaemia-reperfusion injury) to the pulmonary endothelium, impair endothelium-dependent vasodilation, and enhance pulmonary vasoconstriction.
Outcomes of surgery: In patients with recurrent pulmonary hypertensive crisis, residual left-to-right shunts and left atrioventricular valvar regurgitation must be excluded.
Postoperative critical care milieu: Hypoxaemia, hypercarbia, and respiratory and metabolic acidosis promote pulmonary vasoconstriction.

In the current era, early surgical repair, improvement in surgical and perfusion techniques, and intraoperative identification and tackling of residual lesions, prophylactic or early institution of inhaled nitric oxide in at-risk patients, and meticulous intensive care have markedly decreased the incidence of postoperative pulmonary hypertensive crisis.

56.3 Clinical Manifestations and Findings

Factors that trigger an episode of pulmonary hypertensive crisis may be identified (Box 56.1). Signs include tachycardia, hypotension, hypoxaemia, hypercarbia, and increased central venous pressure.

Box 56.1 Triggering Factors of Pulmonary Hypertensive Crisis

- suctioning of endotracheal tube
- inadequate pain relief and sedation of patient
- suboptimal ventilation causing hypercarbia and/or hypoxaemia
- metabolic and/or respiratory acidosis

56.4 Management Strategy

The management should aim at improving patient sedation, ventilation, reducing pulmonary vascular resistance, augmenting right ventricular systolic function, and maintaining systemic cardiac output (Box 56.2). Vasopressors (vasopressin or noradrenaline) improve tissue perfusion and promote the reshifting of the ventricular septum to the right. Compared with noradrenaline, vasopressin may be a better choice as it does not increase and may possibly reduce pulmonary vascular resistance.

Box 56.2 Management of Pulmonary Hypertensive Crisis

- increase sedation and paralyse patient
- hand ventilate with 100% oxygen and inhaled nitric oxide
- increase inhaled nitric oxide up to 40 ppm or initiate inhaled nitric oxide at 20 ppm if not already started
- increase ventilatory support (FiO_2 to 100% and to maintain a low or low normal $PaCO_2$ level)
- increase right ventricular contractility with adrenaline and calcium
- increase systemic vascular resistance with vasopressin
- avoid vasodilators including milrinone
- addition of oral or intravenous sildenafil

56.5 Rebound of Pulmonary Hypertension

Rebound of pulmonary hypertension and recurrence of episodes of pulmonary hypertensive crisis may occur upon withdrawal of nitric oxide and delay extubation. This may be minimized by slow weaning of inhaled nitric oxide, in particular the last 5 ppm of inhaled nitric oxide. Transition to oral sildenafil has been shown to reduce the risk of rebound and shorten the time to extubation. In difficult patients, oral bosentan, intravenous sildenafil, inhaled iloprost, and intravenous prostacyclin analogues may be required.

Cardiac Arrhythmias 57

Cardiac arrhythmias occur commonly after paediatric cardiac surgery with a prevalence of about 10–50%. Tachycardia, bradycardia, and the loss of atrioventricular synchrony constitute important causes of low cardiac output syndrome in the early postoperative period.

57.1 Mechanisms and Risk Factors

Three main mechanisms underlie the development of postoperative cardiac arrhythmias in congenital heart patients: (1) increased automaticity, (2) presence of reentry circuits (e.g. an accessory pathway or areas of scarring), and (3) intrinsic abnormalities of or surgical damage to the conduction at the atrioventricular node (Table 57.1).

Several factors increase the risk of postoperative cardiac arrhythmias. These include: (1) use of inotropes (in particular dopamine and dobutamine), (2) medications that increase QT interval, (3) electrolyte imbalance, (4) anatomic factors (e.g. heterotaxy syndrome, congenitally corrected transposition of the great arteries), and (5) surgical factors (e.g. damage to the sinoatrial node, manipulation around the atrioventricular node).

Y.-f. Cheung, *Congenital and Paediatric Acquired Heart Disease in Practice*,
https://doi.org/10.1007/978-981-99-2862-0_57

Table 57.1 Postoperative cardiac arrhythmias in congenital heart patients

Arrhythmias	Mechanisms	Cardiac conditions
Automaticity		
Junctional ectopic tachycardia	Increased automaticity	Most common cause of tachyarrhythmia, surgical trauma around AV node (e.g. after repair of ventricular septal defect)
Ectopic atrial tachycardia	Increased automaticity	Uncommon, associated with surgery for different types of congenital heart disease in particular TGA
Sinus node dysfunction	Decreased automaticity	Venous cannulation or surgery near the sinoatrial node e.g. Fontan operation
Reentry circuits		
AV reentrant tachycardia	Accessory pathway	Ebstein malformation
AV nodal reentrant tachycardia	Dual AV nodes	Right isomerism, hypoplastic left heart syndrome
Intraatrial reentrant tachycardia	Macro reentrant circuit	Post repair of tetralogy of Fallot, Fontan operation, and atrial switch operation
Atrioventricular nodal block		
Complete heart block	Intrinsic predisposition or surgical damage	cc-TGA, left isomerism, surgical repair of ventricular and atrioventricular septal defects

57.2 Pathophysiology

Bradycardia reduces cardiac output. The effect is more marked in children as their primary physiologic response to augment cardiac output is an increase in heart rate. Significant tachycardia decreases ventricular filling time and hence the stroke volume. Tachyarrhythmias with loss of atrioventricular synchrony reduce ventricular filling further. The role of atrial contraction is particularly important in patients with postoperative diastolic ventricular dysfunction (e.g. patients with restrictive right ventricular physiology after repair of tetralogy and those after Fontan operation).

57.3 Clinical Approach

The approach to patients who develop cardiac arrhythmias after congenital heart surgery includes (1) an immediate clinical evaluation, (2) assessment of 12-lead ECG and performing an atrial electrogram if necessary, and (3) chest radiographic and echocardiographic assessment (Fig. 57.1).

Unstable patients with narrow QRS complex tachycardias and haemodynamic compromise require immediate synchronized cardioversion (although cardioversion is ineffective for junctional ectopic tachycardia and ectopic atrial

Clinical

- assess haemodynamics, if unstable, manage as per paediatric advanced life support guidelines (including immediate cardioversion)
- assess for fever and evidence of low cardiac output syndrome
- assess central venous line waveform (cannon wave suggests atrioventricular dyssynchrony)
- review cardiac diagnosis and details of cardiac surgery
- review earlier ECGs and the need for pacing
- review the use of inotropes and other medications
- check for electrolyte imbalance and lactic acidosis

ECG

- perform 12-lead ECG and atrial electrogram
- determine the type of arrhythmia
- assess the effect of adenosine and atrial overdrive pacing (which may terminate reentrant tachycardias) where appropriate

Imaging

- review the position of central venous line from CXR
- echocardiography to exclude haemodynamically significant abnormalities

Fig. 57.1 Approach to patients with cardiac arrhythmias after congenital heart surgery. Abbreviations: *CXR* chest X ray, *ECG* electrocardiogram

Table 57.2 Clinical and ECG features of two main types of cardiac arrhythmias

Increased automaticity	Reentrant tachycardias
Gradual increase and decrease in rate	Abrupt onset and termination
Rate increases with temperature and sympathetic stimulation	Little beat-to-beat variation
Does not terminate with adenosine, cardioversion, or overdrive pacing (although overdrive pacing may restore atrioventricular synchrony)	Termination with adenosine, cardioversion, or overdrive pacing

tachycardias). Certain clinical and electrocardiographic features provide clues to the mechanism and type of cardiac arrhythmias (Table 57.2). Performance of an atrial electrogram (Box 57.1) with administration of adenosine may aid the diagnosis of the type of cardiac arrhythmias by assessing the relationship between the atrial and ventricular electrical activity. Intravenous bolus of adenosine can both be diagnostic and therapeutic (Box 57.2).

Box 57.1 Performance of Atrial Electrogram

Unipolar atrial recording

- connect the four limb leads as usual
- attach atrial pacing wire to V2
- select three-lead mode (I, aVF, and V2)
- V2 shows atrial ECG (I and avF for comparisons)

Bipolar atrial recording

- connect the two lower limb leads as usual
- attach two atrial wires respectively to the right and left upper limb leads
- lead I shows the bipolar atrial electrogram
- leads II and III show unipolar atrial electrogram (but with the lack of concurrent limb leads for comparisons)

Transesophageal atrial electrogram

- use of an esophageal lead if atrial wires are not available
- connect as per unipolar atrial recording

Box 57.2 Use of Intravenous Bolus of Adenosine

Electrophysiologic effects

- slowing of sinus rate
- increasing atrioventricular nodal conduction delay

Utilization in approaching patients with postoperative narrow QRS complex tachycardias

- inducing transient atrioventricular block unveils morphology and rate of P waves and flutter waves
- termination of arrhythmias is diagnostic of AV reentrant and AV nodal reentrant tachycardias
- continuation of arrhythmias suggests junctional ectopic tachycardia, atrial tachycardias or atrial flutter

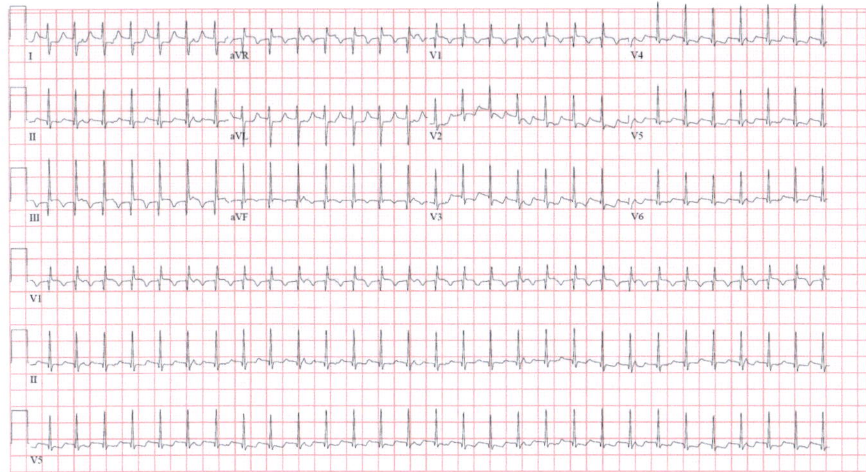

Fig. 57.2 Junctional ectopic tachycardia. ECG showing junctional ectopic tachycardia with atrioventricular dissociation

57.4 Types of Postoperative Cardiac Arrhythmias

57.4.1 Junctional Ectopic Tachycardia

Junctional ectopic tachycardia (JET) is the most type of tachyarrhythmia in infants and children after cardiac surgery for congenital heart disease. This is related to increased automaticity of the atrioventricular node or His bundle and is associated with surgical manipulation around the atrioventricular node. It occurs typically in the early operative period with rewarming of the patients and worsens with increasing dose of catecholaminergic agents.

The characteristic electrocardiographic features are (1) tachycardia with QRS complexes the same as in normal sinus rhythm, (2) regular ventricular rhythm, and (3) atrioventricular dissociation (atrial rate slower than ventricular rate) (Fig. 57.2). Administration of adenosine (especially when performed with an atrial electrogram) unveils atrioventricular dissociation, although occasionally the atrium may be activated in a retrograde fashion with 1:1 ventriculoatrial conduction.

Management aims at rate control, restoration of atrioventricular synchrony, and conversion if possible (Box 57.3). Amiodarone has been the preferred drug in the management of postoperative JET. Emerging data suggest that dexmedetomidine, a selective α-2 adrenoreceptor agonist used for sedation and analgesia, may prevent development of JET after paediatric cardiac surgery through its sympatholytic action. Oral ivabradine, a selective inhibitor of hyperpolarization-activated cyclic nucleotide-gated channels, has also been used as a monotherapy for rate control and to convert JET to sinus rhythm. Junctional ectopic tachycardia resolves usually within 48 h in most of the patients.

Box 57.3 Management of Junctional Ectopic Tachycardia

- general measures: cooling, sedation, pain relief, minimize the use of catecholaminergic agents, maintain electrolyte balance (especially calcium and magnesium), and volume status
- intravenous boluses and infusion of amiodarone may convert JET to sinus rhythm
- esmolol infusion for rate control
- dexmedetomidine infusion for rate control through its sympatholytic action and may convert JET to sinus rhythm
- oral ivabradine for rate control and may convert JET to sinus rhythm
- atrial overdrive pacing to restore atrioventricular synchrony (but a fast heart rate with rapid atrial pacing limits ventricular filling and cardiac output)
- short duration of extracorporeal membrane oxygenation support for JET refractory to all measures in patients with haemodynamic compromise

57.4.2 Ectopic Atrial Tachycardia

Ectopic atrial tachycardia is uncommon after congenital heart surgery. It is related to increased automaticity of an atrial focus and may occur in a paroxysmal or an incessant fashion. It is characterized by an inappropriately increased atrial rate, which is influenced by temperature and autonomic tone.

The ECG features are (1) increased atrial rate with non-sinus or sinus P waves, (2) presence of usually first-degree (atrial rate equals to ventricular rate) or less commonly second-degree heart block (atrial rate faster than ventricular rate), and (3) QRS complexes the same as in normal sinus rhythm. Administration of adenosine (especially when performed with an atrial electrogram) differentiates ectopic atrial tachycardia from atrial flutter, the latter being responsive to cardioversion or overdrive pacing.

Management aims at rate control, restoration of atrioventricular synchrony, and/or conversion if possible and is similar to that described for JET (Box 57.2). Most of the patients do not require specific interventions and the arrhythmia resolves within few days after surgery.

57.4.3 Reentrant Tachycardias

Postoperative macroreentrant atrial tachycardias include intra-atrial reentrant tachycardia and atrial flutter. Atrial flutter involves the anatomical structural barriers in the reentrant circuit, while intra-atrial reentrant tachycardia involves surgical incision sites (e.g. cannulation site), suture lines, patches, and areas of fibrosis. These atrial tachycardias usually have a 2:1 atrioventricular conduction. An atrial electrogram with administration of adenosine is useful in unveiling the P waves and diagnosing these reentrant atrial tachycardias. In atrial flutter, the sawtooth pattern is characteristic. In intra-atrial reentrant tachycardia, the P-wave morphology is more variable and often smaller.

Patients with accessory pathways or dual atrioventricular nodes are predisposed to development of reentrant tachycardias after cardiac surgery. Diagnostic features include: (1) tachycardia with QRS complexes the same as in normal sinus rhythm, (2) retrograde P waves and a short RP interval, and (3) termination with intravenous bolus of adenosine.

Unstable patients with haemodynamic compromise require immediate synchronized cardioversion. In stable patients, intravenous adenosine with 12-lead ECG or atrial electrogram is performed for diagnostic and therapeutic purposes. In stable patients with accessory pathways or dual atrioventricular nodes not responsive to adenosine, conversion to sinus rhythm can be achieved by intravenous esmolol or amiodarone infusion. For these patients, prophylactic treatment after conversion with beta-blockers may be indicated. For patients with intra-atrial reentrant tachycardia, long-term management with sotalol and other beta-blockers or amiodarone may be required.

57.4.4 Complete Heart Block

Postoperative complete heart block may occur as a result surgical damage to the atrioventricular node of bundle of His in patients undergoing surgery for repair of ventricular or atrioventricular septal effect and resection of subaortic fibromuscular tissue. Patients with congenitally correctly transposition of the great arteries and left atrial isomerism are intrinsically vulnerable to development of complete heart block.

Characteristic electrocardiographic findings are (1) atrioventricular dissociation, (2) no conduction of atrial activity to the ventricle, (3) atrial rate being faster than the escape rhythm, and (4) if the block occurs at the atrioventricular node, the escape rhythm may be a junction rhythm (with narrow QRS complex) or ventricular rhythm (Fig. 57.3). The management strategy of postoperative complete or advanced second-degree heart block is described in Box 57.4.

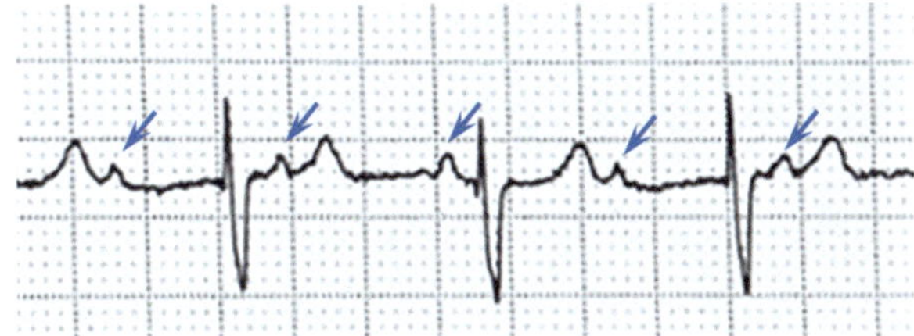

Fig. 57.3 Postoperative complete heart block. ECG showing postoperative complete heart block with atrioventricular dissociation and absence of conduction of atrial activity (arrows) to the ventricle

Box 57.4 Management of Postoperative Complete or Advanced Second-Degree Heart Block

- wait for recovery if haemodynamics are stable and rate of the junctional escape rhythm is adequate
- give isoprenaline to increase the rate of junctional escape
- pace (DDD or VVI) using temporary pacing wires
- permanent pacemaker implantation (2021 PACES expert consensus)
  - persisting for at least 7 to 10 days after cardiac surgery
  - at <7 days if extensive injury to the cardiac conduction system
  - in selected patients with even transient heart block who are intrinsically predisposed to progressive conduction abnormalities

Pleural Effusion

58

Pleural effusion occurs when fluid accumulates between the visceral pleura and parietal pleura. It has been reported to occur in 10–40% of children after cardiac surgery and contributes to an increase in intensive care and hospital stay.

58.1 Pathophysiology

In the postoperative setting, fluid in the pleural cavity can be blood, chyle, exudative effusion, and transudative effusion. Bleeding into the pleural cavity leads to haemothorax and occurs early after cardiac surgery. Chylous effusion is discussed in Chap. 59. Exudative effusion related to increased capillary permeability may occur in association with cardiopulmonary bypass-induced capillary leak, post pericardiotomy syndrome (Chap. 60), and pneumonia (parapneumonic effusion). Transudative effusion is the most commonly type of pleural effusion after cardiac surgery in children. The amount of transudative fluid in the pleural space increases when there is an imbalance among the Starling forces: (1) increased hydrostatic pressure (increased right atrial and systemic venous pressure, right heart failure), (2) decreased plasma oncotic pressure (hypoalbuminaemia), and (3) a more negative intrathoracic pressure (lung collapse and atelectasis). Pleural effusion develops when the increased amount of serous fluid being generated overwhelms the drainage capacity of lymphatic system.

58.2 Risk Factors

Postoperative conditions that are associated with increased systemic venous pressure, right atrial pressure, right ventricular systolic and diastolic dysfunction, and hypoalbuminaemia are predisposing risk factors. Hence, postoperative pleural

Y.-f. Cheung, *Congenital and Paediatric Acquired Heart Disease in Practice*, https://doi.org/10.1007/978-981-99-2862-0_58

effusion occurs most commonly occurs in children after repair of tetralogy of Fallot and in those after Fontan procedure. Prolonged positive pressure mechanical ventilation is also a risk factor as it increases systemic venous pressure and decreases lymphatic drainage of the pleural cavities.

58.3 Clinical Presentation and Findings

Most of the patients are asymptomatic and pleural effusion is detected incidentally on routine postoperative chest radiographic examination. In patients with a residual right-to-left shunt, there may be worsening of central cyanosis. The presence of fever suggests an inflammatory or infective cause of pleural effusion. In patients with significant amount of effusion, symptoms and signs of respiratory distress may be obvious. Significant pleural effusion may compromise haemodynamics by impairing ventricular filling and reducing stroke volume. In Fontan patients, the increase in pulmonary vascular resistance may lead to low cardiac output syndrome.

58.4 Investigations

Markers of inflammation: Erythrocyte sedimentation rate, C reactive protein, and leukocyte count are usually elevated in inflammatory or infective causes of pleural effusion.
CXR: Depending on the severity of effusion, the chest radiographic findings vary from blunting of the costophrenic angle to opacification of the lung field (Fig. 58.1a). Subpleural effusion may mimic diaphragmatic paralysis.

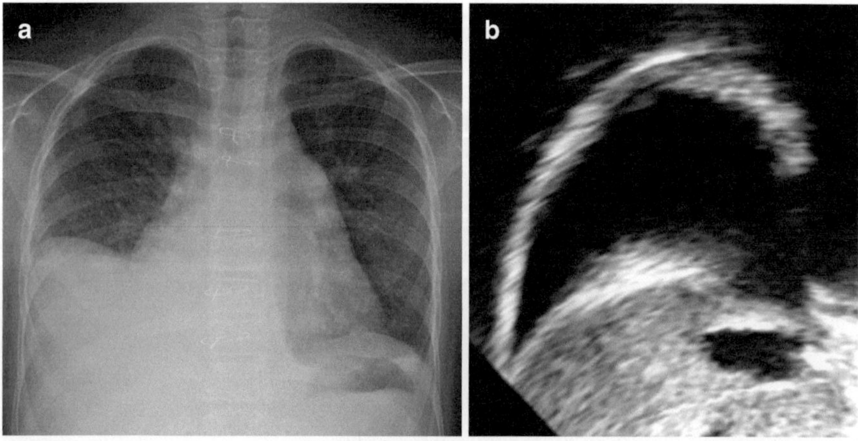

Fig. 58.1 Pleural effusion. (**a**) Chest radiograph and (**b**) bedside ultrasound showing right pleural effusion

Table 58.1 Characteristics of transudative and exudative effusions

Parameters	Transudative effusion	Exudative effusion
Pleural fluid protein/serum protein ratio	<0.5	>0.5
Pleural fluid LDH/serum LDH ratio	<0.6	>0.6
Pleural fluid LDH	<2/3 upper limit of normal for serum LDH	>2/3 upper limit of normal for serum LDH

LDH lactate dehydrogenase

Ultrasonography: Bedside ultrasonography is useful for diagnosing pleural effusion (Fig. 58.1b), assessing the quantity of pleural fluid, differentiating pleural effusion from lung collapse or consolidation, and distinguishing subpleural effusion from diaphragmatic paralysis.

Pleural fluid examination: Diagnostic thoracocentesis is usually not required. When insertion of chest drain is indicated for managing moderate to large amounts of effusion, the fluid should be examined for the appearance, cell count, and biochemistry. A transudative effusion is usually clear or straw-coloured, while an exudative effusion is straw-coloured or cloudy in appearance. Distinguishing features of transudative and exudative effusion (Light's criteria) are shown in Table 58.1.

58.5 Management Strategy

In asymptomatic patents with evidence of postoperative fluid overload, small to moderate amount of pleural effusion usually responds to intravenous frusemide therapy. Symptomatic patients with moderate to large amounts of effusion require insertion of chest drain for management. For patients with transudative effusion, the chest drain can usually be removed if the drain output decreases to less than about 2 mL/kg/day with continuation of oral diuretics. Pleural effusion occurring in association with post pericardiotomy syndrome usually subsides after anti-inflammatory treatment, while parapneumonic effusion generally resolves with antibiotics.

59 Chylothorax

Accumulation of chyle, which is milky lymphatic fluid enriched with fat secreted from the intestinal cells, in the pleural cavity causes chylothorax. The most common cause in children is postoperative chylothorax, which occurs in about 4–9% of children after cardiac surgery. Other causes include congenital malformation of the lymphatics with or without associated syndromic disorders, non-surgical trauma (e.g. blunt force), and tumours.

59.1 Risk factors

Proposed mechanisms for the development of chylothorax after cardiac surgery include (1) direct surgical trauma to the thoracic duct or lymphatic tributaries, (2) increase in central venous pressure, and (3) pre-existing lymphatic malformation occurring in association with syndromic disorders. Risk factors for development of postoperative chylothorax reflect the proposed underlying mechanisms (Table 59.1).

Y.-f. Cheung, *Congenital and Paediatric Acquired Heart Disease in Practice*, https://doi.org/10.1007/978-981-99-2862-0_59

Table 59.1 Risk factors for development of chylothorax in children after cardiac surgery

Risk factors
Surgical procedures with postoperative increase in central venous pressure
Fontan operation
Bidirectional cavopulmonary connection
Repair of tetralogy of Fallot (with restrictive right ventricular physiology)
Complex surgical procedures
Arterial switch operation for transposition of the great arteries
Repair of total anomalous pulmonary venous connection
Repair of truncus arteriosus
Repair of complete atrioventricular septal defect
Heart transplantation
Operations in the vicinity of the thoracic duct
Repair of coarctation of the aorta and interrupted aortic arch
Systemic-to-pulmonary arterial shunt insertion
Ligation of persistent arterial duct
Other surgical factors
Duration of cardiopulmonary bypass
Duration of cross-damping
Patient factors
Low body weight
Genetic syndromes (Turner syndrome, Down syndrome, and Noonan syndrome)

59.2 Complications

Significant chylothorax leads to respiratory compromise, prolongs ventilator dependence and postoperative recovery, and increases the length of intensive care and hospital stay.

High volume of chyle loss is associated with significant morbidity and mortality. Complications include nutritional depletion, hypoalbuminaemia, hypovolaemia, loss of electrolytes (the electrolyte composition is similar to that of serum), increased risk of thrombosis, and secondary immunodeficiency (lymphopenia and hypogammaglobinaemia).

59.3 Clinical Presentation

Some of the patients are asymptomatic and pleural effusion is detected incidentally on routine postoperative chest radiographic examination, while some may present with symptoms and signs of respiratory distress.

In patients with a chest drain in situ, chylothorax is recognized by the increasing amount of milky fluid (Fig. 59.1) being drained as full enteral feeding of breast milk or normal formula for infants and a normal diet for older children is resumed. However, in fasted patients, the fluid may appear less milky and only slightly turbid due to a lower fat content.

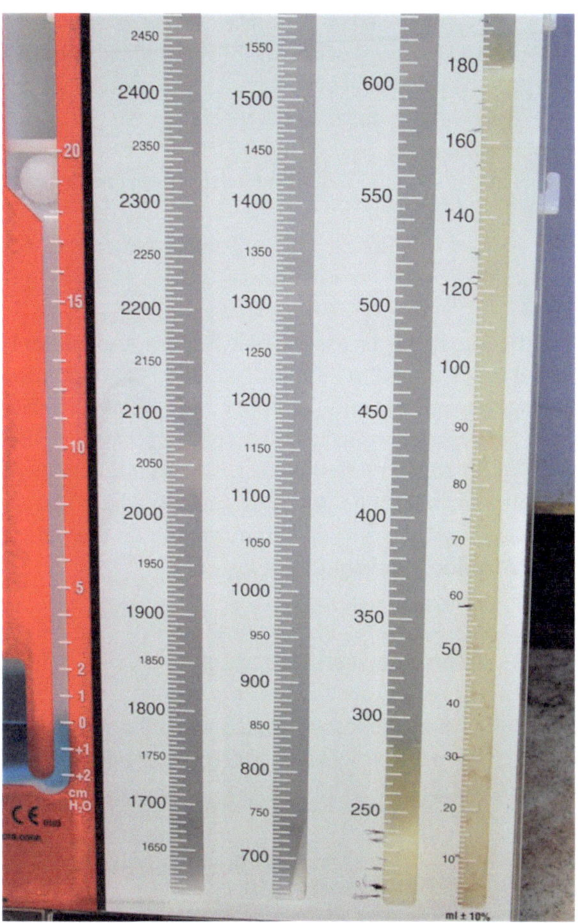

Fig. 59.1 Chylous drainage. Drainage of milky fluid from the chest drain with establishment of milk feeding

When allowed to stand in tube for a while, chyle separates into 3 layers: (1) a creamy upper layer containing chylomicrons, (2) a milky middle layer, and (3) a clearer bottom layer containing mostly lymphocytes.

59.4 Investigations

CXR: Depending on the severity of chylous effusion, the chest radiographic findings vary from blunting of the costophrenic angle to opacification of the lung field.
Ultrasonography: Bedside ultrasonography is useful for diagnosing pleural effusion, assessing the quantity of pleural fluid, and differentiating pleural effusion from lung collapse or consolidation.
Pleural fluid examination: The fluid from the chest drain should be for evidence of chyle (Box 59.1).

Box 59.1 Diagnosis of Chylothorax Based on Pleural Fluid Examination

- triglyceride concentration > 110 mg/dL (1.24 mmol/L)
- total cell count >1000 cells/μL
- lymphocytes >70% of total cell count
- when in doubt, detection of chylomicron using lipoprotein electrophoresis is diagnostic
- Sudan III staining for fat globules (seldom performed nowadays)

Further imaging to assess risk factors and underlying causes: Vascular ultrasound is performed to ascertain patency, stenosis or thrombosis of the central veins and venous return from the upper extremities (superior caval vein, internal jugular vein, innominate vein, and the subclavian veins). Echocardiography enables the assessment of right ventricular systolic and diastolic dysfunction. In patients with chylothorax refractory to dietary and medical management, magnetic resonance lymphangiography provides information on the pattern and site of lymphatic leak and can guide interventions (Chap. 63).

59.5 Management Strategy

A stepwise management approach with incorporation of dietary interventions, medical therapy, and surgical and transcatheter interventions is adopted for management of chylothorax (Fig. 59.2).

59.5.1 Patient Monitoring

Close patient monitoring and early interventions to ameliorate the untoward effects of chylothorax are important (Box 59.2).

Box 59.2 General Management of Patients with Chylothorax

- consult dietician for nutritional support
- monitor fluid balance and chyle output
- replace 50–75% of the excessive chyle loss (>50 mL/kg/day) with 5% albumin every 4 hourly
- replace electrolyte loss
- reduce infection risk and monitor for sepsis
- give intravenous immunoglobulin for management of hypogammaglobinaemia in the presence of active infection
- monitor the side effects of octreotide if given
- educate parents on chylothorax and the need for dietary modification

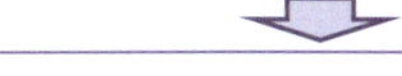

Fig. 59.2 Management of chylothorax. *low fat diet: <5–6 g of fat per day. Abbreviations: *CXR* chest X ray, *TPN* total parenteral nutrition

59.5.2 Octreotide

Octreotide is a synthetic somatostatin analogue with a much longer half-life (1.5–2 h versus 1–3 min) than somatostatin. The physiological actions of octreotide are those of somatostatin, which reduces splanchnic blood flow by vasoconstriction, decreases production of lymphatic fluid, and lowers thoracic lymph flow.

In the management of children with chylothorax, marked variations in the octreotide regimens exist. Despite having a much longer half-life than somatostatin, octreotide is commonly given as an intravenous infusion with reported doses ranging from 7 to 240 μg/kg/day (0.3–10 μg/kg/h). One can start at a dose of 0.1–1 μg/kg/h intravenously, and gradually increase the dose to a maximum of 10 μg/kg/h. Some centres may opt to start at a higher dose and reduce it gradually when there is response. Octreotide can also be given subcutaneously at reported doses ranging from 10 to 70 μg/kg/day in 3 divided doses. Octreotide has been reported to be given up to 1 month or even longer.

Side effects of octreotide are usually minor in infants and children. Reported side effects include hypoglycaemia and hyperglycaemia, nausea, abdominal cramp and pain, hyperbilirubinaemia, and increased risk of necrotizing enterocolitis.

59.5.3 Chemical Pleurodesis

Data on chemical pleurodesis in children after cardiac surgery are limited. Agents including talc, betadine, bleomycin, minocycline, and doxycycline have been administered through the chest drain to induce pleurodesis in adults. In children with postoperative chylothorax, doxycycline is the choice in many centres.

Doxycycline is an inhibitor of matrix-degrading metalloproteinases and promotes deposition of fibrin and collagen deposition in the pleural cavity to induce plural adhesion. A commonly used regimen is 20 mg/kg/dose of doxycycline (based on a dose of 1 g given to adults of 50 kg or more). It is diluted in an adequate volume of normal saline to spread the medication throughout the pleural cavity and administered through the chest drain. After administration, the chest drain is clamped and the patient is rotated every 15–20 min for 2 h. The chest drain is then unclamped afterwards. The process can be repeated for 3–5 consecutive days depending on drain output and chest radiographic findings.

Side effects of doxycycline pleurodesis include fever, pleuritis with pleuritic pain, and worsening of lung compliance.

59.5.4 MR Lymphangiogram and Lymphatic Occlusion

In centres with expertise in magnetic resonance lymphangiography and lymphatic interventions, trial of embolization of the thoracic duct can be attempted (Chap. 63).

Pericardial Effusion

60

Pericardial effusion occurs at two time periods after cardiac surgery in children: (1) immediate postoperative period, and (2) at 1–4 weeks after surgery due to postpericardiotomy syndrome.

60.1 Pathophysiology

Progressive accumulation of fluid in the pericardial cavity increases intrapericardial pressure with compression of the cardiac chambers. With development of pericardiac tamponade, the venous return is decreased, the cardiac chambers (usually right atrium and right ventricle) are collapsed, and systemic cardiac output and blood pressure drops.

Acute bleeding into the pericardial cavity in the immediate postoperative period can result in rapid rise of intrapericardial pressure and early development of tamponade. On the other hand, the relatively slower accumulation of pericardial effusion in postpericardiotomy syndrome allows for gradual increase in the compliance of the pericardium and reduces the possibility of developing cardiac tamponade.

Postpericardiotomy syndrome, reported to occur in 5–40% of patients, is believed to be due to an immune response to surgical injury to the pericardium and the hydrophilic action of blood accumulated in the pericardial cavity. Immune activation leads to an inflammatory response, which usually begins to occur at 1–2 weeks after surgery. It may linger on for 2–3 weeks with a possibility of relapse during tapering of anti-inflammatory treatment.

Y.-f. Cheung, *Congenital and Paediatric Acquired Heart Disease in Practice*, https://doi.org/10.1007/978-981-99-2862-0_60

60.2 Risk Factors

Reported risk factors include female sex, certain types of surgery (repair of atrial septal defect and atrioventricular septal defect, valve surgery, Ross procedure, Fontan surgery), high postoperative pericardial and chest drain output, and warfarin use.

60.3 Clinical Presentation and Findings

Cardiac tamponade due to rapid accumulation of blood in the pericardial cavity in the immediate postoperative period leads to tachycardia, unexpected decrease in cardiac output with systemic hypotension, and increase in central venous pressure. These clinical observations, especially with sudden cessation of the initial significant output from the pericardial drain, should prompt an urgent echocardiographic assessment to diagnose or exclude pericardial effusion and tamponade.

Infants with postpericardiotomy syndrome may present with non-specific symptoms including fever without localizing symptoms, reduced appetite, and irritability. Older children and adolescents may occasionally complain of chest pain. Physical examination may reveal a pericardial rub when the amount of effusion is small. Rarely, in patients with large amount of effusion causing tamponade, signs of low cardiac output, pulsus paradoxus, and elevated jugular venous pressure are evident.

60.4 Investigations

Markers of inflammation: Erythrocyte sedimentation rate, C reactive protein, and leukocyte count usually elevated.
ECG: The changes are suggestive of pericarditis with widespread ST-elevation or PR depression.
Echocardiography: Echocardiogram demonstrates the presence of pericardial effusion (Fig. 60.1), quantifies its size, and provides evidence of pericardial tamponade. Echocardiographic features of tamponade include diastolic collapse of the right atrium, persistence of right atrial collapse in more than one-third of the cardiac cycle, diastolic right ventricular collapse, collapse of the left-sided chambers (only rarely), and dilation of the inferior caval vein.

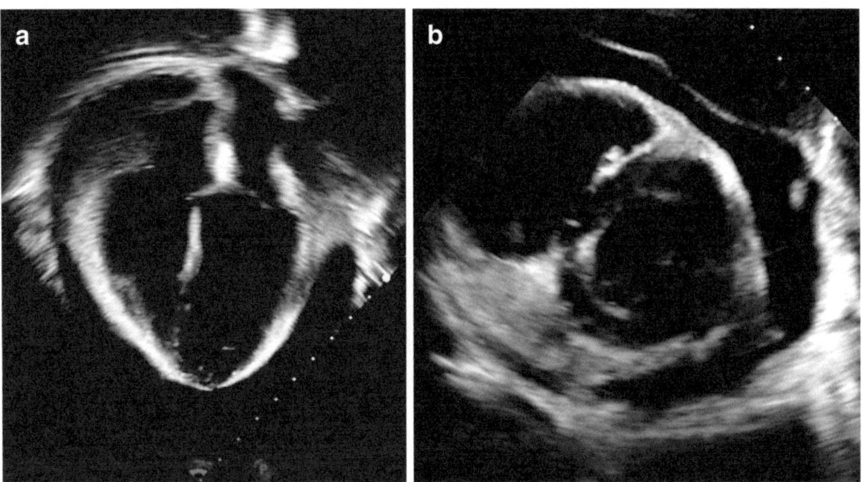

Fig. 60.1 Pericardial effusion. (**a**) Apical four-chamber and (**b**) parasternal short-axis views showing significant circumferential pericardial effusion with right atrial collapse suggestive of cardiac tamponade

60.5 Management Strategy

For acute bleeding into the pericardial cavity causing tamponade early after surgery, immediate surgical drainage is required.

Patients with postpericardiotomy syndrome but without evidence of cardiac tamponade are usually managed by 1–2 weeks of non-steroidal anti-inflammatory drugs and diuretics. Steroid may be considered if the response is incomplete or pericardial effusion recurs after tapering the dose of non-steroidal anti-inflammatory drugs. Data on the use of colchicine for postpericardiotomy syndrome are limited. Significant pericardial effusion not responding to medical therapy requires surgical or percutaneous drainage.

Part XII

Topical Issues

COVID-19 and the Heart in Children

61

The coronavirus 19 disease (COVID-19) infects children of all ages. While most children and adolescents infected with COVID-19 are asymptomatic or having a mild disease (fever with mild respiratory and gastrointestinal symptoms), severe neurological (encephalitis, seizure, stroke) and cardiovascular complications have been described.

The cardiovascular system of children and adolescents may be involved (1) during the acute COVID-19 infection, (2) after the acute infection with development of a severe inflammatory disorder referred to as multisystem inflammatory syndrome in children (MIS-C), and (3) as a rare complication of COVID-19 mRNA vaccination.

61.1 Cardiovascular Involvements in Children During Acute COVID-19 Infection

61.1.1 Pathogenetic Mechanisms

The spike protein of the severe acute respiratory syndrome coronavirus 2 (SARS-CoV-2) binds to the angiotensin-converting enzyme 2 (ACE2) receptor on cell surfaces. ACE2 receptors are expressed in cardiomyocytes, although less so in children than in adults.

Cardiac manifestations in COVID-19 disease have been hypothesized to be due to (1) direct viral invasion of cardiomyocytes, (2) inflammatory damage secondary to the immune response, and/or (3) ischaemic damage related to severe hypoxia. There is, however, no evidence to suggest that treatment with angiotensin-converting enzyme inhibitors or angiotensin receptor blockers increases the risk of COVID-19 infection or developing severe disease.

Y.-f. Cheung, *Congenital and Paediatric Acquired Heart Disease in Practice*,
https://doi.org/10.1007/978-981-99-2862-0_61

61.1.2 Cardiovascular Manifestations

Cardiovascular manifestations are uncommon in children and adolescents during acute COVID-19 infection (Box 61.1).

Box 61.1 Uncommon Paediatric Cardiovascular Manifestations During Acute COVID-19 Infection

- myocarditis with or without cardiogenic shock
- pericarditis
- cardiac arrhythmias (first-degree heart block, atrial tachycardias, ventricular tachycardias)

61.1.3 Cardiovascular Management

Cardiovascular monitoring and supportive care are adequate for most of the patients. Atrial and ventricular tachycardias may subside spontaneously or require the use of antiarrhythmics. Severe cardiogenic shock, although uncommon, may develop in some patients and require support by extracorporeal membrane oxygenation. In critically ill patients, remdesivir should be considered in consultation with a paediatric infectious disease specialist.

61.2 Multisystem Inflammatory Syndrome in Children

Multisystemic inflammatory syndrome in children (MISC-C) develops usually at two to six weeks after acute COVID-19 infection. This postinfectious inflammatory syndrome involves two or more body systems (mucocutaneous, cardiac, renal, pulmonary, haematologic, gastrointestinal, and/or neurological).

61.2.1 Pathogenesis

The pathogenesis is unclear but is probably related to a hyperimmune response in a genetically susceptible child.

61.2.2 Cardiovascular Manifestations and Findings

Cardiovascular symptoms and signs include shortness of breath and respiratory distress, cardiogenic or vasodilatory shock, and mucocutaneous features (rash, conjunctivitis, strawberry tongue, red lips and oral mucosa, and redness and oedema of extremities) that may suggest the diagnosis of classic or incomplete Kawasaki disease. Cardiac arrhythmias and heart block have also been reported.

Differential diagnosis of MIS-C includes Kawasaki disease (including Kawasaki disease shock syndrome), bacteraemic shock, toxic shock syndrome, adenovirus infection, and autoimmune disease.

61.2.3 Cardiovascular and Other Investigations

Inflammatory markers: Laboratory evidence of inflammation (e.g. increased ESR, CRP, procalcitonin, ferritin, and D-dimer) is present.
Cardiac biomarkers: Troponin, brain natriuretic peptide (BNP), or N-terminal proBNP may be elevated.
ECG: Electrocardiogram may reveal non-specific ST and T wave changes, cardiac arrhythmias, and varying degrees of heart block.
Echocardiography: Echocardiographic abnormalities include ventricular dysfunction, mitral regurgitation, pericardial effusion, and coronary arterial dilation and/or aneurysm formation.

61.2.4 Diagnostic Criteria

Diagnostic criteria as proposed by the United States Centers for Disease Control and Prevention (CDC) and the World Health Organization (WHO) are shown in Table 61.1.

61.2.5 MIS-C Versus Kawasaki disease

Several clinical features overlap between MIS-C and Kawasaki disease. On the other hand, there are certain clinical and laboratory features that can help to distinguish between the two conditions (Table 61.2).

61.2.6 Cardiovascular Management

Management of cardiogenic and vasogenic shock requires intravenous infusion of inotropes and vasoconstrictors and mechanical ventilatory support. In severe cases, extracorporeal membrane oxygenation support is required.

Immunomodulation with intravenous immunoglobulin is usually the first-line treatment for MIS-C. Further treatment with glucocorticoids, infliximab (tumour necrosis factor-α antagonist), or anakinra (interleukin-1 receptor antagonist) has also been reported. In patients with coronary artery involvement, antiplatelet therapy and anticoagulation should be given depending on severity of the coronary artery dilation.

Table 61.1 Diagnostic criteria for MIS-C

	CDC criteria	WHO criteria
Age	<21 year	0–19 year
Fever	≥38.0 °C for ≥24 h or subjective fever	Fever ≥3 day
Evidence of inflammation	≥1 laboratory evidence of inflammation: elevated CRP, ESR, fibrinogen, procalcitonin, D-dimer, ferritin, LDH, IL-6, neutrophils, lymphopenia, hypoalbuminaemia	≥1 laboratory evidence of inflammation: elevated CRP, ESR, or procalcitonin
	AND	AND
Multisystem involvement	≥2 organ systems involved: cardiac, renal, pulmonary, haematological, gastrointestinal, dermatological, or neurological	≥2 of the following: mucocutaneous inflammation (rash, bilateral, nonpurulent conjunctivitis, or oral, hands, or feet oedema and redness); hypotension or shock; cardiac involvement; coagulopathy (abnormal PT, PTT, or elevated D-dimer); or acute gastrointestinal illness (diarrhoea, emesis, or pain)
Cardiac abnormalities indicative of involvement	Abnormal biomarkers: elevated troponin or BNP or NT-pro-BNP electrocardiographic changes: conduction block, ST-segment elevation, myocardial ischaemia, low-voltage Echocardiographic findings: z score ≥ 2 in any of the proximal coronary arteries, ventricular dysfunction (right, left, or both), mitral regurgitation, pericardial effusion	Same as CDC MIS-C
	AND	AND
Additional required features	Positive for SARS-CoV-2 infection by RT-PCR, serology, or antigen test or exposure within 4 wk. to a suspected or confirmed COVID-19 case	Positive for SARS-CoV-2 infection by RT-PCR, serology, or antigen test or likely exposure to COVID-19 case
	AND	AND
	No alternative pathology or diagnosis	No alternative pathology or diagnosis

BNP brain natriuretic peptide, *IL-6* interleukin 6, *LDH* lactate dehydrogenase, *PT* prothrombin time, *PTT* partial thromboplastin time, *RT-PCR* reverse transcription polymerase chain reaction

Table 61.2 Distinguishing features of MIS-C versus Kawasaki disease

Feature	MIS-C	Kawasaki disease
Age	Commonly affects older children and adolescents	Infants and young children
Ethnicity	Higher risk in Black and Hispanic children and less common among Asian children	Higher incidence among Asian children
Gastrointestinal symptoms	Common (especially abdominal pain)	Less prominent
Renal involvement	May be present	Extremely rare
Cardiac dysfunction and shock	More common	Less common (the presence suggests Kawasaki disease shock syndrome)
Inflammatory markers (CRP, ferritin and D-dimer)	More elevated than in Kawasaki disease	Elevation is less severe
Troponin, BNP, NT-pro-BNP	More elevated	Usually normal or only mildly elevated
Lymphocyte and platelet count	Lymphopenia and thrombocytopenia may occur	Thrombocytosis and no lymphopenia

Regular cardiovascular monitoring is required during the acute illness and at outpatient follow-up (Box 61.2). Inflammation and cardiovascular abnormalities usually resolve within 1–4 weeks of diagnosis. However, progression of coronary artery aneurysms has been reported and requires long term monitoring and treatment with antiplatelet therapy with or without anticoagulants. In patients with documented ventricular dysfunction, exercise restriction for three to six months is advisable.

Box 61.2 Cardiovascular Monitoring for MIS-C

During the acute illness

- daily ECG
- daily troponin and brain natriuretic peptide (BNP) or N-terminal proBNP levels
- baseline and regular echocardiographic reassessment of coronary artery abnormalities, ventricular function, mitral regurgitation, and pericardial effusion

At outpatient follow-up

- repeat ECG
- Holter monitoring if cardiac arrhythmias are present during the acute illness or if ECG is persistently abnormal on follow-up
- repeat troponin and BNP or N-terminal proBNP levels if still elevated at the time of discharge

- repeat echocardiographic assessment at four to six weeks after discharge, reassess and manage as appropriate for patients with impaired cardiac function and/or coronary arterial abnormalities (similar to guidelines on the follow up of Kawasaki disease)

61.3 Post COVID-19 mRNA Vaccination

Myocarditis, pericarditis, and myopericarditis are rare complications of COVID-19 mRNA vaccinations (Pfizer-BioNTech BNT162b2 and Moderna mRNA-1273), especially in adolescent and young adult males. Overall, the incidence of COVID-19 mRNA-vaccine-related myocarditis is estimated to be in the range of 3–50 cases per million vaccinated individuals. Among boys aged 12–17, about 70–100 cases, and among girls of the same age group, about 6–10 cases of myocarditis per million second dose of the mRNA COVID-19 vaccine administered have been reported.

61.3.1 Pathogenetic Mechanisms

Potential mechanisms include (1) immune reactivity to the mRNA with activation of proinflammatory cascades in the heart and (2) molecular mimicry between the spike protein of SARS-CoV-2 and myocardial contractile proteins. Given the higher prevalence in adolescent and young adult males, the immune reaction is likely to be influenced by age and differences in hormonal signalling.

61.3.2 Cardiovascular Manifestations and Diagnosis

Almost all patients present with chest pain. The onset is usually within the first week after vaccination. Fever may precede chest pain in some patients. The diagnosis of myocarditis and/or myopericarditis should be considered in adolescents and young adults who develop chest pain, shortness of breath, or palpitations after receiving a dose of COVID-19 mRNA vaccine. Fulminant myocarditis resulting in cardiogenic shock has been reported rarely, although a causal relationship needs to be established.

Diagnosis is based on symptoms, blood investigation (cardiac troponin level, inflammatory markers) and non-invasive imaging modalities (echocardiography, electrocardiogram, cardiac magnetic resonance) (Fig. 61.1). Other causes of myocarditis have to be considered. The working case definitions for myocarditis and pericarditis of the United States Centers for Disease Control and Prevention are shown in Table 61.3 and Table 61.4, respectively (MMWR 2021:70;977–982). The term ‘myopericarditis’ may be used for patients who meet criteria for both myocarditis and pericarditis.

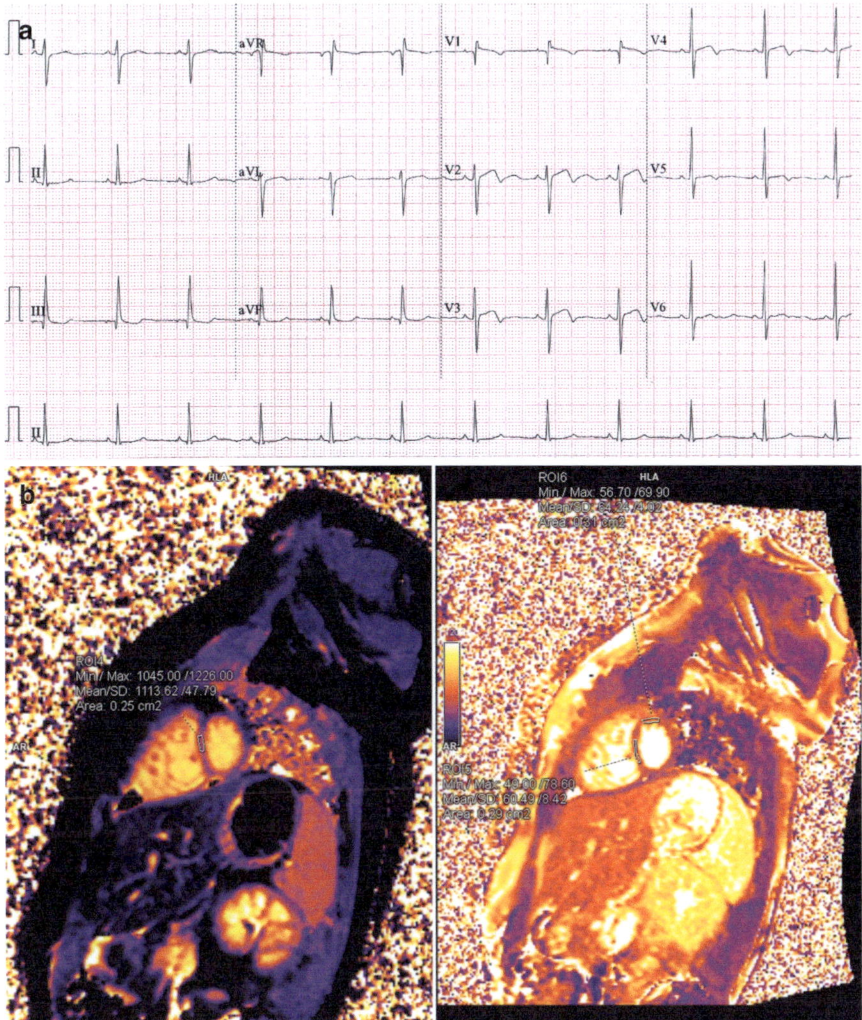

Fig. 61.1 Assessment of myopericarditis after COVID-19 mRNA vaccine. (**a**) ECG showing ST elevation in V2 and V3 and diffuse T wave flattening and inversion (**b**) CMR showing increased T1 (left) and T2 (right) relaxation times at left ventricular apical segment

Table 61.3 CDC working case definition of acute myocarditis

Probable case	Confirmed case
Presence of ≥1 new or worsening of the following clinical symptoms Chest pain/pressure/discomfort Dyspnoea/shortness of breath Palpitations Syncope OR, infants and children aged <12 years might instead have ≥2 of the following symptoms Irritability Vomiting Poor feeding Tachypnoea Lethargy	presence of ≥1 new or worsening of the following clinical symptoms Chest pain/pressure/discomfort Dyspnoea/shortness of breath Palpitations Syncope OR, infants and children aged <12 years might instead have ≥2 of the following symptoms Irritability Vomiting Poor feeding Tachypnoea Lethargy
AND ≥ 1 new finding of Troponin level above upper limit of Normal Abnormal ECG or rhythm monitoring Findings consistent with myocarditis Abnormal cardiac function or wall Motion abnormalities on echo Cardiac MRI findings consistent with Myocarditis (original or revised Lake Louise criteria)	AND ≥ 1 new finding of Histologic confirmation of myocarditis Cardiac MRI findings consistent with Myocarditis in the presence of troponin Level above upper limit of normal (original or revised Lake Louise criteria)
AND No other identifiable cause of the Symptoms and findings	AND No other identifiable cause of the symptoms and findings

Table 61.4 CDC working case definition of acute pericarditis

Probable Case
Presence of ≥2 new or worsening of the following clinical symptoms Acute chest pain (typically described as pain made worse by lying down, deep Inspiration, cough, and relieved by sitting up or leaning forward, although other types of chest pain may occur) Pericarditis rub on exam New ST-elevation or PR-depression on ECG New or worsening pericardial effusion on echocardiogram or MRI

61.3.3 Cardiovascular Management

Cardiovascular monitoring and supportive care are adequate for most of the patients who run a mild clinical course with rapid resolution of symptoms. For more symptomatic patients, the use of nonsteroidal anti-inflammatory drugs, aspirin, steroids, colchicine, and intravenous immunoglobulin has been reported. In patients with left ventricular dysfunction, it is reasonable to consider a short duration of angiotensin-converting enzyme inhibitor or beta- blocker therapy. Inotropic and extracorporeal membrane oxygenation support is required for the rare complication of fulminant myocarditis.

In patients with resolved myocarditis and/or pericarditis, physical activities should be restricted until complete resolution of all clinical and laboratory abnormalities. For patients with impaired left ventricular function, it is reasonable to restrict physical activities for at least 6 months after the onset of the disease and after reassessment for recovery of left ventricular function. The long-term consequences of COVID-19 mRNA vaccine-associated myocarditis remain to be unveiled.

61.3.4 Recommendation on Future Doses of Vaccine

Recommendation on future doses of COVID-19 vaccine depends on the diagnosis (myocarditis, pericarditis, and myopericarditis), certainty of the diagnosis, and its relationship to mRNA vaccination. Options vary among countries but may include deferring any further dose of COVID-19 vaccine until further information is available, selecting an alternative vaccine formulation, or proceeding with the same type of COVID-19 vaccine. Recommendations may change when additional information is available.

Genetics of Congenital Heart Disease 62

With the rapid evolution of genetic testing tools, the understanding of genetics of congenital heart disease has significantly increased. Current genetic testing technologies enable the detection of large genetic variations (karyotyping, array comparative genomic hybridization, and fluorescence in situ hybridization) and, with next generation sequencing, detection of insertion or deletion and single-nucleotide polymorphism (gene panel testing, and whole exome and whole genome sequencing).

62.1 Incidence of Congenital Heart Disease

Congenital heart disease is the most common congenital malformation in newborns. An incidence of 8–10 per thousand live births (0.8–1%) has often been quoted, although this figure does not include non-stenotic bicuspid aortic valves and trivial lesions such as tiny muscular ventricular septal defects and silent persistent arterial duct. The incidence of certain cardiac defects may differ among populations. For example, the high incidence of subarterial ventricular septal defect in Chinese and Japanese is well documented. The relative frequencies of the different types of congenital heart defects are shown in Table 62.1.

Y.-f. Cheung, *Congenital and Paediatric Acquired Heart Disease in Practice*, https://doi.org/10.1007/978-981-99-2862-0_62

Table 62.1 Relative frequencies of different congenital heart defects

Cardiac defects	Frequency
Acyanotic	
Ventricular septal defect	35%
Atrial septal defect	15%
Persistent arterial duct	10%
Pulmonary stenosis	6%
Coarctation of the aorta	4%
Atrioventricular septal defect	3–4%
Aortic stenosis	2%
Cyanotic	
Tetralogy of Fallot	4–5%
Transposition of the great arteries	4%
Hypoplastic left heart (aortic atresia, mitral atresia)	2–3%
Hypoplastic right heart (pulmonary atresia with intact ventricular septum, Ebstein anomaly, tricuspid atresia)	1–3%
Total anomalous pulmonary venous connectionuniventricular hearts	1–2% 1–2%
Truncus arteriosus	1%

Table 62.2 Causes of congenital heart disease

Genetic Cause	% of congenital heart patients
Single gene	3–5
Chromosomal/ aneuploidy	8–10
Copy number variation	3–25 (syndromic), 3–10 (isolated)
Environmental	2
Unknown cause (presumed multifactorial)	estimated to be 70–80

Based on Pierpont et al. Circulation. 2018;138:e653–e711

62.2 Causes of Congenital Heart Disease

Epidemiological studies suggest a genetic or environmental cause in 20% to 30% of congenital heart disease (Table 62.2). With advances made in genetic testing, copy number variations have emerged as important causes of both syndromic and non-syndromic congenital heart disease. On the other hand, single gene mutations found based in families with Mendelian inheritance have not been found to be common in unrelated patients.

Environmental causes of congenital heart defects include antenatal infection, drugs, and maternal disorders (Table 62.3).

Table 62.3 Environmental causes of congenital heart defects

Environmental influence	Risk of heart defects	Cardiac malformations
Infection		
Rubella	35%	PDA, peripheral pulmonary arterial stenosis, ASD, VSD
Drugs		
Alcohol	25–30%	VSD, ASD, PDA
Hydantoin	2–3%	PS, AS, CoA, PDA
Lithium	10–20%	Ebstein anomaly, tricuspid atresia
Exogenous female hormones	2–4%	VSD, TGA, TOF
Maternal disorders		
Diabetes mellitus	3–5%	VSD, CoA, TGA
SLE	20–40%	heart block
Phenylketonuria	25–50%	TOF

AS aortic stenosis, *ASD* atrial septal defect, *CoA* coarctation of the aorta, *PDA* persistent arterial duct, *PS* pulmonary stenosis, *SLE* systemic lupus erythematosus, *TGA* transposition of the great arteries, *TOF* tetralogy of Fallot, *VSD* ventricular septal defect

62.3 Syndromic Congenital Heart Disease

Congenital heart disease is a common feature of syndromic disorders, which are characterized by more than 1 identifying features. Syndromic congenital heart disease, which constitutes at least 25% of all congenital heart disease, can be associated with aneuploidy of the autosomal or sex chromosomes, copy number variants, and single gene variation.

62.3.1 Aneuploidies

62.3.1.1 Down Syndrome

Genetics: trisomy 21, rarely mosaicism.
Phenotypic features: prominent medial epicathic folds, upslanting palpebral fissure, Brushfield spots, flat nasal bridge, low-set ears, protuberant tongue, brachycephaly, short fingers, clinodactyly of little finger, single transverse palmer crease, wide gap between first and second toes (sandal gap deformity), hypotonia and joint hyperflexibility.
Cardiovascular anomalies: occurs in 40–50% of patients, most common malformations are complete atrioventricular septal defect, ventricular septal defect, atrial septal defect, persistent arterial duct, and tetralogy of Fallot.

62.3.1.2 Edwards Syndrome

Genetics: trisomy 18.
Phenotypic features: low birthweight, microcephaly, micrognathia, low-set ears, camptodactyly (overlapping of the flexed middle finger by the index and little fingers), rocker-bottom feet, inguinal or umbilical hernia, hypertonia.

Cardiovascular anomalies: occurs in almost all patients, common malformations are ventricular septal defect, persistent arterial duct, bicuspid aortic and/or pulmonary valve, nodularity of valve leaflets.

62.3.1.3 Patau Syndrome

Genetics: trisomy 13.
Phenotypic features: low birth weight, microcephaly, microphthalmia, coloboma of iris, cleft lip and palate, camptodactyly, polydactyly, rocker-bottom feet, capillary haemangioma, hyper- or hypotonia.
Cardiovascular anomalies: occurs in 80% of patients, common malformations are ventricular septal defect, atrial septal defect, and persistent arterial duct.

62.3.1.4 Turner Syndrome

Genetics: 45,X, and mosaicism.
Phenotypic features: transient lymphoedema of the dorsum of the hands and feet occurs in newborn baby girls, older girls with short stature, webbing of the neck, a low hairline, cubitus valgus, broad chest with widely spaced nipples, and excessive pigmented naevi.
Cardiovascular anomalies: occur in about 20% of girls with Turner syndrome, characteristically left-sided cardiac lesions including coarctation of the aorta, bicuspid aortic valve, valvar aortic stenosis and, less commonly, idiopathic dilation of the aorta at risk of dissection and rupture, mitral valve prolapse, and hypoplastic left heart syndrome.

62.3.2 Copy Number Variants

Copy number variants include insertion, deletion, and duplication of segments of DNA. Deletions, ranging from a single gene to multiple genes, are in general more deleterious than duplications. The two common deletion syndromes commonly encountered in the clinical settings are described.

62.3.2.1 22q11.2 Deletion Syndrome

Genetics: the most common microdeletion syndrome with contiguous gene deletion involving >40 genes, most of 22q11.2 deletions are de novo but can be inherited in an autosomal dominant fashion, associated usually (but not always) with DiGeorge and velocardiofacial syndromes.
Phenotypic features (DiGeorge and velocardiofacial syndromes): flattened facial features, a bulbous nose, upslanting or downslanting palpebral fissures, small rounded or low-set ears, a small mouth, micrognathia, cleft palate.
Cardiovascular anomalies: occurs in about 60–80% of patients, primarily conotruncal defects (tetralogy of Fallot, pulmonary atresia with ventricular septal defect, truncus arteriosus, type B interruption of the aortic arch), ventricular septal defect with a right-sided aortic arch, and an isolated right aortic arch.

Other anomalies: immunodeficiency related to variable degree of thymic hypoplasia, hypocalcaemia related to hypoparathyroidism (both related to abnormal development of the third and fourth embryonic branchial pouches), behavioural and learning disabilities in older children, psychiatric disorders in adolescent and adult patients, and other problems require long-term monitoring and management (Box 62.1).

Box 62.1 Systemic Assessments of 22q11.2 Deletion Syndrome

Systemic evaluation
- cardiac assessment: ECG, echocardiogram
- renal ultrasound
- scoliosis examination
- dental evaluation
- development and school performance
- behavioural and learning problems
- psychiatric disorders (adolescents and adults)

Blood investigations
- ionized calcium, parathyroid hormone
- thyroid-stimulating hormone

Immunologic evaluation
- chest radiograph for thymic shadow
- complete blood cell count and differentials for lymphopenia
- T and B cell phenotyping, T cell function, and immunoglobulin levels

Genetic assessment
- genetic counselling
- genetic studies of parents

62.3.2.2 William Syndrome

Genetics: a contiguous gene deletion syndrome, usually sporadic but can be inherited in an autosomal dominant fashion, microdeletion at chromosome 7q11.23, which encompasses the elastin gene, *ELN*, and nearby genes.
Phenotypic features: intellectual disability, sociable personality, characteristic facies with broad forehead, bitemporal narrowing, full cheeks, flat nasal bridge, anteverted nostrils, long philtrum, prominent lips with open mouth, small and widely spaced teeth.
Cardiovascular anomalies: occurs in about 75% of patients, supravalvar aortic stenosis and peripheral branch pulmonary arterial stenosis are the most common, but narrowing of other arteries (ascending aorta, aortic arch, thoracic and abdominal aorta, coronary arteries, carotid and cerebral arteries, mesenteric arteries, and renal arteries) is also characteristic.

Other anomalies: failure to thrive, hypercalcaemia, hypercalciuria and nephrocalcinosis, hypothyroidism, and other problems require long-term monitoring and management (Box 62.2).

Box 62.2 Systemic Assessment of William Syndrome

- monitoring of growth
- developmental and neurologic assessment
- blood pressure measurement (both upper limbs and one lower limb)
- cardiac assessment: ECG, echocardiogram, CT and MR angiogram
- dental, audiological, and ophthalmological assessments
- renal assessment: renal ultrasound including Doppler assessment, urinalysis for hypercalciuria
- blood investigations: serum calcium concentration, thyroid function test
- genetic assessment

62.3.3 Single Gene Variants

Single gene variants are also associated with syndromic congenital heart disease. Selected entities are described.

62.3.3.1 Alagille Syndrome

Genetics: an autosomal dominant disorder with pathogenic variants in *JAG1*, a gene encoding a transmembrane protein that functions as a ligand for the Notch family of receptors involved in signalling pathways in cell fate specification.
Phenotypic features: facial dysmorphic features include broad forehead, deep-set eyes, bulbous nose, prominent chin, other features include paucity of intrahepatic bile duct causing neonatal cholestatic jaundice, eye defect (posterior embryotoxon, an opaque white-grey ring at the margin of the cornea), vertebral anomalies (hemivertebrae, 'butterfly' vertebrae, spina bifida occulta).
Cardiovascular anomalies: occur in >90% of patients, usually right-sided anomalies (peripheral branch pulmonary arterial stenosis, valvar pulmonary stenosis, and tetralogy of Fallot), other anomalies include atrial septal defect and coarctation of the aorta.

62.3.3.2 CHARGE Syndrome

Genetics: an autosomal dominant disorder with pathogenic variants in *CHD7.*
Phenotypic features: CHARGE is an acronym for Coloboma, Heart defects, cho-Anal atresia, Retarded growth and development, Genital anomalies (cryptorchidism and micropenis in males, and hypogonadotropic hypogonadism in both males and females), and Ear anomalies (involving the external ear canal, ossicles, and cochlea).

Cardiovascular anomalies: occur in 75% of patients, including conotruncal defects (tetralogy of Fallot, interrupted aortic arch, truncus arteriosus, and double-outlet right ventricle), all types of septal defects, persistent arterial duct, and vascular rings.

62.3.3.3 Ellis-Van Creveld Syndrome

Genetics: an autosomal recessive disorder with pathogenic variants in *EVC* or *EVC2.*
Phenotypic features: facial dysmorphic features include short upper lip bound to the alveolar ridge, skeletal dysplasia with postaxial polydactyly, short limbs, and short ribs, dental abnormalities include natal teeth, small teeth, and delayed eruption, other features include hypoplastic nails, and sparse hair.
Cardiovascular anomalies: occur in about 50%, characteristically a common atrium with deficient atrium septum, other cardiac anomalies include persistent arterial duct, ventricular septal defect, hypoplastic left heart syndrome, and abnormalities of the mitral and tricuspid valves.

62.3.3.4 Kabuki Syndrome

Genetics: X-linked and autosomal dominant disorders with pathogenic variants in *KMT2D and KDM6A.*
Phenotypic features: intellectual disability, growth deficiency, dental anomalies, persistent fetal fingertip pads, facial dysmorphic features include long palpebral fissures, arched eyebrows, long eyelashes, eversion of outer one-third of lower eyelid, depressed nasal tip, cleft lip and/or palate, and large prominent ears, skeletal abnormalities include brachydactyly, clinodactyly, scoliosis, kyphosis, and hypermobility of hip and knee joints, other features include cryptorchidism and hypospadias in males.
Cardiovascular anomalies: occur in about 40% to 70%, characteristically left-sided obstructive lesions including hypoplastic left heart syndrome, mitral stenosis, bicuspid aortic valve, and coarctation of the aorta, other cardiac anomalies include atrial septal defect, ventricular septal defect, pulmonary stenosis, and double-outlet right ventricle.
Other anomalies: growth, neurodevelopmental, orthopaedic, urogenital endocrine, immunologic, and other problems require long-term monitoring and management (Box 62.3).

Box 62.3 Systemic Assessment in Kabuki Syndrome

- assessment of feeding and nutritional status
- monitoring of growth
- developmental assessment

- cardiac assessment: ECG, echocardiogram
- dental, audiological, and ophthalmological assessments
- renal ultrasound
- assessment of spine for scoliosis and vertebral anomalies
- endocrine assessment for hypothyroidism, growth hormone deficiency and hyperinsulinism
- neurologic assessment and imaging
- immunologic evaluation for humoral immune deficiency and autoimmune disease
- genetic assessment

62.3.3.5 Holt-Oram Syndrome

Genetics: an autosomal dominant disorder with pathogenic variants in *TBX5*, which encodes a transcription factor and is an important regulator of limb and heart development (hence also referred to as cardiac-limb syndrome).

Phenotypic features: upper limb defects, ranging from thumb hypoplasia to phocomelia, are usually bilateral, although the left is usually more affected than the right.

Cardiovascular anomalies: occur in about 85% of patients, the most common being secundum atrial septal defect, other defects include isolated atrioventricular conduction block, primum atrial septal defect, ventricular septal defect, tetralogy of Fallot, aortic stenosis, mitral valve prolapse, and hypoplastic left heart syndrome.

62.3.3.6 RASopathies

RASopathies comprise several autosomal dominant disorders that are characterized by (1) causative pathogenic variants in genes that encode proteins involved in the RAS/MAPK (mitogen-activated protein kinase) pathway, which plays an important role in the regulation of the cell cycle, differentiation, growth, senescence, and apoptosis, and (2) overlapping phenotypic features including dysmorphic facial features, abnormal growth and neurodevelopment, and cardiac anomalies. These disorders include Noonan syndrome (described below), cardiofaciocutaneous syndrome, Costello syndrome, and Noonan syndrome with multiple lentigines (previous referred to as LEOPARD syndrome), and neurofibromatosis type 1 (although cardiac anomalies are uncommon is this condition).

62.3.3.7 Noonan Syndrome

Genetics: an autosomal dominant disorder with pathogenic variants in *PTPN11* (50% of patients) and variants in other genes in the RAS/MAPK pathway including *SOS1*, *RAF1*, *RIT1*, *KRAS*, *SHOC2*, *NRAS, SOS2*, and *BRAF* (about 30% of patients).

Phenotypic features: transient peripheral lymphoedema may be present during infancy, facial dysmorphic features include ptosis of eyelids, hypertelorism, downslanting palpebral fissures, low-set ears, webbing of the neck, a low hairline, shield-like chest, cubitus valgus, and majority of males have cryptorchidism.
Cardiovascular anomalies: occur in 80–90% of patients, the characteristic cardiac defect is valvar pulmonary stenosis (with thick and dysplastic valve cusps), other cardiac anomalies include peripheral branch pulmonary arterial stenosis, atrial septal defect, tetralogy of Fallot, mitral valve abnormalities, coarctation of the aorta, and hypertrophic cardiomyopathy.
Other anomalies: growth, neurodevelopmental, orthopaedic and other problems require long-term monitoring and management (Box 62.4).

Box 62.4 Systemic Assessment in Noonan Syndrome

- monitoring of growth
- developmental assessment
- cardiac assessment: ECG, echocardiogram
- dental, audiological, and ophthalmological assessments
- haematological: complete blood count and coagulation profile
- renal ultrasound
- assessment of spine for scoliosis
- genetic assessment

62.3.3.8 Heterotaxy Syndrome

Genetics: aneuploidies, chromosomal rearrangements, and copy number variants have been found in patients with heterotaxy syndrome, genetic variants associated with heterotaxy involve genes associated with ciliary defects and left-right organization. About 10% of patients with primary ciliary dyskinesia exhibit heterotaxy.
Cardiovascular and other anomalies: cardiac and extracardiac associations in heterotaxy syndrome are discussed in Chap. 20.

62.4 Non-syndromic Congenital Heart Disease

The list of genetic variants identified in children with non-syndromic congenital heart disease is expanding (Table 62.4). The genes identified encode mostly (1) transcription factors (proteins that bind to DNA and activate its transcription to RNA), (2) signalling molecules (an example is the altered Notch signalling pathway due to *JAG1* mutation that causes Alagille syndrome and nonsyndromic valvar pulmonary stenosis and tetralogy of Fallot), and (3) structural proteins (sarcomeric proteins, elastin).

Table 62.4 Examples of genes involved in nonsyndromic congenital cardiovascular disease

Gene	Cardiovascular malformation
Transcription factors	
CITED2	ASD, VSD
GATA4	ASD, VSD, AVSD, valvar PS, TOF
NR2F2	AVSD, AS, CoA, VSD, HLHS, TOF
NKX2–5	ASD, atrioventricular conduction delay, TOF, HLHS
TBX20	ASD, VSD, MS, DCM
Cell signalling and adhesion proteins	
CRELD1	ASD, AVSD
JAG1	TOF, valvar PS, pulmonary arterial stenosis
NOTCH1	BAV, AS, HLHS, TOF, valvar PS
SMAD6	BAV, CoA, AS
Structural proteins	
ELN	Supravalvar aortic stenosis
MYH6	ASD, HCM, DCM
MYH7	Ebstein anomaly, LVNC, HCM, DCM

Adapted with modifications from Pierpont et al. Circulation. 2018;138:e653–e711
Abbreviations as in Table 62.3; other abbreviations: *AVSD* atrioventricular septal defect, *BAV* bicuspid aortic valve, *DCM* dilated cardiomyopathy, *HCM* hypertrophic cardiomyopathy, *HLHS* hypoplastic left heart syndrome, *LVNC* left ventricular noncompaction, *MS* mitral stenosis

62.5 Recurrence of Congenital Heart Disease

The inheritance pattern of many syndromic congenital heart disease as described above is known. For isolated nonsyndromic congenital heart disease, the recurrence risk in sibling or offspring (in the absence of parental history of congenital heart disease) varies from 1% to 4%. When either of the parents is affected, the recurrence risk increased to 5% to 10%. These is an excess of congenital heart defects in offspring born to affected mothers, about twice the risk, compared to offspring born to affected fathers (Table 62.5).

While the type of congenital heart disease may differ between parents and offspring and among siblings, three categories of congenital heart disease have the highest risk of recurrence with the same phenotype: (1) heterotaxy syndrome, (2) right ventricular outflow obstructive lesions, and (3) left ventricular obstructive lesions.

Table 62.5 Recurrence risks for isolated (nonsyndromic) congenital heart disease

Defect	Father affected, %	Mother affected, %	1 sibling affected, %
Atrial septal defect	1.5–3.5	4–6	2.5–3
Atrioventricular septal defect	1–4.5	11.5–14	3–4
Ventricular septal defect	2–3.5	6–10	3
Aortic stenosis	3–4	8–18	2
Valvar pulmonary stenosis	2–3.5	4–6.5	2
Tetralogy of Fallot	1.5	2–2.5	2.5–3
Coarctation of the aorta	2–3	4–6.5	2
Persistent arterial duct	2–2.5	3.5–4	3
Hypoplastic left heart syndrome	21		2–9
Transposition of the great arteries	2		1.5
Congenitally corrected transposition of the great arteries	3–5		5–6
Ebstein anomaly	NR	6	1
Truncus arteriosus	NR	NR	1
Tricuspid atresia	NR	NR	1
Pulmonary atresia	NR	NR	1

Adapted with modifications from Pierpont et al. Circulation. 2018;138:e653–e711 *NR* not reported/insufficient data)

Lymphatic Abnormalities in Congenital Heart Disease

63

The lymphatic system has been regarded as the 'forgotten third circulation'. Recent advances in the imaging of the lymphatic system and lymphatic interventions have led to an increasing interest in lymphatic abnormalities. In patients with congenital heart disease, the alteration of haemodynamics, pre-existence of lymphatic malformation associated with syndromic congenital heart disease, and surgical trauma can significantly impact on the structure and function of the lymphatic system.

63.1 Lymphatic System

63.1.1 Lymph

'Lymph' is derived from the Latin word 'lympha', which means 'water'. Lymph is produced as the affluent of interstitial fluid (an ultrafiltrate of the capillary circulation) from the parenchyma of different organs with subsequent addition of circulating lymphocytes as the lymphatic vessels pass through the lymph nodes. The composition of lymph is similar to that of plasma. Additionally, proteins derived from extracellular matrix processing, tissue growth and remodelling, cellular metabolic and catabolic activities, and cell death in the tissues are enriched in the lymph. Lymph is also the medium for the transport of nearly all dietary lipid in the form of chylomicrons absorbed through the lacteals (lymphatic vessels in the intestinal villi).

63.1.2 Lymphatic Circulation

Lymphatic capillaries drain into larger collecting lymphatic vessels, which are lined by smooth muscle cells. About 75% of the lymph drains via the thoracic duct, while the remaining drains thorough the lymphatic duct into the systemic venous system.

Y.-f. Cheung, *Congenital and Paediatric Acquired Heart Disease in Practice*, https://doi.org/10.1007/978-981-99-2862-0_63

From the lower part of the body and abdominal organs, the lymphatic vessels drain into the cisterna chyli. The thoracic duct originates from the cisterna chyli, ascends anterior to the vertebrae, passes through the aortic hiatus of the diaphragm into the posterior mediastinum, and runs in the superior mediastinum posterior to the aortic arch and left subclavian artery. It empties as a single or multiple lymphatic channels into the junction between the left subclavian and the left internal jugular vein.

From the right arm, right side of the head, and the right lung, the lymphatic vessels drain into the right lymphatic duct, which empties into the right subclavian vein usually near its angle of junction with the right internal jugular vein.

63.2 Lymphatic Disorders in Congenital Heart Disease

Patients with congenital heart disease are at risk of lymphatic disorders due to several reasons: (1) easy traumatization during cardiac surgery of lymphatic vessels due to their close proximity to the surgical field, (2) postoperative alteration of haemodynamics that causes acute or chronic increase in central venous pressure (the latter typically found in Fontan patients,) and (3) pre-existing lymphatic malformation associated with syndromic congenital heart disease (e.g. Noonan syndrome, Turner syndrome, Down syndrome).

Certain congenital heart populations are hence vulnerable to development postoperative chylothorax, protein-losing enteropathy, and plastic bronchitis; the latter two lymphatic complications being primarily seen in Fontan patients,

63.2.1 Postoperative Chylothorax

Risk factors for development, diagnosis, and management of postoperative chylothorax are discussed in Chap. 59. The potential roles of lymphatic imaging and interventions in the management of postoperative chylothorax are discussed in the next section.

63.2.2 Protein-Losing Enteropathy

Protein-losing enteropathy in Fontan patients results in excessive leakage of protein from the intestine and hypoalbuminaemia. Its diagnosis carries prognostic implication as only about 50% of patients survive for more than 5 years once diagnosed to have protein-losing enteropathy.

63.2.2.1 Pathophysiology

Multiple factors have been hypothesized to contribute to protein-losing enteropathy after Fontan operation: (1) chronic venous congestion, (2) altered lymphatic architecture with lymphatic congestion and increased obstruction to lymphatic flow (due to high central venous pressure) promote retrograde lymphatic flow into the gut, (3) reduced cardiac output leading to decreased mesenteric flow and increased gut permeability, (4) chronic inflammation, and (5) loss of heparin sulfate and syndecan-1 proteoglycans affecting intestinal epithelial barrier function, which is worsened by inflammation and elevated central venous pressure.

63.2.2.2 Clinical Presentations and Findings

Protein-losing enteropathy can present from weeks to years after the Fontan operation, often preceded by viral prodromal symptoms few weeks before its onset. Presenting symptoms include diarrhoea, mild periorbital or ankle swelling, abdominal distension due to ascites, and shortness of breath due to pleural or pericardial effusion. Growth and wound healing are impaired due to malabsorption and protein loss. Vitamin D deficiency and hypocalcaemia cause osteoporosis. Lymphopenia and hypogammaglobulinaemia predispose to recurrent sepsis. Imbalance between pro- and anticoagulants due to enteric loss and/or impaired synthesis may increase the risk of either thrombosis or bleeding.

Although the clinical manifestations are usually obvious in most of the patients with protein-losing enteropathy, there are some patients with subclinical protein loss from the gut (with normal serum albumin and total protein levels) and some with transient protein loss and an alternating symptomatic and asymptomatic clinical course.

63.2.2.3 Diagnosis and Further Investigations

Protein-losing enteropathy should be suspected when patients present with diarrhoea, oedema, or effusions together with serum hypoalbuminaemia and hypoproteinaemia. Exclusion of differential diagnoses requires assessment of urinary protein loss (e.g. due to nephrotic syndrome) and referral to gastroenterologist for assessment of other causes.

Diagnosis is based on the clinical features as described above, laboratory findings of increased faecal alpha-1-antritrypsin (spot level or 24-h clearance), serum hypoalbuminaemia and hypoproteinaemia, and exclusion of differential diagnoses. Patients with normal serum albumin and protein levels are regarded as having subclinical protein-losing enteropathy. Whether subclinical protein-losing enteropathy is always followed by full-blown protein-losing enteropathy remains to be clarified. Further assessments and workup are shown in Box 63.1.

Box 63.1 Further Workup for Protein-Losing Enteropathy

- blood investigations: haemoglobin, lymphocyte count and immunoglobulin level, left and renal function test, serum calcium level
- evaluation of Fontan haemodynamics and structural lesions: ECG, 24-h Holter monitoring, echocardiography, cardiac catheterization, CT, and CMR
- imaging of central veins: for stenosis and occlusion, and in preparation for further interventions
- lymphatic imaging (including intrahepatic dynamic contrast MR lymphangiography)

63.2.2.4 Management Strategy

The management strategy is stepwise and is based on the initial assessment of haemodynamics and structural lesions of the Fontan circuit, severity of protein loss, and its response to various therapeutic interventions. Therapeutic options include: (1) nutritional support, (2) medical therapies based on possible pathogenesis of protein-losing enteropathy in Fontan patients, and (3) surgical and/or transcatheter interventions (Fig. 63.1).

Confirmation of diagnosis

Nutritional support: high protein and low-fat diet, MCT supplementation, correct anaemia
Medical therapy: diuretics, intermittent intravenous albumin replacement, sildenafil, angiotensin-converting enzyme inhibitor (in the presence of ventricular dysfunction), control of arrhythmias
Interventions: balloon dilation and stenting of Fontan circuit and branch pulmonary arteries

If albumin level remains low,
Medical therapy: trial of subcutaneous heparin (unfractionated or low molecular weight heparin), oral midodrine, oral budesonide
Interventions: counselling patient and family regarding the possibility of further surgery or lymphatic interventions if condition worsens

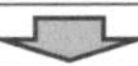

If albumin loss remains very severe,
Medical therapy: trial of intravenous octreotide therapy and inotropes
Interventions: lymphatic embolization, surgical (innominate vein turn-down procedure) or transcatheter lymphatic decompression, creation of fenestration, Fontan takedown (surgical or transcatheter), surgical repair of atrioventricular valvar regurgitation and relief of systemic ventricular outflow obstruction, mechanical circulatory support to bridge to heart transplant

Fig. 63.1 Management algorithm of protein-losing enteropathy in Fontan patients. Abbreviation: *MCT* medium-chain triglyceride

63.2.3 Plastic Bronchitis

Plastic bronchitis is characterized by expectoration or bronchoscopic finding of proteinaceous cast in the airways due to pulmonary lymphatic disorder. Its occurrence in Fontan patients is thought to result from decompression of lymphatic vessels with spillage of lymph into the lumen of airways.

63.2.3.1 Pathophysiology

Increased central pressure after Fontan operation may cause lymphatic congestion. Lymphatic insufficiency leads to spillage of lymph into the airways. The presence of superimposed inflammation and/or respiratory tract infection may lead to the formation of proteinaceous bronchial casts and promote development of lymphatic-to-bronchial communications. These bronchial casts can obstruct the airways and cause hypoxaemia.

63.2.3.2 Clinical Presentations and Findings

Plastic bronchitis can present at two to three years or earlier after Fontan operation. Patients may present with cough, wheezing, and shortness of breath. There may or may not be expectoration of bronchial-shaped casts. Occasionally, the presentation may be acute with severe hypoxaemia and respiratory failure. Physical examination may reveal signs of respiratory distress, wheeze, and decreased air entry.

63.2.3.3 Diagnosis and Further Investigations

The diagnosis should be strongly suspected in Fontan patients with chronic cough and episodes of wheezing, which may initially be diagnosed as asthma. Diagnosis is made by visual assessment of airway cast being expectorated or removed by bronchoscopy. Further dynamic contrast magnetic resonance lymphatic imaging substantiates the diagnosis and guides lymphatic interventions.

63.2.3.4 Management Strategy

The management strategy is in part similar to that described for protein-losing enteropathy in terms of (1) dietary modification, (2) medical therapies including diuretics and pulmonary vasodilators, and (3) optimization of the Fontan circuit to minimize the central venous pressure by transcatheter and surgical interventions and control of cardiac arrhythmias (Fig. 63.1).

Further management should include (1) therapies that facilitate expectoration of the airway cast, (2) preparation for the management of respiratory emergencies, and (3) more definitive treatment to reduce or abolish cast formation (Fig. 63.2).

Facilitation of expectoration of proteinaceous bronchial cast: chest physiotherapy, mucolytics (dornase-α, N-acetylcysteine), bronchodilators, nebulized fibrinolytics (tissue plasminogen activator, urokinase), heparin, and hypertonic saline, steroid use (oral steroid, inhaled budesonide) has mixed results

Management of respiratory emergencies: bronchoscopic removal of airway casts to relieve airway obstruction

More definitive management options: lymphatic embolization, lymphatic decompression (innominate vein turn-down procedure, transcatheter decompression), heart transplantation

Fig. 63.2 Specific management options for plastic bronchitis in Fontan patients. General management of plastic bronchitis is similar to that described for protein-losing enteropathy

63.3 Lymphatic Imaging and Interventions

Conventional imaging of lymphatics by injection of contrast agent into the cannulated small lymphatic ducts in the dorsum of foot is challenging and provides little information on lymphatic flow dynamics. The introduction of noncontrast magnetic resonance lymphangiography, dynamic contrast magnetic resonance lymphangiography, and computed tomographic lymphangiography has changed the landscape of diagnosis and intervention of lymphatic disorders in congenital heart patients (Fig. 63.3).

Dynamic contrast magnetic resonance lymphangiography, with integrated intranodal lymphangiography using gadolinium and imaging of lymphatics, has provided insights into the pathophysiology of lymphatic disorders through understanding of lymphodynamics and identification of possible causes of lymphatic failure (e.g. traumatic leakage, non-traumatic leakage of lymph into the pleural cavities and the gut, retrograde lymphatic flow, absence of central flow). The findings provide further guidance for lymphatic interventions.

Interventional procedures include lymphatic embolization and, in selected patients, surgical lympho-venous anastomoses. In Fontan patients with protein-losing enteropathy and plastic bronchitis, lymphatic decompression with incorporation of the thoracic duct into a lower pressure venous circulation has also been achieved by the surgical innominate vein turn-down procedure (drainage of the innominate vein to the left atrium that has a lower pressure) or transcatheter intervention (puncture from the innominate vein to the left atrium with placement of a covered stent). The long-term outcomes of these lymphatic interventions remain to be seen.

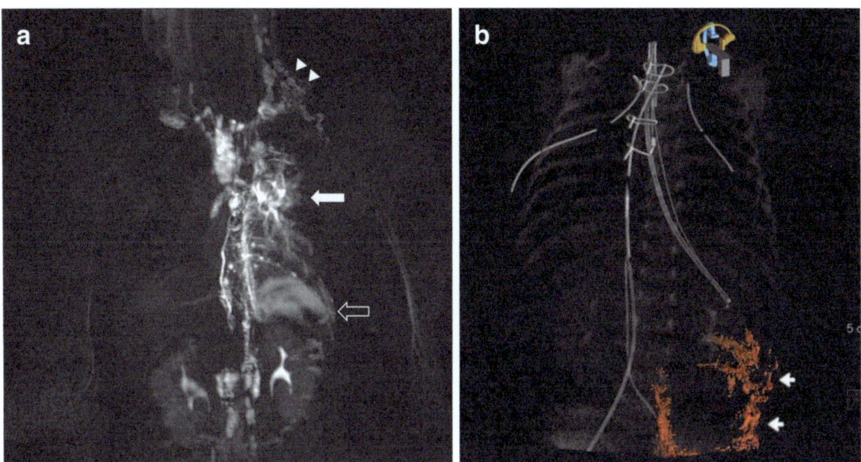

Fig. 63.3 Magnetic resonance and computed tomographic lymphangiography. (**a**) Dynamic contrast enhanced magnetic resonance demonstrating gadolinium-based contrast leak in the mediastinum and left hilar region into the left lung (solid arrow) and left pleural cavity (hollow arrow), and lymphatic reflux at the left supraclavicular region (arrowheads) in an adolescent with non-traumatic chylothorax (**b**) 3D volume-rendered image of cone-beam CT lymphangiogram acquired at 20 min post-contrast injection highlighting dermal backflow (arrows) significantly suggestive of central lymphatic flow disorder in an infant after arterial switch operation for transposition of the great arteries

Paediatric Heart Failure

64

The syndrome of heart failure represents an imbalanced state, in which the heart fails to provide an adequate output at a rate to meet the demand of the body. The clinical manifestations of heart failure as a mode of presentation in infants and children with heart disease are discussed in Chap. 1. In this chapter, the aetiology in terms of the structural and functional abnormalities, pathophysiology, the approach to diagnosis of the underlying cause, and management strategy are discussed.

64.1 Aetiology

The syndrome of heart failure may result from (i) an extra demand posed on the heart by an abnormal volume or pressure load with preservation of function of the myocardium, which is the most common cause in infants and children, and/or (ii) impaired myocardial contraction (systolic dysfunction) or impaired myocardial relaxation or diastolic filling of the ventricle (diastolic dysfunction) (Table 64.1).

In neonates presenting with early-onset heart failure, severe left ventricular outflow obstruction with duct-dependent systemic circulation (critical aortic stenosis, severe coarctation of the aorta, interrupted aortic arch) must be excluded. In infants and children, heart failure is most commonly caused by left-to-right shunts with preservation of myocardial function. Isolated pulmonary and aortic stenosis does not usually cause heart failure in childhood.

Systolic dysfunction of the left ventricle is usually related to disease of the myocardium without structural cardiac abnormalities. Myocardial ischaemia or infarction in infants and children can be caused by congenital (e.g. anomalous origin of the left coronary artery from the pulmonary artery) or acquired (e.g. thrombosis of coronary artery aneurysm complicating Kawasaki disease) conditions.

Systolic dysfunction of the subpulmonary right ventricle (e.g. in patients with repaired tetralogy of Fallot, Ebstein anomaly, systemic pulmonary hypertension),

Y.-f. Cheung, *Congenital and Paediatric Acquired Heart Disease in Practice*,
https://doi.org/10.1007/978-981-99-2862-0_64

Table 64.1 Causes of paediatric heart failure

Normal myocardial function	Impaired myocardial function
Volume-overloading conditions	**Myocardial disease**
Left-to-right shunts	Cardiomyopathies
Valvar regurgitation	Myocarditis
Extracardiac shunts (systemic Arteriovenous malformation)	Myocardial ischaemia or infarction due to Kawasaki disease or ALCAPA
High-output conditions (anaemia, thyrotoxicosis)	Cardiac arrhythmias (heart block, supraventricular and ventricular tachycardias)
Pressure-overloading conditions	**Congenital heart disease**
Severe left ventricular outflow	Subpulmonary right ventricle
Obstructive lesions	Systemic right ventricle
Severe right ventricular outflow	Functional single ventricle
Obstructive lesions	**Pulmonary hypertension**
Pulmonary hypertension	**Secondary causes**
	Sepsis
	Acid and electrolyte imbalance
	Renal failure

systemic right ventricle (in patients with congenitally corrected transposition of the great arteries and those after atrial switch for complete transposition of the great arteries), and functional single ventricle are discussed in the respective chapters.

Diastolic dysfunction can occur in association with systolic dysfunction of the ventricle. Isolated diastolic heart failure is uncommon in childhood. The occurrence of heart failure symptoms and signs in the presence of normal ventricular size and ejection fraction suggests diastolic dysfunction. Diastolic ventricular dysfunction can be related to impairment of myocardial relaxation, reduction of ventricular compliance, and, in the setting of congenital heart disease, hypoplasia of either the right or the left ventricle. The clinical phenotype of diastolic dysfunction is most obvious in children with restrictive cardiomyopathy. Chronic increase or decrease in preload, increased afterload, alteration of myocardial architecture, myocardial fibrosis, and hypoplasia of the ventricular cavity in congenital heart disease predispose to impairment of ventricular filling during diastole (Box 64.1).

64.2 Pathophysiology

The pathophysiologic consequences characteristic of each of the conditions included in Table 64.1 are discussed in the respective chapters. The relative inadequacy (due to the extra demand) or absolute reduction (due to myocardial dysfunction) of cardiac output activates the sympathetic nervous system and renin–angiotensin–aldosterone system to maintain blood pressure and blood flow by causing vasoconstriction and fluid retention. At the same time, the natriuretic peptide system is activated with increased release of atrial and brain natriuretic peptides to attenuate the effects of excessive vasoconstriction and sodium retention.

Box 64.1 Congenital Heart Conditions Associated with Impaired Diastolic Function

Right ventricular (RV) diastolic dysfunction

- repaired tetralogy of Fallot (restrictive RV physiology)
- pulmonary atresia with intact ventricular septum (RV hypoplasia and fibrosis)
- critical pulmonary stenosis (transient and usually resolve with regression of RV hypertrophy)
- Ebstein malformation (non-functional RV myocardium impairs contraction and filling of the right ventricle despite repair of the tricuspid valve)
- transposition of the great arteries post atrial switch (impaired atrioventricular transport with decreased systemic RV preload)

Left ventricular (LV) diastolic dysfunction

- Shone complex (LV hypoplasia and hypertrophy)
- subvalvar and valar aortic stenosis (LV hypertrophy and increased afterload)
- repaired aortic coarctation or interruption (LV hypertrophy and increased afterload)
- repaired tetralogy of Fallot (RV volume overloading with adverse diastolic ventricular-ventricular interaction)
- Ebstein malformation (RV dilation with adverse diastolic ventricular-ventricular interaction)

64.3 Clinical Presentation and Findings

The symptoms and signs of heart failure are discussed in Chap. 1. The clinical presentation and findings unique to each of the conditions included in Table 64.1 are discussed in the respective chapters.

64.4 Investigations

CXR: The chest radiograph enables the assessment of cardiomegaly due to ventricular and/or atrial enlargement, pulmonary plethora due to left-to-right shunts, and pulmonary venous congestion due to left ventricular systolic and/or diastolic dysfunction, and monitoring of the effectiveness of heart failure management.

ECG: Electrocardiogram enables the evaluation of ventricular and atrial enlargement or hypertrophy, cardiac arrhythmias, and myocardial ischaemia and infarction.

Echocardiography: Echocardiographic assessment provides structural evaluation of congenital and acquired heart disease and coronary arterial anomalies, systolic

and diastolic functional evaluation of the ventricles (Chap. 6), and haemodynamic assessment of obstructive and regurgitant lesions and pulmonary arterial pressure.
CMR: Cardiac magnetic resonance is performed when indicated for assessment by ventricular volumes and ejection fraction, myocardial inflammation and fibrosis, and cardiac structures (Chap. 8).
Cardiac catheterization: Cardiac catheterization is performed when indicated for assessment of coronary arterial anomalies, ventricular filling pressures, and pulmonary vascular pressure and resistance, differentiation between constrictive pericarditis and restrictive cardiomyopathy (Chap. 46), and endomyocardial biopsy.
Cardiac biomarkers: Elevation of troponin I and troponin T levels suggests myocardial injury due to myocarditis or myocardial ischaemia. The level of brain natriuretic peptide (BNP) or N-terminal proBNP provides an assessment of the severity of heart failure due to structural and functional cardiac abnormalities and provides monitoring of response to the treatment of heart failure.
Other blood investigations: Hyponatraemia, renal dysfunction, and impairment of liver function are common in children with severe heart failure. Elevated lactate level and metabolic acidosis signify decompensated heart failure with decreased tissue perfusion.

64.5 Management Strategy

64.5.1 Acute Heart Failure

Acute heart failure can be due to de novo presentation of a newly diagnosed cardiac condition (e.g. myocarditis, dilated cardiomyopathy) or decompensation of known underlying cardiac disorders.

Initial management include diagnosis of the underlying disorder or the cause of decompensation in patients with a known cardiac diagnosis, infusion of prostaglandin E in neonates diagnosed to have a duct-dependent systemic circulation (Chap. 13), and institution of medical therapies including diuretics, inotropes, calcium sensitizers, and other vasoactive medications (Chap. 52). Other measures include ventilatory support, correction of anaemia, electrolyte imbalance, metabolic acidosis, and treatment of infection when present.

64.5.2 Heart Failure Due to Unrepaired Congenital Heart Disease

Structural congenital heart defects should be surgically repaired. Preoperative general management includes nutritional supplementation, ventilatory support, correction of anaemia, electrolyte imbalance, and metabolic acidosis, and treatment of infection when present. Specific management strategies for left-to-right shunts and severe left and right ventricular outflow obstruction are discussed in the respective chapters.

64.5.3 Heart Failure in Association with Repaired Structural Heart Disease

Specific management strategies for patients with systolic dysfunction of the subpulmonary right ventricle (after repair of tetralogy of Fallot, Ebstein anomaly, systemic pulmonary hypertension), systemic right ventricular dysfunction (in congenitally corrected transposition of the great arteries, post atrial switch for complete transposition of the great arteries), and dysfunction of the single ventricle are discussed in the respective chapters. Medical management of chronic heart failure in these patients are discussed below.

64.5.4 Chronic Heart Failure with Impaired Myocardial Function

Chronic heart failure with impaired myocardial function occurs in functional and structural heart conditions (Table 64.1). Staging of heart failure (Table 64.2) provides guidance to therapy.
General management: Supportive treatment includes nutritional supplementation, ventilatory support, correction of anaemia, electrolyte imbalance, and metabolic acidosis, and treatment of infection when present.
Medical treatment: The commonly used medications and emerging drug therapies for paediatric heart failure are shown in Table 64.3.
Clinical trials in paediatric heart failure are limited and challenging due to small number of patients, heterogeneity in the underlying cardiac conditions, overlapping phenotypes of heart failure, and difficulties in defining clinical endpoints. Most of the paediatric recommendations are extrapolated from adult guidelines that focus on systemic left ventricular systolic dysfunction. There is no conclusive evidence to date of beneficial effects of medical therapy for dysfunction of the subpulmonary and systemic right ventricles and functional single ventricle. Guideline-directed

Table 64.2 Stages of heart failure in infants and children based on the International Society for Heart and Lung Transplantation (ISHLT)

Stage	Definition	Examples
A	Patients with normal cardiac function and chamber, but with increased risk of development heart failure	Post chemotherapy family history of cardiomyopathy
B	Patients with abnormal cardiac morphology or function, with no past or present symptoms of heart failure	Post chemotherapy or left ventricular noncompaction with impaired left ventricular systolic function
C	Patients with structural or functional heart disease, with past or present symptoms of heart failure	Dilated cardiomyopathy, structural heart disease with ventricular dysfunction
D	Patients with end-stage heart failure requiring specialized interventions	Inotrope-dependent end-stage cardiomyopathy

Table 64.3 Medical treatment of children with chronic heart failure

Class	Drug	Beneficial effects
Diuretics[a]	Loop diuretics; frusemide thiazides: hydrochlorothiazide, metolazone	Reduce volume overloading
ACE inhibitors[b]	Captopril Enalapril	Inhibit RAAS Decrease myocardial fibrosis
Angiotensin receptor blockers	Losartan, valsartan (paucity of data on the use in paediatric heart failure)	Inhibit RAAS Decrease myocardial fibrosis
ARNI	Sacubutril-valsartan	Inhibit RASS and neprilysin (inhibition of the latter prevents breakdown of natriuretic peptides)
Mineralocorticoid receptor antagonists[b]	Spironolactone Eplerenone	Diuresis with potassium sparing Decrease myocardial fibrosis
Beta-blockers[b]	Carvedilol Metoprolol	Counteract effect of activation of sympathetic nervous system Decrease myocardial fibrosis Reverse ventricular remodelling
Glycoside	Digoxin (not routinely used in the present era)	Inhibit Na+/K+ ATPase and increase intracellular calcium enhance contractility Vagotonic effect
SGLT2 inhibitor	Dapagliflozin (limited data in paediatrics)	Unclear
HCN channel blocker	Ivabradine	Reduce heart rate through regulating the voltage-regulated inward funny current (If)

[a] For treatment of systolic or isolated diastolic dysfunction to achieve euvolaemia
[b] Recommended by ISHLT for treatment of symptomatic left ventricular systolic dysfunction
ACE angiotensin-converting enzyme, *ARNI* angiotensin receptor-neprilysin inhibitor, *HCN* hyperpolarization-activated cyclic nucleotide-gated, *RAAS* renin-angiotensin-aldosterone system, *SGLT* sodium-glucose cotransporter

medical therapy for paediatric heart failure is not available. In practice, worsening of the stage of heart failure informs the need to escalate heart failure therapies (Fig. 64.1).

Device therapy: Cardiac resynchronization therapy can be contemplated in patients with stage C and D heart failure not responding refractory to medical therapy. This has been applied to children with dilated cardiomyopathy and structural heart disease with varying degrees of success. Nonetheless, evidence-based criteria for cardiac resynchronization therapy in paediatric heart failure are lacking.

Mechanical circulatory support and heart transplantation: Mechanical circulatory support, in the form of extracorporeal membrane oxygenation or ventricular assist device, is used to bridge patients with end-stage heart failure refractory to medical therapy to heart transplantation.

Stage A: usually observe with regular follow-up assessment, pre-emptive therapy with ACE inhibitor has also been suggested (though empirical and not evidence-based)

Stage B: ACE inhibitor, addition of mineralocorticoid receptor antagonist can be considered

Stage C: ACE inhibitor or sacubutril-valsartan inhibitor, mineralocorticoid receptor antagonist, and diuretics (for fluid overload), gradual introduction of beta-blocker, addition of ivabradine can be considered for better control of heart rate, can consider addition of dapagliflozin in older adolescents

Stage D: intensive care management with intravenous diuretics, inotropes, calcium sensitizers, and other vasoactive medications, ventilatory support if indicated, heart transplant evaluation, and mechanical circulatory support as a bridge to transplant

Fig. 64.1 Treatment of heart failure based on the stage of heart failure. *ACE* angiotensin-converting enzyme

Correction to: Congenital and Paediatric Acquired Heart Disease in Practice

Yiu-fai Cheung

Correction to:

Chapters 13 and 35 in: Y.-f. Cheung, *Congenital and Paediatric Acquired Heart Disease in Practice*, https://doi.org/10.1007/978-981-99-2862-0_13, https://doi.org/10.1007/978-981-99-2862-0_35

The book was inadvertently published with the wrong placement of figures 13a and 13b and now they are swapped in the correct order. And additional content as L or E in Figure 35.3 on page 338 of the print PDF, and now it has been removed.

The updated version of these chapters can be found at
https://doi.org/10.1007/978-981-99-2862-0_13
https://doi.org/10.1007/978-981-99-2862-0_35

Y.-f. Cheung, *Congenital and Paediatric Acquired Heart Disease in Practice*,
https://doi.org/10.1007/978-981-99-2862-0_65

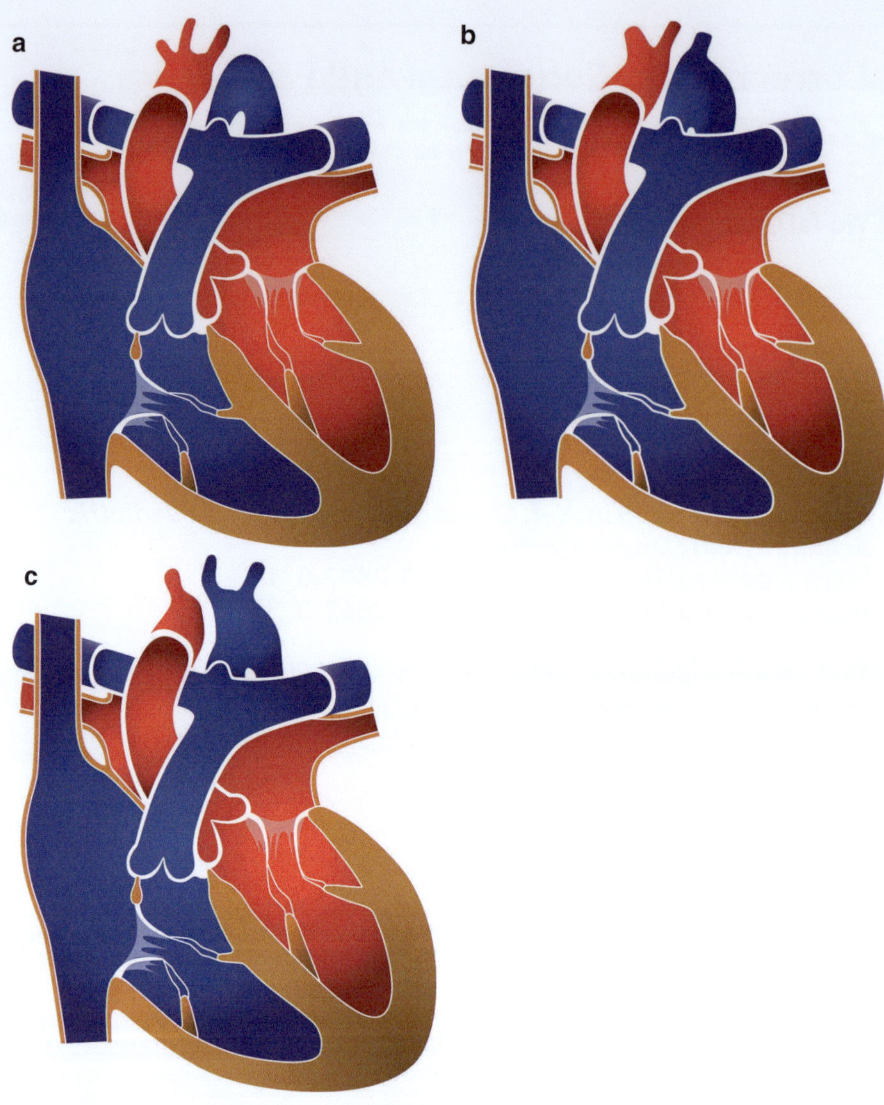
a
b
c

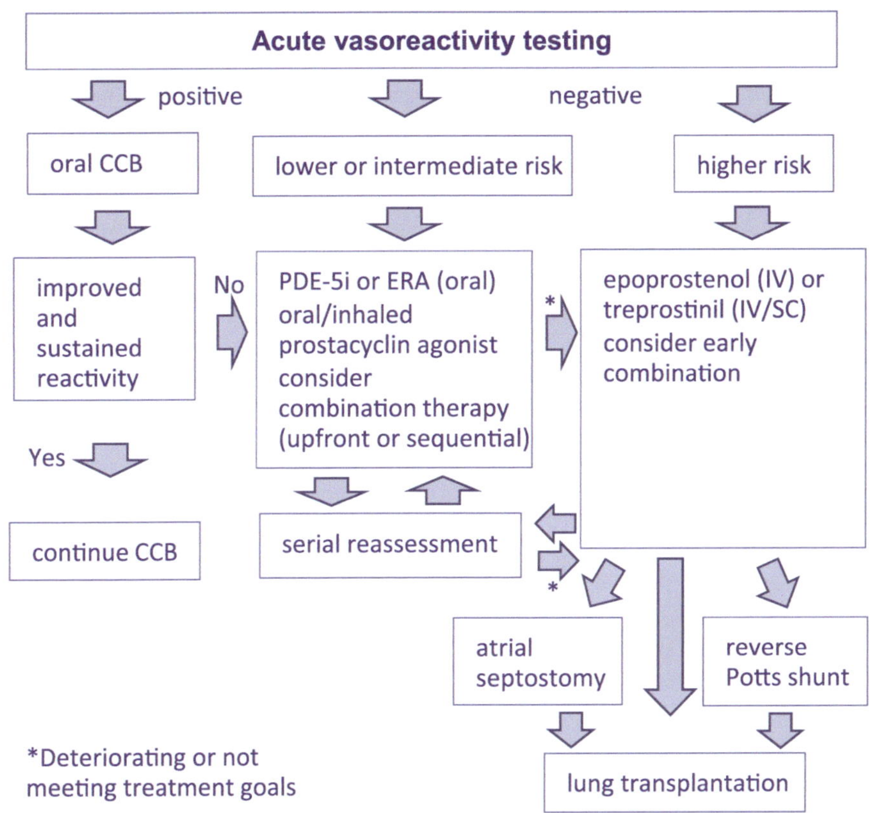
Acute vasoreactivity testing
positive
negative
oral CCB
lower or intermediate risk
higher risk
improved and sustained reactivity
No
PDE-5i or ERA (oral) oral/inhaled prostacyclin agonist consider combination therapy (upfront or sequential)
*
epoprostenol (IV) or treprostinil (IV/SC) consider early combination
Yes
continue CCB
serial reassessment
*
atrial septostomy
reverse Potts shunt
lung transplantation
*Deteriorating or not meeting treatment goals

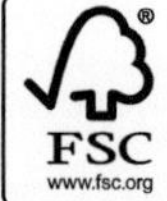

MIX
Papier aus verantwortungsvollen Quellen
Paper from responsible sources
FSC® C105338

If you have any concerns about our products,
you can contact us on
ProductSafety@springernature.com

In case Publisher is established outside the EU,
the EU authorized representative is:
Springer Nature Customer Service Center GmbH
Europaplatz 3, 69115 Heidelberg, Germany

Printed by Libri Plureos GmbH
in Hamburg, Germany